PRAISE FOR
Ancient Map for Modern Birth

"For modern women, navigating the maze of pregnancy tests, results, and risks can distance us from the emotional and spiritual journey of childbearing. The exceptional journey from conception to early motherhood and beyond gifts us with opportunities for profound healing, growth, and transformation on every level. *Ancient Map for Modern Birth* offers warmth and wisdom, as well as deep compassion, and invites us into the awe-inspiring emotional and spiritual terrain that lies at the heart of childbearing."

—Sarah Buckley, MD, MB, ChB, Dip Obst
Author of *Gentle Birth, Gentle Mothering*

"I would have loved this book when I was pregnant! *Ancient Map for Modern Birth* offers practical wisdom for natural birth and yet honors the strength in every birth journey. Pam England blends psychological, mythical, and an insider's knowledge to bring birth confidence to the next generation of birthing women and their partners."

—Gail Tully, CPM
www.SpinningBabies.com

"*Ancient Map for Modern Birth* is based on the concept of giving birth as something a woman's body intuitively knows how to do even though many of us today are disconnected from this ancient wisdom. Its soothing guidance, enchanting stories, and creative exercises pave the ideal first steps along the parenting journey."

—Amity Hook-Sopko
Executive editor of *Green Child Magazine*

"Pam England has devoted her career to facilitating the birth process and empowering women giving birth. As such, *Ancient Map for Modern Birth* represents the accumulation of a lifetime of work. The layering of the book—with the Call, the Tasks of Preparation, the Gates of Laborland, and the Warrior's Return—provides a solid organization, and even a sense of heroic journey. The many exercises make the presentation quite experiential and very useful for both practitioners and pregnant families."

—Lewis Mehl-Madrona, MD, PhD
Author of *Narrative Medicine* and
Healing the Mind through Story

"As a midwife, mother, and artist, Pam England brings a one-of-a-kind perspective to childbirth. Because her own personal birth transformations laid the foundation for her ancient map, we can follow her advice confidently. Her book prepares us for a successful birth in a deep and powerful way."

—Peggy O'Mara
Former editor and publisher of *Mothering Magazine*
and author of *Natural Family Living, Having a Baby Naturally,*
and *A Quiet Place*

"Though our female bodies naturally know how to birth our babies, the collective culture has largely forgotten how to hold the women while they become mothers. *Ancient Map for Modern Birth* is a companion guide reminding you that birthing and mothering are passages into the heart and soul of what it means to be alive. With *Ancient Map for Modern Birth*, Pam England has created a book worthy of this sacred journey."

—Tami Lynn Kent
Author of *Wild Feminine, Wild Creative,* and
Mothering from Your Center

"*Ancient Map for Modern Birth* is a soulful, authoritative, and exquisitely written guide for the heroine's journey we call childbirth. I highly recommend this beautiful gift of insight and knowledge."

—Christiane Northrup, MD
Author of *The New York Times* bestsellers
Goddesses Never Age, Women's Bodies, Women's Wisdom, and
The Wisdom of Menopause

"The childbirth rite of passage holds potential for powerful transformation and self-growth. Women are beginning to reclaim this ancient and sacred aspect of mothering. *Ancient Map for Modern Birth* offers a guide for transformation within the context of a modern maternity system and honors all women as birth warriors regardless of the choices they make or the type of birth they have."

—Rachel Reed, BScHons Midwifery, PhD
MidwifeThinking

Also by Pam England, cnm, ma

Birthing From Within
An Extra-Ordinary Guide to Childbirth Preparation
(coauthored)

Our Birthing From Within Keepsake Journal

Inanna's Descent
Initiation & Return—A Journal

Labyrinth of Birth
Creating a Map, Meditations and Rituals for Your Childbearing Year

Preparation, Passage, and Personal Growth during Your Childbearing Year

Ancient Map
for MODERN BIRTH

PAM ENGLAND, CNM, MA

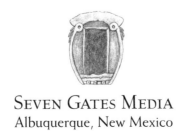

SEVEN GATES MEDIA
Albuquerque, New Mexico

Published by

SEVEN GATES MEDIA
PO Box 27406
Albuquerque, New Mexico 87125
www.sevengatesmedia.com

Copyeditor: Ellen Kleiner

Interior design by Karen Stroker and Angela Werneke

Cover design and page production by Angela Werneke

Printed in the United States of America

First Edition

PUBLISHER'S CATALOGING-IN-PUBLICATION DATA

Names: England, Pam, author.

Title: Ancient map for modern birth : preparation, passage, and personal growth during your childbearing year / Pam England.

Description: Albuquerque : Seven Gates Media, [2017] | Includes index.

Identifiers: ISBN: 978-0-998-1202-0-1 (paperback) | 978-0-998-1202-1-8 (eBook) | LCCN: 2015919810

Subjects: LCSH: Pregnancy—Psychological aspects. | Childbirth—Psychological aspects. | Natural childbirth. | Pain—Psychological aspects. | Mind and body. | Mindfulness (Psychology) | Meditation. | Childbirth—Study and teaching. | Holistic medicine. | BISAC: Health & Fitness / Pregnancy & Childbirth. | Women's Health.| Parenting/General.

Classification: LCC: RG661 .E53 2017 | DDC: 618.4/5—dc23

1 3 5 7 9 10 8 6 4 2

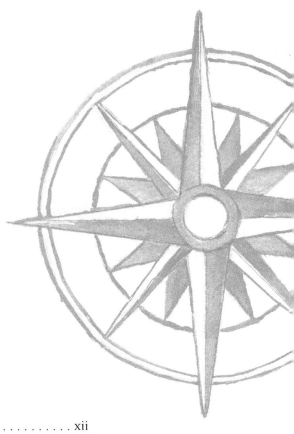

Contents

INTRODUCTION

*A*ncient Map for Modern Birth is a coherent vision and model of childbirth preparation, a colorful tapestry that weaves together art, science, meditations, ceremonies, and the telling of mythic stories. Every pregnant woman has within her a personal compass. Yet if she has never been to Laborland she needs a map that highlights her tasks of pregnancy, birth, and the postpartum transition. This book offers that map.

My first book, *Birthing From Within*, has been more popular than I ever dreamed possible when it was self-published in 1998. Many people have said, "Why are you writing a new book? We love the old book!" adding, "Don't change it too much." There is a part of us that likes to cling to favorite places, customs, and books associated with warm feelings. And yet change is inevitable and necessary for the healthy evolution of ideas and of humanity.

In the last eighteen years, a lot has changed in our fast-paced world, including the expectations and knowledge of birthing couples, as well as the culture and practice of obstetrics and midwifery. Women are also benefiting from the successful revival of a centuries-old birth custom—emotional support during labor and postpartum (in the form of doulas)—and a resurgence in home births, which have increased 29 percent in the last nineteen years.[1] While there are now fewer episiotomies, there are more cesareans. Labor induction, occurring in a whopping 23 percent of all births, has become an epidemic.[2] Obstetricians are quitting in droves, while midwives are slowly gaining ground and now attend 8 percent of all births, up from less than 1 percent in the mid-1970s.[3] And there are new questions regarding the safety of fetal ultrasound.

Ancient Map for Modern Birth sheds light on important blind spots in childbirth education that were not addressed in *Birthing From Within*, including inductions, ultrasound, vaginal birth after cesarean, postpartum ceremonies, and birth stories. This book also introduces many new processes inspired by our unwavering commitment to balancing evidence-based information with art and personal awareness in childbirth preparation. In addition, you will experience the power of mythic stories that teach in a way nothing else can and that highlight archetypes of birth and how they live within us. Hopefully this book will also dispel two misconceptions about the *Birthing From Within* model that came from the first book: that it is a crunchy granola approach focusing on birth art to the exclusion of practical information and that it is only useful to mothers planning natural births.

When I wrote *Birthing From Within*, I was eager to share the birth art process, which was then novel, so I dedicated an entire section to it. This emphasis gave some the impression that our classes focused on making drawings and sculptures at the expense of sharing information. While the birth art process is still an integral part of preparing mothers emotionally, in the model introduced by *Ancient Map for Modern Birth* only a few birth art assignments are included, sprinkled throughout the book. In the past decade, I began painting my own birth art and mandalas, a few of which are in this book for you to enjoy.

Regarding the second misconception—that the Birthing From Within model is only useful to mothers having natural births—parents and journalists have repeatedly asked about Birthing From Within's "natural birth classes." During interviews I explain that we don't teach *natural* birth classes; we teach *birth* classes. There are many ways to give birth; the natural way is just one. Because there is no crystal ball to know who will experience which kind of labor, today's women and men need to be emotionally and mentally prepared to participate in a range of birth experiences, from spontaneous to medically managed.

Stories are maps and teachers. The mythic story that has inspired Birthing From Within classes more than any other during the past two decades, the golden thread that runs through this entire book, is the ancient Sumerian myth known as "Inanna's Descent."[4] I initially read about the goddess Inanna around the time of my first birth. In Inanna, I saw a reflection of myself and my personal birth journey, as well as a glimpse of how childbirth can become a heroic journey for women. In recognizing that my preparation for, and descent into, labor paralleled the warrior queen's preparation and passage through the seven gates of the underworld, I realized that by following in Inanna's footsteps I would—and did—find my way out of my postpartum underworld.

Two decades ago I became curious about how pregnant couples would respond, and what they would learn, if I told them a mythic story during childbirth classes. I began by telling parents a modified version of the story I called "Inanna's Descent into Laborland." I quickly discovered that pregnant women are riveted by Inanna's journey because they, too, are answering their hearts' calls, leaving behind comfort, certainty, and even friends to enter the unknown. Countless parents have shared with me that in the midst of their labor, when all the facts they had learned and the plans they had made had been forgotten, this story became their inner map that helped them get through their birth and return.

Another ancient, universal map of birth is the labyrinth. The labyrinth symbol not only provides the perfect map of the inner journey of pregnancy, labor, and postpartum but has been used in childbirth meditations for centuries to help women cope with pain. I experienced my first labyrinth—an outdoor walking one—while leading a workshop in 1999 at Grailville, in Loveland, Ohio. Around 2002, I began showing parents in my childbirth classes how to draw a labyrinth, or, as we call it, a "Laborinth." The popularity of this addition to the Birthing From Within birth art and pain-coping practices led me to publish *Labyrinth of Birth: Creating a Map, Meditations and Rituals for Your Childbearing Year* in 2010.

One more change, perhaps the most significant and welcome, is that I am no longer alone in working or experimenting with the Birthing From Within paradigm. This approach, which was first developed in my small childbirth classes in Albuquerque, New Mexico, is now being used by childbirth mentors, doulas, and mothers around the world. Since 2006 I have been privileged to work with Virginia Bobro of Santa Barbara, California, who is now co-owner and managing director of Birthing From Within, LLC, as well as a dynamic facilitator inspiring birth professionals globally to utilize this unique approach. As a result of Virginia's dedication, Birthing From Within has grown into an international practice with a presence in eighteen countries. This expanding number of dynamic, intelligent, and visionary women and men who share a commitment to personal and professional growth is engaged in a continuous dialogue, taking us on a journey of the heart we never imagined.

All these changes have been significant enough to warrant an entirely new book. Read this book and get involved.

My Map

It's been some thirty years since I first envisioned a philosophy and system of holistic childbirth preparation that would validate, motivate, educate, initiate, and celebrate women and men during their life-changing passages of pregnancy, birth, and becoming parents. That vision began in a most unlikely place: lying on a table in a cold operating room having cesarean surgery. At the time, I was a home birth midwife who had planned to birth at home, but after a long, difficult labor I was transferred to the hospital. As I lay on the table utterly exhausted, a question arose: "What is it that I needed to know as a mother that I didn't know as a midwife?" That question took hold in my heart and became my North Star, leading me on a lifelong pilgrimage. I am still walking, and the answer is still evolving.

During my second pregnancy, I realized that my greatest task was to forget all I knew as a nurse-midwife so I could remember my instincts as a pregnant woman. I believe the personal work I did between my first and second births made all the difference. My second son, Lucien, was born peacefully at home. My two very different birth experiences resulted in a balanced understanding of what birth can be and how to prepare for it.

My training as a certified nurse-midwife and my master's degree in psychology-counseling have enabled the ongoing exploration of topics in this book and continued development of the Birthing From Within model. My role as birth story listener and mentor to other birth story listeners around the world through an online course has further enhanced my experiences in this field. I also still work and paint in Albuquerque, New Mexico, and offer long-distance teaching and birth story sessions.

Ancient Map for Modern Birth is organized into six sections, taking you from your prenatal Call through your postpartum Return. It's best to orient yourself to this approach by reading Part I first. Then you can decide to either read the book straight through or choose chapters in any order. Be sure to read the chapters about topics you want to avoid—which are often those most feared—to strengthen yourself as a Birth Warrior and perhaps help reduce your worry. Listening to the audio recordings at www.sevengatesmedia.com and completing the Tasks of Preparation in Part IV of the book will further help you cultivate the skills and mindset needed to give birth from within. However, all the knowledge and information gained from the book and recordings cannot replace the kind of learning and healing possible through contact with a trained and compassionate childbirth mentor. So consider taking a Birthing From Within childbirth class from a mentor in your community or arranging private sessions by phone or Skype.

Ancient Map for Modern Birth is essential to birth professionals. After *Birthing From Within* was published, many birth professionals were inspired by our philosophy and eager to incorporate the innovative exercises, pain-coping practices, and birth art assignments into their own classes. When they later came to one of our trainings, they expressed how much more they understood of the philosophy and how to make the processes work even better. Maps are not static, and neither are our workshops for professionals. Even if you have taken a workshop or online course in the past, our offerings continue to evolve to keep pace with the changing birth world and to reflect the new material presented in these chapters. So read this book, try out the processes, and, if you wish to deepen your understanding, sign up for a workshop, webinar, or online course. *Please note*: words throughout the book that are followed by an asterisk appear in the glossary for easy reference.

May you find here what you are looking for.

Pam England
Albuquerque, New Mexico

Part 1
ANCIENT MAP

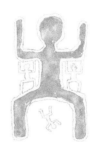

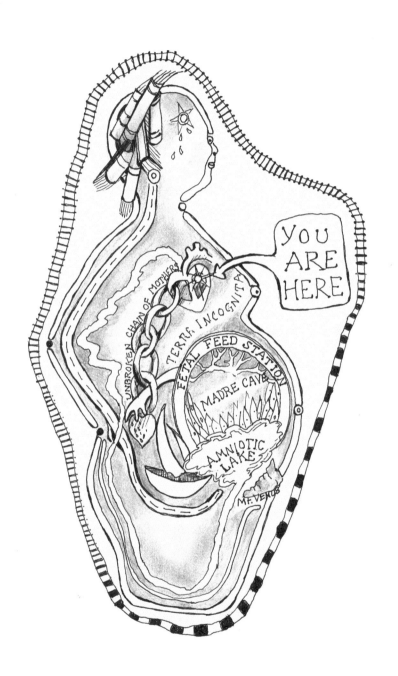

ANCIENT MAP FOR MODERN BIRTH

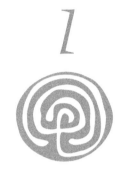

To envision living your childbearing year as a Birth Warrior changes everything. This radical, heart-opening map will change how you prepare for giving birth.

*I*t is human nature to want to know how to get from "here" to "there" without getting lost. As a pregnant woman, you will be handed our culture's "modern map" of birth, which is useful for navigating routine medical and consumer tasks. And yet, many women have told me that something is missing from that modern map—that there is something more. When shown the ancient map, which reveals hidden terrain, they intuitively feel their inner compass pointing to their true self.

While the modern map of birth is accessible through common knowledge, the ancient map must be actively sought. If you are searching for an inner map as you prepare to become a mother, you are in luck: you are holding it in your hands.

The journey you are making this year is personal and unique to you. By following the ancient, universal map of the mythic journey, the one that humans have been making for millennia, your childbearing year links you to all mothers who have come before you.

This ancient map—the map of the Birth Warrior—is not a simplistic road map to achieving a perfect birth or any other specific outcome. Instead, it guides you across countless inner thresholds, over unforeseen hurdles, beyond your edge, and into the unknown and uncharted territory. This map shows you ways to keep going—and to find your way "home" again.

Because birth is a rite of passage, you can expect to encounter mystery, uncertainty, and even a loss of control. The ancient map—tried and true—reassures you that you are not lost. With this template, women and birth workers, whether just beginning their journeys or approaching the ends, find that their complex modern experiences suddenly "click." They express gratitude and surprise when they hear, see, and feel their personal stories mirrored in ancient wisdom and knowing.

> *For years, my experience of becoming a mother felt fragmented and confusing. Birthing From Within's map brought the pieces together at last.*
> —EMILY

During your childbearing year, you will be traversing two paths at once: the inner path of personal, spiritual, and psychological awareness, and the outer path of practical learning about birth. This book integrates both paths, providing you with sustenance, information, inspiration, and tasks for finding your way through the experience whole and integrated.

The journey of the Birth Warrior is reflected in a complex map made up of many layers. Within the body, a living map flows through our veins. Within the soul, a timeless map guides our intuition. Within the mind, an ever-changing map is ingrained in our values and beliefs. Within the heart, a personal map connecting thousands of stories informs us. Mindful preparation for birth and parenting means becoming aware of the multi-layered map within you.

Have you ever seen the cellophane overlays of human anatomy in the old Encyclopedia Britannica? Each system of the body (skeletal, muscular, circulatory, and so on) was drawn on transparent pages, so, as you turned the pages, you watched the human body built layer by layer from skeleton to skin. In the same way, as you turn the pages of this book each new discovery and each task you complete will build a new self that is fully ready for birth. This map, like the book itself, is layered in five parts: the Call, Awaken the Mother, the Tasks of Preparation, Gates of Laborland, and the Warrior's Return.

Answering Your Call

Throughout your life, you have heard many calls: calls to travel, to pursue a career, to choose a life partner, and now perhaps a call to motherhood, or to give birth in a particular way or place. We are called not merely to do something new but to restore our internal balance and fulfill our soul's fundamental needs. Answering your Call is more than making a silent promise to yourself or a proclamation of intent. Infused with fierce and unswerving determination, you begin by taking small, practical, necessary steps toward realizing what you are called to *do*. In the process, a maturation and reorientation of the mind and soul inevitably take place.

A circle divided into three parts represents the phases of the Birth Warrior's journey: Preparation, Descent, and Return. These phases correlate to pregnancy, labor, and postpartum, respectively, although some mothers experience Descent in pregnancy or postpartum.

> *Prenatal preparation begins with a Call,*
> *which comes not from your mind, but from your heart.*

Prenatal Preparation

Even though countless women have gone to Laborland* before you, if you have never given birth or become a parent, remember that there are two distinct phases of preparation: unintentional and intentional (or unconscious and conscious).

Unintentional Preparation

Your earliest prenatal preparation was unintentional, even accidental; it began passively, in childhood. You absorbed and created assumptions and beliefs about life, relationships, religion, birth, and ways of thinking while living through the ordinary activities of growing up. As a child, you did not get to choose the assumptions, beliefs, images, and stories that created your internal compass, which still points you in certain directions—even when you "know better."

Intentional Preparation

Your intentional prenatal preparation begins now as you thoughtfully question assumptions, beliefs, advice, and authority while actively gathering and assessing new information from a variety of sources. Dare to look in every direction, including points of view that challenge your own long-held opinions.

You can't do this alone. It is impossible to prepare yourself fully for a journey you've never made before. Ideally, in addition to following your intuition, you, along with your birth companions, will be guided by mentors and engage in dialogue with professionals and peers.

Entering the Terra Incognita of Laborland

Terra incognita, Latin for "unknown land," was a term scrawled across old maps before the interiors of continents had been meticulously explored and charted. With GPS and satellite imagery, we have solved most of our world's geographical mysteries, so we no longer see this term on maps. However, in rites of passage, such as childbirth, a terra incognita still lies within. Before labor, as a first-time mother you can only imagine what labor will be like. Then at some point during labor you will cross a chasm and enter your terra incognita—the place beyond which your conscious mind could not have envisioned. It is in crossing this threshold that birth becomes a rite of passage.

No matter how many times you go to Laborland and give birth, or how familiar some of the landmarks become, you will encounter something unexpected, a new territory to explore. Even when you complete your journey through Laborland, a part of your map will always remain terra incognita.

BIRTH, DEATH, AND REBIRTH

Initiation involves a kind of psychic death and rebirth. What "dies" is naïveté, habits, plans, fears, or deeply held assumptions. At least one old belief or assumption will not survive the descent. What dies is never something you choose or plan to let go of. It is done *for* you; circumstances shake loose or take from you what is no longer needed or true. This kind of death creates uncertainty, an opening into not-knowing, and ultimately a metamorphosis. The heroic task in this sacred void, which endures well into your Return, is the continuous challenging of your beliefs and assumptions about birth, mothering, and self.

CALL TO RETURN

Your journey does not end with giving birth or even with completing six weeks of postpartum recovery. Until you complete the tasks of the Return and pass through its nine gates, your journey is not complete. It may take a year (or two, or even three) for you and your partner to fully inhabit your new roles as parents and integrate the birth and your new sense of self.

When the Maiden dies, the Mother is born.

Our culture emphasizes learning about labor, while giving little, if any, thought to guiding mothers and their partners through their transition into parenthood. The Birth Warrior map aims to return this piece to the modern birth map.

When your childbearing year becomes a heart journey, you will not just be birthing your child; all along the way you will be birthing a new self. The Birth Warrior map and model described here will change the way you see yourself as a woman and mother, how you prepare to give birth, how you think and feel about labor, and how you tell your birth story.

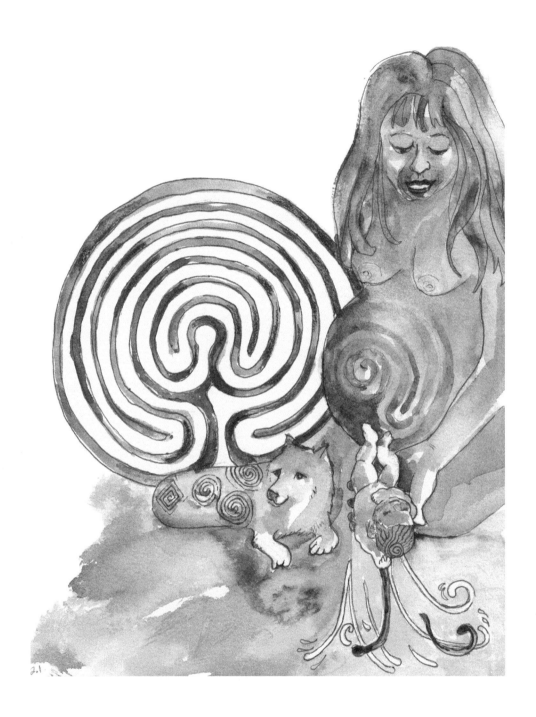

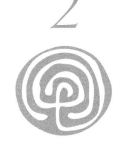

LABORINTH
THE BIRTH WARRIOR'S MAP

You come to the threshold of a great rite of passage with a map, but it is incomplete. Everyone comes with tattered fragments of maps made from stories and information from other travelers. You may be trying to figure out which way to turn the fragments and how to fit them together.

A map cannot tell you everything. No matter how detailed it is, it cannot predict or prepare you for everything you could experience—not the weather, not a beautiful sunset, and not the allies or detours you will encounter along the way. Your Birth Warrior's map is incomplete until you have lived your journey. It is only through immersing your body and mind in the territory of birth that you can have a direct experience of it and complete your map.

You can study another's map or show someone yours, but remember: no two landscapes of labor are the same.

THE LABYRINTH AS MAP

For centuries the labyrinth has been regarded as a symbol of our journey through life. In our Birthing From Within childbirth classes, we show parents how to draw or sculpt the classic seven-circuit labyrinth because it is a perfect metaphorical "map" of a woman's journey through labor and postpartum. The labyrinth is an accessible and visual snapshot that parents connect to. Here is one way that labor is like a labyrinth:

Once you enter a labyrinth, the continuous, winding, twisting-and-turning pathway eventually leads to the center and out again. Unlike a maze, a labyrinth has no dead ends or choices to be made. Yet, hairpin turns in the labyrinth disrupt your sense of direction, inducing doubt and confusion. Unpredictable, sudden changes in direction in the labyrinth parallel unexpected, unwished-for surprises that are part of every labor and postpartum. You may begin thinking that you are back where you started, or that you are getting nowhere, or that you are moving away from the "end." In a labyrinth (and in labor), you cannot see how far you've come, or how close you are to the center or to exiting (or to giving birth). You can learn how to make your own Laborinth by following the instructions below.

To use the labyrinth as part of your birth preparation, see index listings. To learn more about the labyrinth of birth, meditations, and rituals, read Labyrinth of Birth by Pam England.

HOW TO DRAW A CLASSIC LABYRINTH

1. First draw the "seed." Many labyrinths begin with a seed, a simple pattern from which the rest of the labyrinth grows. The seed shown here is the beginning of a classic seven-circuit labyrinth.

2. Draw the seed about one-third from the bottom of your paper because labyrinths grow upward and outward as you draw them.

3. Draw the corridors. Begin by drawing an arc from the vertical centerline (in the "+") to the first vertical line on the "corner" in the upper left. Continue to follow the step-by-step illustrations. Extend lines or dots as needed to keep the widths of the corridors fairly even and at least as wide as your finger so you can finger-trace it later. You can choose to make the corners round or square.

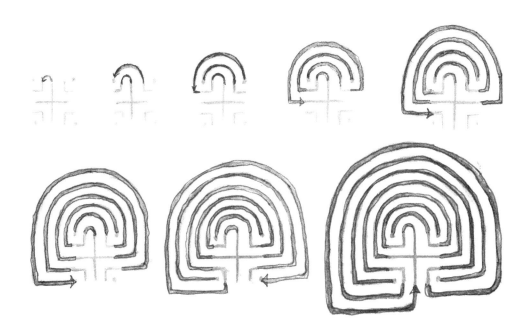

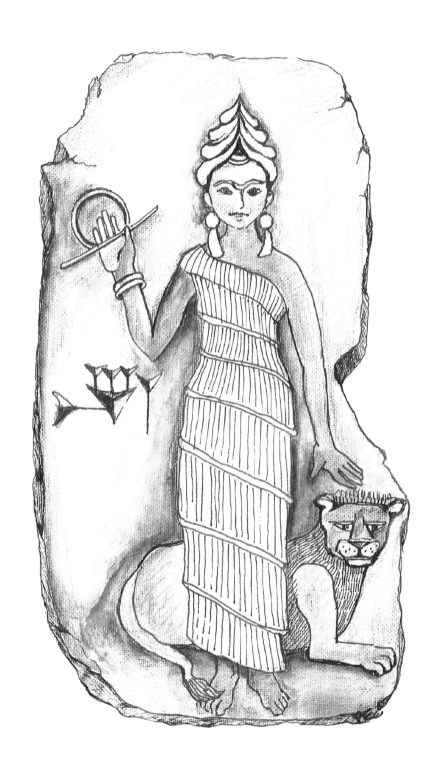

INANNA'S DESCENT
A MYTHIC STORY

Combining the ancient art of teaching through storytelling with evidence-based information fuses different kinds of knowing and makes for meaningful and holistic preparation.

Perhaps the best way to learn about the journey you are now on is the original way: through hearing a great story—not just any story, or even a personal story, but a mythic story. For centuries, hero myths have been told to entertain, but more importantly to teach, inspire, and prepare initiates for their rites of passage. It is through identifying with a character who is larger than life that you internalize your heroine. Her mythic story—her Call, her hardships, her determination, her cleverness, and her triumph—will become an inner map guiding you through and beyond your own rite of passage. The ancient Sumerian myth of the journey of Inanna (pronounced ee-NA-na) has proven to be especially powerful for parents because the warrior queen's preparation, ordeal, and return parallel modern women's experiences during the childbearing year.

It is customary for a storyteller to begin by introducing the roots of the story, that is, the place it comes from and the people who first told it. "Inanna's Descent," as the myth is known, has roots that run deep, for it is the oldest story ever written. It was first set down (around 2300 BCE) in Sumer, which occupied some of the land that is now Iraq. It is a mythic story about a warrior-queen-mother who made the classic heroic journey.

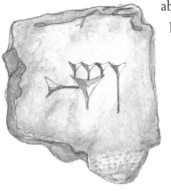

"Inanna's Descent" was written and preserved for us by a woman named Enheduanna, a high priestess at the temple of Ur for some forty years. She wrote the story in cuneiform (the first written language) by pressing a reed stylus into hand-held clay tablets.

For centuries, oral storytelling has connected individuals to their communities' history. In traditional cultures, this led to stories that explain the origins of the first people and everything in the natural world, including what brings rain and what makes the sun rise and set. There are teaching stories about planting, herding, weaving, getting along with others, healing, dying—and about birthing. Before initiates undertook a rite of passage or a vision quest, stories informed them about what to eat and drink, how to find herbs for healing, and landmarks to look for to ensure completion of their personal tasks.

You can read about Inanna's journey yourself or allow the story to slowly enter you while listening to your partner or a friend read it aloud. Afterward, have a cup of tea. Then make a drawing of a scene from the story that spoke to you. A mythic story, rooted in the heart, will nourish, guide, and inspire.

Tribute to Diane Wolkstein and Samuel Noah Kramer

We would not be able to read the epic poem "Inanna's Descent" were it not for the painstaking efforts of two people—storyteller Diane Wolkstein and cuneiformist Samuel Noah Kramer—who collaborated on a scholarly translation of the ancient Sumerian work. The translation appears in their book *Inanna: Queen of Heaven and Earth*.

"This is what we know about our stories. They go to work on your mind and make you think about your life."

—NICK THOMPSON[1]

INANNA WAS A WOMAN OF POWER—a warrior, a queen, a poet, and the priestess of seven temples. Inanna heard her Call from the Great Below. She knew that answering it would disrupt her life's rhythms and relationships and bring uncertainty. Like hearing a drum beating in the distance, it's possible to ignore such a Call for a while, but they persist until answered. When Inanna's heart was ready, she accepted her Call. From that moment on, there was no turning back. With her whole body and mind, she began preparing for her inner journey.

Inanna was the priestess of seven temples, a time-consuming vocation as Sumerian temples were bustling community centers with markets, gardens, social gatherings, and ceremonies. To free up time to retreat from her ordinary life, Inanna's first task was to abandon her seven temples.

Her next task was gathering seven royal articles imbued with power that would offer her protection as she journeyed through the unknown. Inanna dressed for her rite of passage in her finest royal warrior clothes, arranged her hair, and donned her crown. Around her neck she tied a lapis necklace and blessing beads. To protect her heart, she tied on her warrior breastplate. Over her hand, she slipped a gold bracelet. Around her shoulders, she wrapped a royal robe. Lastly, she took up her lapis measuring rod and ring.

Inanna called on her trusted advisor, Ninshubur (pronounced neen-SHU-ber), Queen of the East, to help her prepare for her descent into a place from which no one returns unchanged. All the while, Ninshubur fretted. If anything went wrong or Inanna suffered too much during her descent, Ninshubur would feel responsible for not having dissuaded her queen from taking this risk. She also worried that Inanna's powerful transformation might change their friendship. So she tried to talk Inanna out of answering her Call, but Inanna would not be deterred.

Although Ninshubur and Inanna had fought side by side in other battles, Inanna knew she had to fight this one alone. She also knew she could trust her faithful advisor Ninshubur above all others with the task of ensuring her safe return. She said, "My dearest friend and advisor, if I do not return in three days by my own efforts, go to the three wise elders and ask them to help me complete my return. Do not abandon me in the underworld."

Having completed her Tasks of Preparation, Inanna walked away from the comforts of her ordinary life. In due time, she arrived at the First Gate of the underworld (Laborland).

Bidu, the Gatekeeper, whose name meant "to open," demanded, "Who are *you*?"

"I am Inanna," she answered, "queen of heaven and earth. I am a poet, warrior, priestess, and wife. I have learned the body ways of birth, yoga, herbs, dances, and breathing, and I have my birth plan right here in my lapis measuring rod. Let me enter."

Bidu asked, "Why has your heart led you here, to a place from which no one returns unchanged or unscathed?"

Inanna gave her reasons and demanded to be let in.

"Come," he said, "you may enter."

As Inanna crossed the first threshold, Bidu took her crown. Inanna protested, to which Bidu explained, "The ways of the underworld are ancient and proven. Its ways may not be bargained away or questioned."

Inanna continued her descent through a labyrinthine passage. Gate after gate, Inanna encountered Bidu, the Gatekeeper. Each time, Bidu asked Inanna, "Who are you? Why has your heart led you to this place, a place from which you will not return unchanged?"

Each time Inanna passed through a gate Bidu took something of value, something she had brought or worn for protection, comfort, or as a sign to let others know she was special. At the Second Gate, Bidu took her lapis necklace and blessing beads. At the Third Gate, he took her breastplate. At the Fourth Gate, he took her royal robe, leaving her cold and exposed. At the Fifth Gate, he removed her gold bracelet. At the Sixth Gate, he took her shoes. And at the Seventh Gate he took from her hands the lapis measuring rod and ring.

With each small loss, the queen protested, "It isn't fair! Give it back! I didn't agree to this!"

Bidu reminded Inanna, "The ways of the underworld are ancient and may not be questioned. Keep going, Inanna. Find out who you really are."

Gate by gate, Inanna descended deeper and deeper into the underworld. The underworld was an unfamiliar place. She did not know her way. Only her resolve lit the path through the dark and twisting labyrinth, across thresholds of mercy, terror, and doubt.

Naked, humble, sweaty, and exhausted, Inanna crawled on her hands and knees toward the last threshold. She had given her all. Finally, she arrived at the Seventh Gate. By now the Gatekeeper had seized everything except the one thing he could not take: Inanna's determination to do what needed to be done next. Reaching deep inside herself, she mustered up a great push, and then another and another until the Gatekeeper opened the last gate.

And there, in the deepest, most sacred place of all, she saw the one who had been calling her and who was still calling to her (her newborn baby). In this transformative moment, the person Inanna had died. In the next breath, she was reborn (as a Mother).

Three days and three nights passed. Inanna was suspended between two worlds. She could not make it home. Three days is a long time to wait while someone you love is out of reach in the underworld. Ninshubur went to the elders. The first two would not help, blaming Inanna for her predicament. The third elder listened carefully and came up with a plan. Of the three, only he knew the way out because he had gone to the underworld and returned. He created two allies and gave them the Water of Life and the Food of Life, and instructed them to take these to Inanna.

⑤

Once she had gathered her strength, Inanna began to hear another Call, this time from the Great Above, to return to her life. She began her slow ascent.

At each gate on her return, Bidu asked, "Who are you? What do you know now that you did not know before you made this descent?"

At each gate, the Gatekeeper took from Inanna something that belonged to the underworld. At the First Gate, he took self-absorption from her and gave her gratitude. At the Second Gate, he took worry from her and gave her relief. At the Third Gate, he took sleep from her and gave her stamina. At the Fourth Gate, he took old relationship dynamics and gave her renewal. At the Fifth Gate, he took the weight of blame of self and others and gave her understanding. At the Sixth Gate, he stopped her mind from spinning. At the Seventh Gate, he took pride and gave her humility. At the Eighth Gate, Bidu took her gathering basket and turned her attention inward. At the Ninth Gate, he lifted the weight of the whole story and gave her wisdom.

The warrior-priestess who had left on this journey was surely not the one who returned, for the descent and return had transformed Inanna's mind, body, and heart.

"That story is working on you now. You keep thinking about it. That story is changing you now, making you want to live right. That story is making you want to replace yourself."

—Nick Thompson[2]

Where and how to listen to the story

You might enjoy hearing me tell the story "Inanna's Descent into Laborland," a version adapted for childbirth preparation.

Part 2
THE CALL

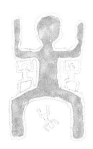

Your Call
Is an Invitation

4

*When the student is ready to start, Don Juan says,
"It is not so simple as that. You must be ready first."*

"I think I am ready," Carlos answers.

*"This is not a joke. You must wait until there is no
doubt. . . . You may give up the whole idea after a
while. You get tired easily. Last night you were ready
to quit as soon as it got difficult. [The warrior's
journey] requires a very serious intent."*

—CARLOS CASTANEDA

A Call is an invitation from your soul compelling you
to do something you have not done before, something that
may not make sense or come easily to you. Hearing your Call
awakens a deep hunger. You can't sleep. There is a quickening
in you.

Troubles are calls from the gods.

—JAMES HILLMAN

There is not just one Call in a lifetime or even during the
childbearing year. In a sense, every important moment of your

life and every decision you face is a small invitation to love yourself, to be open instead of hiding or retreating, to speak your truth, and to do what needs to be done next.

A Call may come to you suddenly or gradually. Sometimes it is a subtle inner whisper, so you have to be listening. Sometimes it comes in a vision or dream, so keep a dream journal and pen by your bed to record dreams before they fade. A Call may come to you during an ordinary conversation, a scene in a movie, a song, or while viewing art that seems to ignite a glowing ember in your being and awakens you to a new yearning.

> Inanna heard the Call from deep in her belly
>
> Inanna heard the Call from her longing heart
>
> Inanna heard the Call from the Great Unknown.

When you become aware of a Call, you may be eager to act at first, until the difficulty of doing things in a new way becomes evident and takes you beyond your ordinary limitations. For example, for someone who has always insisted on being organized suddenly being spontaneous or not planning can be a leap out of her comfort zone. Agreeing to do something unfamiliar means risking failure, disapproval, or disagreement with loved ones or authority figures. It takes courage to deal with necessary conflict, to do the thing you don't yet know how to do and face the unknown. Consequently, after taking a step or two in a new direction it is natural to experience doubts, second thoughts, or to want to postpone making decisions or taking further action. Your inner voice of doubt may be asking: "Is this a good idea? Are you strong enough, smart enough, or brave enough to do this? What will people think of you if you do this? What will people think of you if you fail? Is there another way?" This is not a phase of the heroine's journey in which you should remain.

If you do go through a refusal, a phase of hesitation to act on the invitation, you are not necessarily resisting or doing nothing. During this time, you are likely gathering and sorting

information, and assessing assumptions and opinions, sometimes unconsciously.

Even during this phase the soul is persistent and will keep
calling you. Every Call answered wholeheartedly, no matter how
small and quiet the steps, is part of the preparation for your quest.

YOUR HEART'S QUESTION

Knowing your heart's question is central to preparing for
birth as a heroic journey. You might have many cerebral questions about labor or your birthplace, but it is your heart's question that will help you know yourself and thus deepen your
preparation for labor and transition to parenting.

You cannot answer this question with words and logic but
must manifest the answer with your whole being through the
way you live. Living the answer to your heart's question will
cause you to form new habits of thinking and responding.

To find your heart's question, ask yourself, "What is it I need
to know to give birth as a mother (not as a health consumer)?"
Or ask, "What is it I need to do or know to enjoy my pregnancy
more?" Listen intently for what your heart wants to know. When
your heart's question comes to you, jot it down.

LIVING THE ANSWER
TO YOUR HEART'S QUESTION

To authentically answer your heart's question, you have to
live the answer. So as you go about each day, from time to time
recall your heart's question and manifest the answer in how you
take your next step, slice a carrot, or answer the phone.

If your heart's question involves being more loving, ask yourself, "How am I bringing love to *this* moment?" Live the answer
by bringing your full attention to what is at hand. For example,
while making a salad ask your heart's question. In living the
answer, you might feel gratitude for the healthy food and its
colors and textures, arranging the vegetables in a pleasing way.
Or you might sprinkle in sunflower seeds or some new ingre-

dient. Even though no one else knows that you asked your heart's question while preparing the food, upon tasting it people may notice it was prepared with love.

When living the answer to your heart's question, you might notice that you walk more mindfully, wash the dishes a little more quietly, or drive more calmly. This is because living the answer to your heart's question focuses your attention and nourishes your relationship with everything you touch.

Tips for living the answer to your heart's question:

- Ask your heart's question in the present tense to make it easier to live the answer. For example, instead of asking, "How will I open in labor?" ask, "How am I opening in this moment?"

- Keep your heart's question short so you can ask it often throughout the day. For example, "What does this moment need?"

- You can't live the answer to a question about someone else's behavior. For example, instead of asking, "How can I make the doctor listen to me?" you might ask, "Am I willing to risk conflict to ask for what I want?"

- Avoid asking your heart's question in such a way that it can be answered with a yes, no, or maybe. For example, asking, "How can I avoid a cesarean?" leaves you open to others' opinions and invites mental chatter.

- Write your heart's question on an index card with a bold-colored marker and post it where you will see it every day to remind you to live the answer.

- Hold your question in your heart. Ask it silently when you wake up, during ordinary day-to-day activities, and as you fall asleep. Look for the answer from every angle until your conscious mind is exhausted, which is when your heart is most receptive to answers. Listen deeply. Answers often come after you give up trying to understand them.

THREE WAYS OF KNOWING

5

Holistic preparation for birth and parenting requires cultivating a balance among three ways of knowing: intuitive, modern, and personal. It is important to explore how you know what you know and how to know when to follow your intuition or the advice of others.

Philosophers have struggled for thousands of years to answer the questions "What is knowing?" and "How do you know what you know?" Knowledge is a complex subject often oversimplified, particularly by those in the birth world. Picking a flower off a plant and ignoring the seed from which it grew is like isolating one part of birth knowledge and claiming it alone is the truth. This is represented in catchphrases such as "Your body knows how to give birth," "Trust the experts," and "Make evidence-based choices." Thinking in this simplistic and fragmented way diminishes the nuanced nature of a pregnant woman's knowing. Much like a plant is composed of seeds, roots, stems, and leaves in addition to the flower, knowing about birth arises from many sources.

Holistic preparation for birth requires knowing about the normal course of labor; birth physiology; nutrition; how to prepare for all kinds of possibilities, including inductions and cesarean birth; and navigating postpartum conditions. Just as one cannot understand how scissors cut by looking at a single blade, no decision should be based on one kind of knowing. Consider these three ways of knowing and seek a balance between them.

INTUITIVE KNOWING

Intuition is knowing the truth before you have the proof.

Maternal instinct or intuition is in your gut and in your bones, not in your thinking mind. Intuitive knowing bypasses thought and defies logic. Decisions based on intuitive knowing are sometimes better than those made from information overload. Trying to decide which bits of advice to follow, especially when many are in conflict with one another, can lead to befuddled overthinking and anxiety. With intuitive knowing, there is an absence of foreboding: you just know, although you may not be able to explain how you know.

Because we come from a culture that especially values rational and scientific knowing, we are prone to doubt or dismiss intuitive knowing, especially when it conflicts with modern knowing. Intuitive hunches inform us in everyday situations. Sometimes we tune in; sometimes we intentionally ignore them in favor of pleasing others, avoiding conflict, or overthinking the situation. Social conditioning has taught us not to trust or act on instinct until we have researched its implications or checked to see what others think.

Accessing intuitive knowing does not come easily to people who are fearful, busy, or reliant on scientific knowledge Once you think you know what is going on or what to do, your intuition may cease to speak to you; being in a place of not knowing makes you more intuitive. A decision arising from intuitive knowing should not be any more fixed than a decision based on information. Remember to keep listening as the situation unfolds and as you take in new information; a Birth

Warrior is flexible and ready to change her mind if that is what the situation calls for.

MODERN KNOWING

Get your facts first, then you can distort them as you please.

— MARK TWAIN

Modern knowing involves being savvy about hospital and medical norms and how to give birth within this framework. Modern knowing also includes being aware of when cultural norms and social pressures are informing your decisions and when you are ignoring your intuition in favor of doing what seems most socially acceptable or common even if it is not necessary or valuable. Unfortunately, modern knowing, which necessitates being "in your head," is essential to navigate birth in today's society.

Sometimes modern knowing is based on a belief that the only truth is an objective one derived from logic. We tend to assume that medical recommendations arise purely from science, when often advice and management come from a variety of belief systems and motivations, including the need to be right, the desire to avoid a potential lawsuit, the need to conform with one's medical culture, having limited perspective or knowledge of alternatives, and sometimes simply fatigue and burnout. Thoughtful analysis of your specific situation is required to guide your decisions.

PERSONAL KNOWING

When you reach the end of what you should know,
you will be at the beginning of what you should sense.

—KAHLIL GIBRAN

Personal knowing is about being intimately familiar with your habits, assumptions, and beliefs. This is necessary because the

Gaslighting

"Gaslighting" is a term referring to a type of manipulation depicted in the classic movie *Gas Light* (1944). In this suspense thriller, a husband convinces his wife, whom he wants to get rid of, that she is losing her mind; he does this by making frequent subtle changes in the house, including slowly dimming the gaslights, but denying the changes, thereby creating so much doubt in his wife's mind that she no longer trusts her own perceptions and gradually comes under his control.

In prenatal care, gaslighting happens when a pregnant woman's self-confidence is incrementally eroded by having her intuitions or choices discounted by experts who profess to see perfectly through the lens of scientific knowledge. A variation of this can occur during a home birth when a birthing woman intuits that she should do something different or go to the hospital but her midwives tell her not to let fear get in her way or that she is buying into the bias of the patriarchy. In either case, the mother may begin to doubt her inner compass, relinquish self-trust, and put her fate in the hands of others.

Experts can explain the past by creating a story that fits with observation, but they can never be certain about the future. Later, based on the outcome, we can second-guess ourselves. Don't use hindsight to judge yourself or your decision-making process.

Experience creates blind spots. Once you think you know the answer or what to expect, your eyes stop seeing both internal and external possibilities. Once you believe the limits of what is possible for you, your mind stops searching or imagining. Doing something for the first time, you may think to yourself, "What do I know?" While experience can inform you in helpful ways, it can also inhibit you if it reminds you of mistakes and failures. Second-time mothers may assume that a potential solution won't work because it didn't before, or they may become attached to a narrower range of possibilities. One benefit of being a "rookie mother" is that you make up for lack of experience by being open to solutions and optimistic. Whether you are a rookie or a seasoned mother, find ways to mix knowledge from past experiences with the vitality and imagination of a beginner.

—Inspired by the book *Rookie Smarts* by Liz Wizeman[1]

way you listen to, integrate, and act on both factual information and intuition is influenced by past experiences. Without personal awareness, habitual ways of thinking and responding can suppress both your intuition and your ability to objectively assess a situation. Sometimes determination and wishful thinking can be confused with intuition. Overreacting, making assumptions, and having a strong attachment to an outcome can interfere with personal clarity as decisions are being made. Knowing yourself in the context of your past experiences and setting aside time to be still and introspective may help you clarify how best to interpret information and act on it.

Mixed Messages

As a modern pregnant woman, you may receive conflicting messages regarding knowing. In one ear you may be told that everything you need to know is within you and you should trust your intuition; in the other ear you may be told to become informed and rely on evidence-based research. One moment you may be told to trust your body, and the next moment you may be told that birth is risky and therefore you should rely on experts and technology.

Tasks for the Birth Warrior

1. Think of knowing as a continuum. Imagine one end labeled "intuitive knowing," which includes personal knowing (internal knowledge), and the other end labeled "modern knowing," which refers to what experts know, data from tests, and evidence-based research (external knowledge). Mark the central point on this trajectory as the "point of balance" where you have equal access to internal and external knowledge.

When gathering information or making a decision,

notice where your pointer is on the internal-external knowledge continuum. Sometimes one kind of knowing is needed more than the others. Be aware if you tend to tune in to one kind of knowing to the exclusion of the others. If you have become too trusting of one kind of knowing, then be open to the other ways of knowing. Remaining fixed in a familiar position limits the degree to which you can see the big picture and benefit from a creative solution-focused mindset.

2. As you go about your routine and are faced with choices, notice your intuitions and act on them. Discern which circumstances or conditions allow you to best listen to your intuitions.

3. Before learning what is "out there" in the birth world, ask yourself:

• What do I believe or assume to be true about birth, pain, babies, mothering, and hospitals?

• What assumptions are motivating me to make—or not make—certain decisions?

• What is inspiring me to read about one topic but not another? Am I choosing to read material that matches familiar assumptions?

4. Whether you are planning to birth at home or in a hospital, one of the modern tasks of birth preparation is to learn about the hospital birth culture in your community.

5. When you sense or know that action is needed, "take the bull by the horns" instead of waiting to see what happens or beating around the bush. This is what the brave Greek warrior Theseus did when he confronted a savage bull. The bull bellowed, lowered his head, and rushed him, intending to gore him, but Theseus grabbed the bull by the horns and held its head to the ground until the bull grew too tired to fight, then tied a rope around it and led it away. A Birth Warrior does what needs to be done.

Breath Awareness

There is a way of breathing that's a shame and a suffocation. And there's another way of expiring a love breath that lets you open infinitely.

—RUMI

Throughout the day and night, countless physiological processes occur without any conscious effort on your part. Your body makes continuous adjustments to balance hormones, heart rate, blood pressure, and breathing. Breath Awareness is being aware of how your body is breathing naturally, without making any effort to influence it by slowing it down or imposing a pattern. Notice whether your next exhalation is long or slow, shallow or deep, and exactly when it begins and when it ends. Be aware of whether you are breathing in or breathing out when you wake up, when you open a door, when you cross the threshold, and how your breathing changes spontaneously and subtly during "ice contractions."

"Breath is the bridge which connects life to consciousness, which unites your body to your thoughts. Whenever your mind becomes scattered, use your breath as the means to take hold of your mind again."

—THÍCH NHAT HANH [2]

Become aware of how bringing your full attention to your exhalations centers and calms your mind. In labor, witnessing how your body breathes your baby out also engages your mind and intention.

Hold an ice cube during an "ice contraction" to practice coping with pain during pregnancy.

INNOCENCE AND TRUST

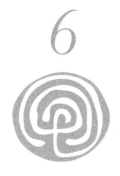

Trust can mean different things to different people. Sometimes trust means waiting; yet trust is also required to question, seek, and take action. When a mother tells me that she "trusts," I ask her: "What do you trust? What or who is worthy of your trust?"

—BRENNA ROTHSCHILD, MOTHER AND DOULA

It is almost inevitable, if not necessary, to begin your childbearing year in a place of innocence, trust, positivity, and optimism—idealistically imagining having a particular kind of birth and holding your sweet little baby in your arms—while minimizing or overlooking challenges in getting there. Having a positive outlook is an important predictor of future resilience and resourcefulness.

Yet a pregnant woman who expresses a positive attitude about birth and mothering may be judged for being too trusting and naïve. Some people may assume that if she is relaxed or making birth art she must be out of touch with reality and not really getting ready for the changes to come. In an attempt to "wake her up" or save her from disappointment later, people may respond by reciting horror stories, bombarding her with advice, or issuing dire warnings. However, if the woman finds these responses unsupportive, not only can this harm relationships but she may tune out people close to her or become fearful or closed-minded.

TRUST BIRTH?

Because of the uncertainties of birth, promises about how to achieve a "positive birth" (from individuals, methods, books, or affirmations) are rampant and seductive but may reinforce idealism or fixed expectations, especially in a first-time mother who tends toward innocence and hopefulness. In response to high intervention rates and the increased use of technology in birth, many who feel passionate about natural birth try to inspire women to have more faith in their bodies and in the normalcy of physiological birth. Yet to a woman pregnant for the first time these simplistic assurances can be confusing. When hearing them as promises, she may narrow her expectations and engage in passivity, magical thinking, and denial of real concerns.

When you imagine your birth experience, do you have realistic goals or are they pure fantasy? Do you have a plan to achieve what you hope for or is it just wishful thinking?

Such "promises" may turn out to be the seed of a mother's later disappointment in her birth or in herself. When a woman who "trusted her body" and expected an easy natural birth does not "progress" or is induced, she may enter motherhood feeling shame, confusion, or betrayal because she believes she "failed" or her body "failed" her. This kind of birth trauma may be lessened by being mindful about the language we use to inspire, support, and educate pregnant women—in particular, by avoiding absolute or outcome-focused messages. It is essential that any conversation about trust and birth be honest, compassionate, and realistic, not idealized, horrific, or oversimplified.

Trusting your body is helpful and important; the problem arises when you believe that if you just trust in the right way you will achieve an ideal or natural birth. No amount of trust or preparation can guarantee an easy birth. In the real world, some women's bodies are not able to give birth. So instead of focusing on the adage "Trust your body," trust that you can meet whatever challenges come your way.

FINDING
THE MIDDLE GROUND

There is a fine line between too much trust and too little trust. Try to balance achieving your goals with maintaining your emotional well-being. Too little trust in your ability to make a difference or to make good decisions can lead to hopelessness, passivity, and obedience. Also distrust of others can lead to a distancing from external sources of information or obsessive researching.

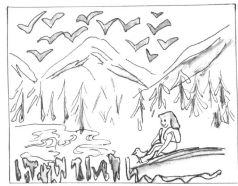

Positive feelings about pregnancy and mothering are expressed by Lilly in her drawing.

You cannot simply build trust, tuck it in your basket, and carry it with you on your entire journey. Certainly some things you trust will see you through. But because birth is a rite of passage, there will be twists and turns, even detours. No matter how trusting and informed you are, it is impossible for you to know what to expect and what to do every step of the way. You can count on this:

At some point you will be surprised, the unexpected will happen, one thing you trust now will get taken or shaken (you won't get to choose what that one thing is), and when it does you will lose your innocence. It is the price of wisdom.

Tips for establishing trust:

- Utilize the power of innocence to encourage imagination and visualization.

- Be aware of the warning signs of having too much trust: denying or ignoring problems or hunches; seeking simplistic solutions; wishing birth were simple "like in the old days"; buying into promises that if

Inspiring and Helpful Affirmations That Can Be True in Any Moment

I trust that birth is a deep and unknowable mystery.

I know what to do when I don't know what to do.

My body may surprise me.

I am learning how to trust myself and others.

The labyrinth of my birth journey is uniquely mine.

I am ready to pass through Gates of Great Doubt and Great Determination.

I am opening to each moment.

Labor is hard work, and I can do it.

you just do _____ your birth will be easy; or hoping everything will magically work out.

- Be aware of the warning signs of having too little trust: micromanaging; long, detailed birth plans; over-researching; and frequently changing care providers.

- Question the birth-related promises and predictions of authority figures.

- Trust your intuition and address concerns rather than dismissing them, hoping they will go away or expecting others to take care of them.

- Be realistic: don't strive for an "ideal" birth or to be a "perfect" parent.

- Be mindful of the company you keep and the birth stories you listen to since what you trust or distrust about birth will be reinforced or not by the attitudes and beliefs of people around you and the resources, such as books and documentaries, to which you are exposed.

"This is your time, and it feels normal to you. But really, there is no 'normal.' There's only change, and resistance to it, and then more change."

—MERYL STREEP[1]

- Practice discerning when, whom, and how much to trust—or not to trust.

- Maintain a healthy balance between trusting yourself and trusting others.

Part 3

AWAKEN THE MOTHER

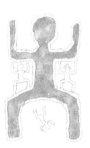

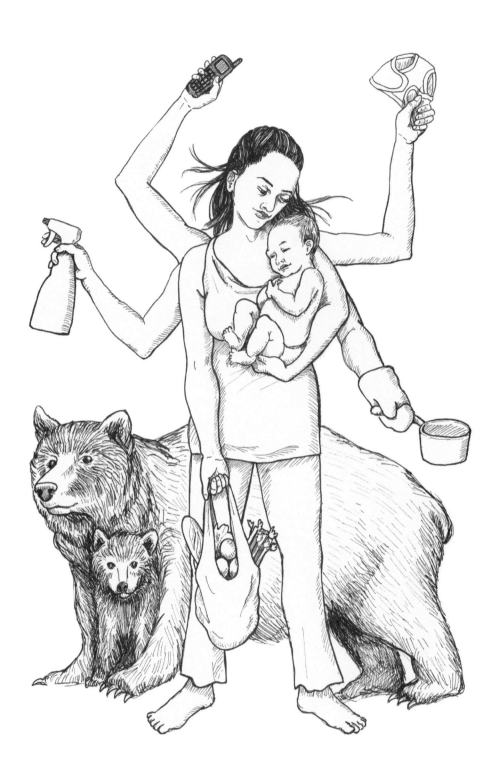

THE MOTHER

7

The relationship of mother and child is so simple that every peasant woman takes it for granted; so full of emotional content that artists, poets and story-tellers have been lured by it in every age.

—M. ESTHER HARDING

You are on the threshold between being a daughter and becoming a mother. Realizing yourself as a mother might dawn on you the moment you see your positive pregnancy test, or when you feel the baby kick for the first time, or maybe when you first hold and comfort your child. Throughout the child-bearing year you are evolving from an archetypal Maiden to a Child-Mother to a mature Mother. Becoming a mother is one of the most complex and profoundly life-changing transformations, so it often unfolds gradually over time.

To touch such enormous wealth of experience is to be penetrated by the holy. Something so beyond the limitations of our own small personality enters us and leaves its imprint.

—TONY CRISP

The Mother archetype is ancient, universal, and complex. She is found in cave art, fairy tales, mythology, religion, literature, and art. This Mother, in all her manifestations, is already within you when you are imagining what being a mother will be like; wondering if you are having a boy or girl; or making lists of names. It is the Mother in you who worries if the baby will be healthy, wants to give your baby a good start in life, eats certain foods while avoiding others, buys or makes things for your baby, creates a special space for your baby. You will also discover the many faces and expressions of the Mother.

The Mother

Accepts her place in the timeless chain of mothers
    throughout time and space.
Sees the vast presence and countless expressions
    of the Mother in nature and humanity.
Embodies her role as the giver of life,
    as both nurturer and teacher.
Releases perfection and rigid expectations
    of her child and herself.
Grows in compassion
    for herself and for all mothers.

Mixed messages to pregnant women about becoming a mother abound. Many assume that, by virtue of conceiving a child, they will immediately experience a maternal instinct. Yet thousands of books, websites, and experts tell you the "right way to mother." Which is correct? Perhaps the truth lies in the middle: maternal instincts are both inborn and learned. You learn how to collect information and guidance from mother-mentors while also listening to your inner voice. This task begins in pregnancy and will follow you throughout your life-long relationship with your child.

Nurture Your Emerging Mother-Self
Taking Baby on a Color Walk

When you feel your child move in your belly, your connection to nature and the mystery of life awakens. For the first time in years, you may notice birds making their nests in the spring, feel especially tender toward baby animals, or be aware of buds unfolding. You may enjoy quiet moments during a busy day communing with your growing child.

A color walk is a lovely practice that fits naturally with this awakening to nature and your baby, still cocooned in his dark, watery world. Once a week, take a leisurely walk and describe to your baby the world of color and beauty that is waiting for him. Choose a different color each week. Wherever you take your walk—through a city park, on a beach, along a river, on a mountain path, or down a bustling street—be your baby's eyes and tell your baby about everything of the chosen color. Your narration might sound like this: *"Look, this shirt is red.…There are hundreds of roses bursting in red.…The petals are very soft, like your velvet-soft skin.…Can you hear the red truck?…There's our red mailbox. I wonder what the letter carrier is bringing."*

Even before your baby is born, taking him on a color walk builds a playful relationship with him. On a color walk, you are not just walking to get from here to there or performing an exercise routine. Even before birth, nurturing your relationship with your child helps you see as a child sees and be delighted with the smallest miracles in nature.

Green

Black

Yellow

Red

White

Silver

Blue

Brown

Red

Orange

Gold

Purple

HUMANIZING YOUR MOTHER

Even if your relationship with your mother is not what you would have liked it to be, in becoming a mother yourself it is beneficial to connect even the finest thread of "wholesome mothering" you experienced. To do this, it may help to supply the missing phrase in the following sentence:

One thing my mother did that I treasure and that I want to continue doing as a mother with my children is _____.

SEEING MYSELF AS A MOTHER

Seeing yourself as a mother may evoke complex or ambiguous images that can be better understood when expressed in artwork. Draw, paint, or sculpt what becoming a mother means to you. Your image should be in human form, not an abstraction. Add as many symbols or colors as needed to express your idea fully. Even when you think you are done, keep working, adding one, two, or three more details, ideas, or symbols. If one picture can't capture everything you feel about becoming a mother, make another or a series of drawings, paintings, or sculptures.

Take time to journal and share your artwork with a trusted friend. What surprised you? What do you know now about yourself or about motherhood?

When I speak to my own mum,
she says where we lived in Warrington
everyone mucked in.
If you were having a bad day, it was OK to
hand the baby over to a neighbor and get your head down.
Nobody judged you.
Now I think the ideal of being a good parent has been supplanted
by this idea that you have to be the best and excel at everything
and that's impossible for anyone to live up to.

—HELEN WALSH

Tapu'at: Mother and Child

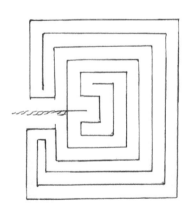

"As you bring your child into the world, your child brings you into your adult-self."

—LUCIEN HOROWITZ

The Hopi, Native American people who live in northeastern Arizona, designed a square labyrinth called Tapu'at, which means "mother and child." It is unique because it has two entrances and contains two labyrinths, one within the other. The outer labyrinth holds the inner labyrinth, like a mother holding her child, or a womb enveloping the unborn baby. The unattached center line emerging from the entrance of Tapu'at represents the umbilical cord. Its two ends symbolize the two stages of life—the unborn child within the womb of Mother Earth and the child after it is born. The U-shaped lines on the outer edges represent the fetal membranes that enfold the child within the womb. The outside lines represent the mother's arms, which will later hold the child.[1]

PLACENTAL CLOCK

8

People have long wondered what starts labor and why this can vary so widely from mother to mother. Many factors influence the timing of birth, including nutrition, smoking, infection, and socioeconomic status. One interesting new line of research relates to what is called the "placental clock," a theory that the placenta's production of stress hormones impacts the timing of birth. This theory suggests it is not the normal ups and downs of daily living that may cause the placental clock to tick faster but rather a single traumatic event (such as Hurricane Katrina or a sudden death in the family), chronic stress, anxiety, or the combination of an anxious disposition and a series of stressful events, especially when the mother is lacking internal or external resources for coping with stress.

Stressful situations cannot always be avoided in life. The good news is that the placental clock is more influenced by how the pregnant woman perceives and responds to stress in her life than by the amount of stress she faces. Her resourcefulness and ability to cope with stress can decrease the levels of stress hormones in her body and lower her risk of preterm birth.

A little primer on how stress hormones work during pregnancy

When a situation is perceived as catastrophic or life threatening (whether it is or not), a stress hormone called CRH (corticotrophin-releasing hormone) is secreted in the brain and signals the release of more stress hormones (adrenaline and cortisol), which are necessary for the fight-flight-freeze response. After the stressor or threat has passed, stress hormones return to baseline.

During the first trimester, CRH levels are typically low. Studies have shown that mothers with low stress and low CRH in the first trimester are less likely to miscarry or to have a preterm birth.[1, 2]

Around 20 weeks there is a normal increase in CRH even when pregnancy is not particularly stressful, because the placenta begins producing CRH, which is secreted into the mother's blood. Ordinarily, a prolonged surge of CRH would stimulate a surplus of stress hormones. However, an amazing change in a pregnant woman's physiology occurs around 20 weeks: large quantities of a CRH-binding protein are produced, which prevents CRH from being recognized, so the body does not go into fight-flight-freeze response.[3] This explains why women tend to feel euphoric—even in otherwise stressful situations—during the second and third trimesters.

During the last three weeks of pregnancy, just when CRH levels reach their peak binding proteins suddenly decrease.[4] Unbound CRH is active and recognized by the body, which induces a spike in maternal cortisol two to three times the normal level.[5] This normal late-term cortisol surge helps prepare both the baby and the mother for the upcoming birth. It stimulates the baby's brain development and maturation of the lungs[6] and it increases the mother's estrogen levels, which makes her uterus more sensitive to oxytocin, the hormone responsible for uterine contractions.[7]

It seems contradictory that a stress hormone would contribute to "nesting," the compulsion to clean the house and organize the nursery just before going into labor. However, right on cue, with motherhood just around the corner, this perfectly timed surge in cortisol alters the brain and awakens maternal attentiveness, instinct, and sympathy for the baby.[8]

The scientific thinking
behind anxiety, stress, and preterm birth

When a woman is experiencing excessive, ongoing stress and unrelenting worry and anxiety, her body releases more cortisol. Remember, in the first half of pregnancy CRH and cortisol-binding protein are normally low. Constant stress releases active cortisol, which passes freely through the placenta and into the baby's circulation. If a mother's stress is not relieved and stress hormones remain high, the baby begins to produce its own cortisol and stress hormones, as much as twenty times the normal level. Elevated CRH and cortisol in the first trimester may signal the fetus to adjust the timing of its birth[9] and increases the chance of miscarriage[10, 11] and preterm labor.[12]

TASKS OF EARLY PREGNANCY

We must have a pie. Stress cannot exist in the presence of a pie.

—DAVID MAMET

In general, when a person ignores a problem or hopes that someone or something "out there" will intervene on her behalf, her CRH and stress hormone levels tend to be higher.[13] So be aware of early signs of tension, avoidance, or stress, especially regarding any decision you have to make. Instead of freezing, which can create more stress, take a small step toward resolution or a solution. Ask yourself, "What needs to happen next?" Stress is reduced when you act decisively and avoid second-guessing or judging yourself.

> *How might our perception of a stressful situation change*
> *if we viewed it as "a portal to a redefining moment,"*
> *an opportunity to "step into a deeper knowing of who we truly are . . .*
> *or to re-invent ourselves."*
>
> —DENNIS MERRITT JONES

Stress can also be reduced by making small adjustments in your daily activities, such as eating breakfast sitting down rather than on the go. Organize your week so you do fewer errands and less driving. If possible, take a day off in the middle of the week and work on Saturdays instead, to lessen the fatigue of a long workweek. Unplug from online pregnancy and birth sites and opt for watching funny movies instead. Practice yoga, tai chi, or meditation, and take long walks in nature, without your phone. Making small adjustments to your routines and allowing yourself to be "lazy" can actually be the most healthful choices for you and your baby.

RELEASE STRESS
Laugh, cry, dance—often.

Group prenatal care reduces preterm birth

Assigned randomly to participate in either a yoga group or a walking group, women assigned to yoga had fewer preterm babies, fewer birth complications, and babies with higher birth weights.[14]

Centering Pregnancy groups, led by midwives, consist of small groups of pregnant mothers or couples who meet regularly for prenatal sessions instead of private appointments. Pregnant women receive routine prenatal checkups then participate in a facilitated group discussion or class. Such groups are fun, offer social support, reduce stress, and significantly lower the numbers of preterm births.[15] Expectant parents report feeling more prepared for birth and breastfeeding. Find out if there is a Centering Pregnancy group near you. Rosanna Davis, one of our Certified Mentors who is a midwife in California, has started a program called Village Prenatal Care that offers her home birth clients a group prenatal experience using the Birthing From Within model.

Mother-to-Be Retreat

Is there a part of you that yearns for solitude or a few hours of quiet reflection to hear your own thoughts, connect with your baby, or stop the clock and just rest? Whether or not you think you have time, make a weekly appointment with yourself for a mother-to-be retreat. If necessary, let everyone concerned know in advance that during your retreat you will "go offline" and avoid email, telephone, social media, household responsibilities, and errands.

9

Is Ultrasound
Safe for My Baby?

*New information on fetal ultrasound and its po-
tential effects on the developing fetal brain returns
fetal ultrasound to its original purpose as a diagnostic tool for specific obstetric concerns. One of
the first responsibilities of parenthood is to become
informed and ask questions before consenting to
routine or frequent ultrasounds that may affect the
baby's long-term health.*

Gathering Tidbits for Your Fact Basket

Humans hear sound waves that cycle between 20 and
20,000 hertz (vibrations per second).* The frequency of
prenatal ultrasound is between 1 million and 10 million
vibrations per second, which is too high for the human ear
to hear and why the procedure is called "ultrasound." This very
high-pitched sound both shakes and heats up whatever it
passes through. Even though you cannot hear it, your baby
experiences the vibrations and heat. Some parents think it's cute
when their baby covers his ears, or jumps, or tries to move away
during an ultrasound. But the baby's movements could be a sign
of discomfort.

How does ultrasound make a picture of your baby?

The instrument that a sonographer holds and glides over your belly is called a "transducer." It emits high-frequency sound waves in short pulses lasting one millionth of a second. The sound travels through the baby's tissues then bounces back during the pause. Like sonar used by submarines or bats, the echoes of the pulse are "heard" by the transducer, and the signal is integrated into a picture on the computer screen.

Potential benefits of diagnostic ultrasound

Faulty transducers give inaccurate readings

In a study of 676 transducers, 40 percent were found to malfunction, potentially giving incorrect results that could lead to misguided medical recommendations.[1] It is not known if a malfunctioning transducer sends a higher acoustic beam to the baby or if it takes longer to get a good picture, but in either case the dosage to the baby is increased. Rather than retesting a baby to confirm results, it is critical that transducers are tested several times a year and replaced when necessary.

Ultrasound can be a useful tool in diagnosing ectopic pregnancy or fibroids; confirming multiple gestation; estimating the due date (when done between 16 and 20 weeks' gestation); detecting some genetic anomalies such as Down syndrome; and assessing the level of amniotic fluid and position of the placenta.

Limitations of diagnostic prenatal ultrasound

Ultrasound gives us a peek inside a once-hidden, mysterious world, but the readings are not always accurate. Sometimes the image is not clear, so the reading is ambiguous, and there can also be human error. Sometimes an ultrasound reports a problem that does not exist (this is called a "false positive"), which causes unnecessary anxiety and an urgency to do something, usually conduct more tests or induce labor. At other times a scan misses an actual problem.

*Isn't it wonderful that even with technology
there is mystery in the womb?*

Estimating Your Baby's Weight

Surprisingly, research has found that a pregnant woman's estimation of her baby's birth weight is more accurate than either ultrasound or a caregiver's estimation,[2] so get in the guessing game. How much do you feel your baby weighs?

Ultrasound is not a reliable predictor of birth weight

Careful hands-on abdominal palpation to assess fetal growth, position, and weight used to be part of every prenatal exam and has been found to be as accurate as ultrasound.[3] Nevertheless, many obstetricians now rely solely on ultrasound to assess fetal weight and position. Unfortunately, 40 percent of fetal weight predictions by ultrasound in the third trimester have a 10 percent margin of error, which means the prediction can be off by a full pound—an error that may lead to unwarranted anxiety, inductions, and cesareans.[4]

Elizabeth, a healthy first-time mother was transferred out of midwifery care after an ultrasound predicted her baby weighed over ten pounds. The consulting doctor convinced the woman not to labor, not even in the hospital, and to have a cesarean. In the operating room, a nurse called out the baby's weight: "Seven pounds." Elizabeth was devastated. Her first words were, "Seven pounds! I could have had that baby!"

Once a "big baby" is predicted, the medical snowball begins to roll

When a woman is told that her baby is "big" after an ultrasound (even if a doctor tries to reassure the woman that the estimate could be wrong), her vivid and fearful imagination of trying to birth a huge baby undermines her confidence and allows her anxiety to take over. This explains why 67 percent of such mothers agree to induction and the rest try to self-induce.[5]

When ultrasound predicts a big baby, the induction rate triples.[6] There is an increased perception by birth attendants that labor is not progressing, resulting in a cesarean rate two to three times higher compared to women whose babies were predicted to be of average weight but at birth were actually "big" (8 lb. 13 oz. or more).[7, 8] Also, these mothers experience four times more complications from the interventions.[9]

On the other hand, another study found that the average birth weight of suspected big babies is only 7 lb. 13 oz.[10] The increase in inductions and cesareans for suspected big babies did not improve maternal or fetal outcomes. Perhaps it is better not to seek or know the prediction of a machine that 7 percent of the time is off by 20 percent.[11, 12]

How Safe Is Ultrasound for My Baby?

Initial confidence in the safety of prenatal ultrasound for babies was established from studies published before 1992. No correlation between prenatal ultrasound and long-term health of a baby was found, except for an increase in left-handedness. However, the validity and relevance of those studies was undermined for two reasons. First, the researchers did not accurately measure or compare ultrasound dosages or the amount of time babies were exposed. Second, in 1992 the Food and Drug Administration (FDA), without first researching the effect of added dosages on fetal development, increased the allowed maximum power of fetal ultrasounds roughly eightfold so doctors could get better pictures. This increase in dosage adds to the risk of overheating the developing baby's tissues and makes former studies performed at lower power levels obsolete.[13] The steady rise in the incidence of autism and other neurological disorders began after 1992 and coincides with the steady increase in the use of prenatal ultrasound.

Routine prenatal ultrasound is the biggest uncontrolled experiment in history.

—Beverly Beech

From one pregnancy to the next, what was considered safe or necessary can change rapidly as new research and interventions arise. Learning about potential consequences of ultrasound for the first time after having had ultrasound in a previous pregnancy or earlier in this pregnancy can be unsettling. Unfortunately, such information was not available earlier so that parents and professionals could make more informed decisions and be more cautious.

Bioeffects* of elevated temperature and ultrasound

Neurological fetal tissue is sensitive to any rise in temperature, including maternal fever, which may result in neurological problems.[14, 15] It is for this reason that you have been cautioned not to take hot baths, use saunas, or soak in hot tubs during pregnancy. If a pregnant woman develops a fever, she is treated to reduce her temperature quickly.

Fetal ultrasound also creates a rise in core temperature. Ultrasound waves are converted to heat when absorbed by your baby's body. This is just as true whether the scan is for medical diagnosis, finding out gender, or as a keepsake memento. When low-intensity ultrasound was applied to prepubescent rat testicles, serum testosterone increased 62 percent.[16] If testosterone rises in young rats, could it also surge in human male fetuses? Is it worth the risk to find out the gender of your baby?

If you do have a medical ultrasound, get it done quickly rather than prolonging exposure while you watch your baby on a monitor or take pictures. This is because, while as much as 70 percent of the total temperature increase associated with ultrasound occurs within the first minute of exposure,[17] the temperature continues to rise as exposure time is prolonged. Thus minimizing the exposure time is probably the single most important factor for ensuring patient safety from thermal injury.[18] Ultrasound heats bone faster than muscle, soft tissue, or amniotic water. As pregnancy advances and fetal bones calcify, they absorb and retain more heat. During the third trimester, the baby's skull can heat up fifty times faster than the surrounding tissue,[19] which subjects the part of the brain closest to the skull—the cortex—to secondary heat that persists after the ultrasound has stopped.[20]

DO MORE ULTRASOUNDS IMPROVE MATERNAL AND FETAL OUTCOMES?

Ultrasound was originally intended to assess specific medical indications. Now almost every American woman has at least one routine ultrasound between 16 and 20 weeks' gestation even when there is no medical indication. Low-risk women often receive five or more, with little to no medical justification other than to satisfy parental curiosity. Women who are over thirty-five years old carrying twins, overdue, or considered high risk may have five to ten ultrasounds during pregnancy. However, research shows that early screening and more ultrasounds do not improve outcome[21] but do increase anxiety, uncertainty, inductions, cesareans, and consequently, increased infant and maternal morbidity.[22] Most of the problems detected in

If your caregiver suspects your baby is small or growing slowly . . .

Keep in mind two things:

1. Ultrasound is a diagnostic picture, not a treatment, so it won't magically help your baby grow.

2. Since hands-on assessment of the baby is usually as accurate as ultrasound, if there is concern about your baby's growth being slow, then before exposing your baby to ultrasound assess your diet. A mother's diet deficient in protein and calories is the most logical reason a baby grows slowly. After eating very well for several weeks or a month, you can look forward to your next appointment to see how much your baby has grown.

early pregnancy are congenital and are impossible to fix, but detection allows parents to consider terminating the pregnancy.

Placenta previa

Do not worry if you are told you have a low-lying or marginal placenta in the first half of pregnancy. The placenta naturally migrates upward, away from the cervix, as the uterus elongates in the second half of pregnancy. By the end of pregnancy, 85 percent placentas are in the upper half of the uterus.[23] And yet an early misdiagnosis creates enough worry and anxiety to expose the baby to a series of unnecessary ultrasounds to keep checking when, in fact, all women with persistent low-lying placentas (placenta previa) develop the classic symptom of bleeding between 28 and 34 weeks, which is how this condition was diagnosed and managed long before the dawn of ultrasound. Depending on how much of the cervix the placenta covers, a woman may give birth vaginally or by cesarean.

The bottom line: whether true placenta previa is discovered early by ultrasound or later, there are no differences in management or outcome and there's no need to do repeat ultrasounds.[24]

Ultrasound and Peace of Mind

The technology of prenatal diagnosis is usually presented to us as a solution, but it brings with it problems of its own. . . . The technology of prenatal diagnosis has changed and continues to change women's experience of pregnancy.
—Barbara Katz Rothman

One of the emotional consequences of fetal surveillance is that with every ultrasound, and even the anticipation of an ultrasound, some women subtly dissociate from their body, baby, and intuition. Ultrasound terminology affects the way mothers talk about their babies, sharing and comparing notes on the circumference of the babies' heads or levels of amniotic water. Not so long ago a pregnant woman daydreamed about her healthy baby, perhaps asking what she could do to ensure his health and well-being. Now a pregnant woman seeking assurance through ultrasound tends to ask, "Is there anything wrong with my baby?"

While many women claim ultrasound accelerated bonding, others have experienced a disruption in prenatal bonding with "false positive" and "soft marker" findings. Even after a follow-up ultrasound rules out an initial misdiagnosis, many mothers never view their pregnancy or baby the same again, and the anxiety and disconnect can continue into motherhood.[25]

Questions for Your Huntress

There are risks to not knowing and there are risks to knowing. There are no risk-free choices; there are no guarantees. Which unknowns are you willing to live with? Does the illusion or comfort of knowing something from a digital image make you more dependent and trusting of technology and therefore more readily accepting of medically routine and unnecessary procedures in labor?

Love Warrior To-Do List

There is nothing intrinsically wrong with heroic discovery. However, it is as much subject to criticism as anything else. This is to say, it may be good or bad, depending on what is discovered and what use is made of it. Intelligence minimally requires us to consider the possibility that we might well have done without some discoveries, and that there might be two opinions about any given discovery . . .

—Wendell Berry

We have become trusting and comfortable with technology in childbirth. This is one reason why people tend to overlook possible long-term risks. I asked Dr. Manuel Casanova, of the University of South Carolina Greenville, how confident he was that ultrasound is linked with our present epidemic of autism spectrum disorders. "Ninety percent," he answered. Time will tell. Research will eventually answer this question.

"I have had five ultrasounds—the first at 8 weeks and the next at 11, 16, 20, and 24 weeks—and I can't wait till next week, when I get to have a 3-D. I already have thirty-two pictures and a video of my baby."

—Krystal

Until we know for certain what dosage and frequency of exposure is safe for the developing fetus, use caution and restraint in exposing your baby to prenatal ultrasound. Here's what you can do to reduce potential risks:

1. Limit the total number of medical ultrasounds, and eliminate all scans done for social reasons or out of curiosity.

2. Avoid ultrasound imaging in your first trimester.

3. Avoid routine ultrasound between 16 and 20 weeks when clinical findings are within normal range and you would not seek an abortion if the baby is discovered to have a congenital anomaly.

4. Do not expose your baby to long scans.

5. Do not get an ultrasound every time it is recommended. Instead, make an informed choice every time ultrasound is offered. Ask why it is being recommended and what, if anything, can be done based on the results.

> As a parent, you don't want to put your baby at risk by avoiding a needed test and you don't want to do extra testing that could put your baby at risk.

6. Postpone ultrasound if you have a fever because your core temperature is already elevated. If ultrasound is absolutely necessary, limit ultrasound exposure as the baby is already being heated.[26]

7. Ask the ultrasound tech to avoid directing the ultrasound beam into your baby's face and eyes. The lens in the eyes have diminished circulation and therefore reduced capacity for heat dissipation.[27] The permissible pulse intensity for the fetal eye is up to 1.9 as part of overall exposure regulatory limits. For ophthalmic ultrasound following birth, it is 0.23.[28]

8. Do not expose your baby to additional ultrasound by purchasing or borrowing a Doppler to hear the heartbeat or a portable ultrasound machine for home use to see what the baby is doing and how she is growing.

户

BRAIN DEVELOPMENT AND AUTISM

Autism spectrum disorders are characterized by ineffective verbal or nonverbal communication, abnormal social behaviors, and other symptoms that range from mild to severe. There is no single cause of autism. It is believed to be caused by a number of interacting factors that interfere with brain development, including genetic predisposition, or untimely environmental influences and events that include pesticides and chemical toxins, drugs, nutrition, untreated maternal fever, and prenatal ultrasound.

During normal formation of the brain, brain cells divide in the center of the brain (ventricles) and migrate to the surface of the brain (cortex) at a precise time, where they organize into columns of 80 to 100 cells. Normal brain cells mature in sync with inhibitory cells. Inhibitory cells accompany migrating brain cells en route to the gray matter and contain the minicolumns. In the absence of inhibitory cells, brain cells can divide when they are not supposed to, and the information organized and intended for a particular minicolumn can spread to, or permeate, other minicolumns.[29]

In autism there is a higher rate of cell division in the center of brain, so more cells try to migrate to the cortex. Autistic people's brains have 10 to 12 percent more minicolumns compared to nonautistic brains. Ultrasound damages brain cell membranes and accelerates cell division and the formation of too many minicolumns.[30, 31]

In autism, mental retardation, epilepsy, and schizophrenia, many brain cells do not complete their migration to the gray matter (cortex) because something in the environment on a particular day, possibly ultrasound, disturbed or slowed down their migration.[32] In autistic brains, there are islands of gray within white matter where migrating cells were interrupted before reaching their normal destination (gray matter). When and where damaged brain cells cluster may explain the different types and expressions of autism and other brain disorders.

Autism was first described as a disorder in the 1940s. In the

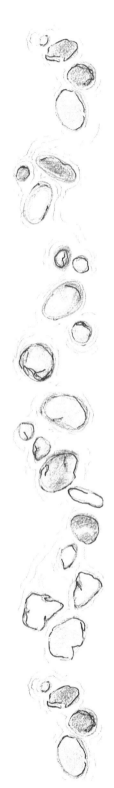

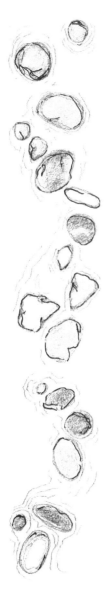

1970s and 1980s, autism was reported at a rate of one 1 per 25,000. Between 1992 and 2003, the Centers for Disease Control reported an 800 percent increase in autism.[33] In 2012, the incidence was one 1 in 88; in 2014, it was one 1 in 68.[34] Twenty-six percent of the increase can be attributed to more inclusive diagnostic criteria.[35, 36]

When the rate of autism began to rise, some people wondered if thimerosal, a mercury-based preservative added to vaccines in the 1930s, was responsible. During the 1990s, babies and toddlers received multiple vaccines with thimerosal. Since 2001 the preservative has not been used in routine childhood vaccines, with the exception of flu vaccine. Research has not found a link between vaccines and autism.[37]

In September 2016, researchers from the University of Washington published findings that link the severity of autism to ultrasound exposure in the first trimester. Ultrasound is frequently ordered in the first trimester to estimate the length of gestation and anticipated due date (instead of, or in addition to, performing a pelvic exam) to confirm fetal heartbeat or to assess status of a threatened miscarriage. Whenever possible, avoid using ultrasound in the first trimester when time and patience will make the due date or other diagnosis clear.[38]

The debate in brain development is not one of nature versus nurture, but of how many factors interact during the brain's development to render particular traits, behaviors, and disorders.

—ANN MCDONALD

WOMB WITH A VIEW (SEEING YOUR BABY)

For the human, necessity is not just to know, but also to cherish and protect the things that are known, and to know that a thing can be known only through cherishing.
                                                            —WENDELL BERRY

Ultrasound has become a technological ritual of prenatal bonding. Seeing a moving image of the baby can enkindle positive feelings about becoming parents, and yet throughout history mothers have always bonded with their unborn.

Want a picture? Draw a picture of your baby in your womb.

Imagine that you could peek through a window in your womb. What do you see your baby doing in her watery womb all day? What does she look like? Imagine what your baby sees, hears, or feels while growing in your womb. Using pastels or watercolors, make a picture of your baby. Include as many details as possible, and if you like, write your baby a personal message on the image. Your picture can be small enough to carry in your purse or glue in a baby book, or big enough to hang on a wall. You might even make a series of these drawings or paintings as your baby grows.

Here are a few more ways to connect and bond with your unborn baby:

♥ Knit or sew something for your baby, such as a stuffed animal or a small quilt.

♥ Ask a massage therapist to help you get in touch with your baby using guided imagery during a prenatal massage.

♥ Ask your birth attendant, while she palpates the position of the baby, to guide your hands so you can feel how he is curled up inside you.

♥ Sing a lullaby or special song to your baby within. Some parents even write their own lullaby. During the last six weeks of pregnancy, mothers in a study were instructed to read aloud *Cat in the Hat* by Dr. Seuss every day. After their babies were born, when the mothers read aloud *Cat in the Hat* their babies suckled harder, but when a stranger read the story aloud the babies showed no change in suckling, suggesting that a baby knows and likes his mother's voice best, even before birth.[39]

♥ Invite your partner to listen to the sound of the baby's heartbeat by pressing an ear to your belly. The natural sound of a baby's heartbeat is different from the mechanical sound produced by a Doppler scan or heartbeat monitor.

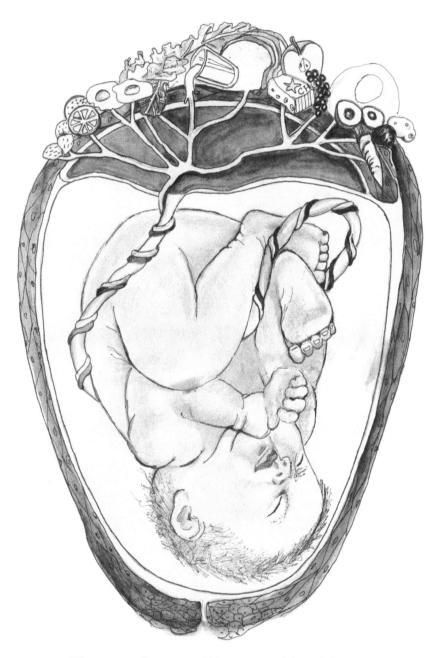

When you eat well, you are nourishing your uterus, baby, and placenta.
As your baby grows, so does your placenta.

NOURISHING THE LIFE WITHIN

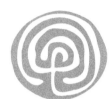

With all the changes to our food and lifestyle, eating well during pregnancy may not be instinctive anymore. Prenatal care and childbirth classes rarely include information on prenatal nutrition or provide regular dietary checkups. Therfore, this chapter has been designed to be used as a comprehensive "home study class," complete with a daily prenatal diet chart.

Your first task of mothering is to eat well. Eating three good meals a day with a couple of snacks in between is not a radical idea; it is common sense. When prenatal nutritional needs are met, you and your baby will be healthier and happier. And if complications arise, your body will be better able to respond and heal. Make sound nutrition and healthy cooking habits during pregnancy the cornerstone for your well-being and that of your baby.

This chapter was meticulously coauthored by Lyn Jones, a friend who began doing prenatal nutritional counseling with me over thirty years ago.

Technology is no substitute for good nutrition....Blood sampling, urine testing, ultrasonography...are for diagnostic information only....They do not treat....They do not nourish. They do not prevent ... complications.
—DAVID STEWART

YOUR PRENATAL DIET IS NOURISHING YOU

By eating a healthy prenatal diet, you are not only nourishing your baby but also ensuring your own well-being. What you eat directly affects six major changes in your body, making certain that you are:

1. Growing a healthy placenta

2. Making plenty of flavorful amniotic fluid

3. Meeting the increased demand on your liver

4. Expanding your blood volume

5. Growing a roomy and strong uterus

6. Gaining about 28 to 40 pounds

Growing a Healthy Placenta

Your placenta is an amazing organ. Your baby and placenta developed from a single cell—so the placenta is part of your baby! It takes twelve weeks to establish the blood supply between you and your baby via the growing placenta. From then on, the placenta functions as your baby's lungs, kidneys, liver, and stomach, and it produces hormones. Until about the sixteenth week of pregnancy, your baby's placenta will be bigger than your baby.

The placenta is composed of mostly protein and thus depends on adequate protein intake to get a good start in the first trimester. At birth, a healthy placenta is about an inch thick and weighs between 1.5 and 2 pounds. When a mother is undernourished, the growth of her placenta and baby slows down. Babies weighing less than 5.5 pounds at birth have more health problems before and after birth. A small placenta may have a diminished capacity to deliver oxygen to the baby during labor, or it may abrupt—separate from the womb before the baby is born. Good nutrition often prevents such conditions.

Your baby is not a parasite

It used to be thought that if the mother did not have enough food her baby would magically extract protein from her muscles, calcium from her bones, and calories from her fat stores.[1] This is not the case. Nutrients are also sent through the umbilical cord to nourish and grow your baby. If nutrients are not in your blood, your placenta and baby cannot receive them.

Another commonly heard myth is that an overweight mother does not have to eat as much or gain as much weight because her body's fat "stores" will metabolize into nutrients to feed the baby. In actuality, a mother's fat cannot be metabolized into protein, vitamins, minerals, and enzymes. Therefore, adequate calories from nutrient-dense food is essential for all pregnant women, regardless of their weight.

Making Plenty of Flavorful Amniotic Fluid

The amniotic sac, or "bag of water," forms and fills with water about two weeks after conception. At first, your body provides the amniotic fluid. After the 20th week, your baby continuously produces amniotic fluid. In her watery world, your baby is cushioned from bumps and tumbles and is able to move around and develop her muscles while her umbilical cord floats freely. She also begins to practice "breathing." By the third trimester, she will "inhale" and "exhale" twice as much amniotic fluid as she swallows, which will help her lungs develop normally.

When your baby and her placenta are well nourished and growing, there is usually plenty of amniotic fluid. Food deprivation and dehydration decrease the amount of amniotic fluid. Other conditions, too, may cause low levels of amniotic fluid, so it is essential that you eat well and drink plenty of fluids.

Building a flavor bridge for your baby

Amniotic fluid comes in sweet, sour, salty, bitter, and savory flavors depending on what you are eating. Your baby's sense of smell and taste form in the early weeks, so she is already "tasting" and "smelling" what you eat as she drinks and breathes in the flavorful amniotic fluid.

A child's preference for certain foods may be formed before she is born. One study of three groups of pregnant women

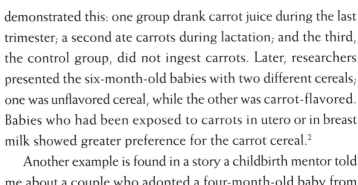

demonstrated this: one group drank carrot juice during the last trimester; a second ate carrots during lactation; and the third, the control group, did not ingest carrots. Later, researchers presented the six-month-old babies with two different cereals; one was unflavored cereal, while the other was carrot-flavored. Babies who had been exposed to carrots in utero or in breast milk showed greater preference for the carrot cereal.[2]

Another example is found in a story a childbirth mentor told me about a couple who adopted a four-month-old baby from India. The baby was crying from hunger but would not drink formula. The worried parents consulted their pediatrician, who suggested they add a sprinkle of curry to the formula. The baby happily began to eat.

Meeting the Increased Demand on Your Liver

Your liver performs five hundred metabolic functions, one of which is purifying and detoxifying your blood. By the end of pregnancy, daily progesterone levels are a hundred times greater than the amount contained in birth control pills. Your liver has to be healthy to metabolize and excrete extra pregnancy hormones. Your liver also functions as a factory where nutrients from the food you eat are combined to synthesize special proteins. The proteins grow and repair cells, boost your immune system, and give you energy. One of these special proteins, called albumin, plays a critical role in increasing your blood volume.

Expanding Your Blood Volume

To send enough oxygen, nutrients, and hormones to your baby through the placenta during the second half of pregnancy, your blood volume must increase by 40 to 50 percent. The extra blood also protects you by helping to maintain normal blood pressure and by preventing shock from normal blood loss during birth. Your blood volume will not expand automatically just because you are pregnant; this change is dependent on an adequate intake of salt and protein to increase the production of albumin. Albumin acts like a little sponge, absorbing and holding water in your bloodstream, thus increasing blood volume. Increased blood volume means more nutrients and hormones are carried to your baby.

Three hundred quarts of blood per day pass through the umbilical cord to your baby.

When a pregnant woman's diet is protein deficient, her liver cannot produce enough albumin. If her albumin level is too low during the second half of pregnancy, her kidneys will try to compensate by reabsorbing sodium (salt) and water to increase her blood volume. However, when there is not enough albumin in her blood to hold that extra water it leaks out into the tissues and causes swelling in the feet and eventually in the hands and face. Although not all researchers agree, many believe additional consequences include elevated blood pressure (pre-eclampsia, or HELLP syndrome*) and other problems for mother and baby.

How can you be certain your diet and albumin levels are adequate? To maintain an adequate albumin level, eat well. Also check your daily food intake against the chart on page **70**. If you are still not confident, get a blood test to check your "serum albumin." Blood tests for hematocrit and hemoglobin, routinely done for pregnant women, determine whether you have anemia, but these tests cannot determine whether you are eating enough protein; only a serum albumin test can do this. The normal range for albumin is between 3.5 and 5.5 gm per 100 cc serum. The serum albumin test is standard in the monitoring of mothers after they develop pre-eclampsia, but it has not become a standard part of preventative prenatal care. You'll have to ask for it.

Salt your food to taste with whole salt

During pregnancy, salting your food to taste helps expand your blood volume. Recent studies show there is no benefit from restricting salt in pregnancy, and indeed it may cause complications.[3] We all begin life swimming in our own little salty Amniotic Ocean. The composition of ocean water is almost identical to that of the amniotic water and the blood, lymph, and extracellular fluids in your body. When taken from the sea, unprocessed and unbleached sea salt contains eighty-six trace minerals on which every function in your body depends. The table salt we've become accustomed to has lost eighty-

"Normally I do not salt my food much or crave saltier snacks. When pregnant, however, I do find myself adding salt and opting for more savory items. It was nice to learn that I should not only honor this instinct but also be mindful to include enough salt in my diet."

—ADRIENNE

four of its original eighty-six minerals during intensive processing, bleaching, demineralizing, and the addition of chemicals to make it white and shaker-ready. Using whole sea salt is preferable to consuming processed salt, and it also tastes better. A lot of salt is labeled "sea salt" even though it has been processed. To determine if salt is whole, read the label carefully.

Growing a Roomy and Strong Uterus

Before you became pregnant, your uterus was the size of a pear and weighed about two ounces. For your uterus to expand during pregnancy and contract strongly in labor, it needs extra protein and vitamin C to make new muscle fibers and connective tissue. By the end of your pregnancy, your womb will have grown thirtyfold to hold your baby, placenta, and a quart of amniotic fluid.

Gaining about 28 to 40 Pounds

Weight gain patterns during pregnancy vary widely, depending on food choices, caloric intake, and metabolism. Some women have a fear that eating more or gaining weight will lead to a "big baby" and more complications in birth; but actually, mothers with poor diets and underweight babies have more complications during birth and postpartum. So instead of worrying about gaining a certain amount of weight monthly, focus on eating a wholesome diet each day that includes ample calories from whole foods. Reduce refined carbohydrates and sugars.

Women who are very active or athletic during pregnancy need to increase their caloric and protein intake.

Healthy pregnant women who neither restrict nor overindulge at mealtime can expect to gain about 28 to 40 pounds by the end of pregnancy. Women who gain this amount are less likely to have a cesarean and more likely to have a baby with a healthy birth weight (between 5 lb. 8 oz. and 8 lb. 14 oz.).

Gaining weight during pregnancy and increasing your caloric intake while nursing might go against years of dieting for controlling weight gain. Some women (and sometimes their partners) worry that they'll keep the weight on after the baby is born. Commit yourself to maintaining a balanced diet during pregnancy, nursing, and beyond. At the end of this important time, you can choose to keep the positive nutrition habits you cultivated as you begin to feed your new family and lose the weight when it's time.

Tribute to Dr. Tom Brewer, an obstetrician who researched the metabolic and nutritional cause of pre-eclampsia and developed standards for sound prenatal nutrition.

"Programming" Your Baby's Organs and Metabolism for Life

Since the 1930s, research has consistently shown that what mothers eat is the single most important factor in growing a healthy baby and placenta. Recent research reveals irrefutable evidence that the mother's prenatal diet literally programs her baby's lifelong appetite, weight-gain patterns, and metabolism at a cellular level.

When a pregnant mother eats healthy food in normal amounts and at regular intervals, her baby's metabolism is programmed for a healthy appetite and body weight as a child and as an adult. On the other hand, when a fetus is grown on a high but empty calorie prenatal diet composed largely of processed or fast food containing lots of bad fats, artificial chemicals, and sugar, the baby's appetite and metabolism are programmed accordingly. A fetus undernourished before birth has an increased chance of developing lifelong challenges with obesity, insulin resistance, type 2 diabetes, coronary heart disease, and hypertension.[4]

There is a common assumption that whatever the fetus needs the mother will instinctively crave and that if she loses her appetite she can trust that, too. These assumptions are not always true. Maternal cravings may be due to dietary habits or high levels of pregnancy hormones and unrelated to satisfying real nutritional needs of the mother or fetus.

Prenatal Nutrition and Type 2 Diabetes

Researchers have found a link between prenatal nutrition and diabetes. Normally the pancreas secretes the right amount of insulin in response to varying blood sugar levels. Type 2 diabetes, which is on the rise in young people, even when they are of normal weight or have no family history of diabetes, occurs when the pancreas does not secrete sufficient amounts of insulin to regulate the blood sugar.

Pregnant mice fed low-protein diets in the third trimester gave birth to low-birth-weight pups. Fed a healthy diet after birth, the pups gained weight and appeared as healthy as the pups fed a high-protein diet prenatally. Later, as adult mice, the majority of the low-protein group developed diabetes. According to the study, the pancreases of mice in the low-protein diet group could secrete insulin, but they could only do so in limited amounts regardless of the blood sugar levels. When the prenatal diet was low in protein, pancreatic cells were smaller and fewer in number. Even when fed a good diet after birth, the abnormal pancreas development and cellular damage was irreversible.[5]

Brain Power and Visual Acuity

When it comes to brain cells, 70 to 80 percent are developed before a baby is born. All told, 100 billion neurons are formed before birth.[6]

Your baby's brain development begins three weeks after you conceive and goes through three growth spurts between 18 weeks of gestation and your baby's fourth birthday. Over the first year, an estimated 2 million connections form between neighboring brain cells every second, totaling 173 billion synaptic connections a day.[7]

During the second trimester, there is a rapid increase in brain cells; billions of neurons, which process and analyze information, are formed. One month before birth, there is another major growth spurt. Although brain development and adaptations continue throughout life, this is no time to restrict food or weight gain.[8]

Nutrients essential to your baby's brain, retina, and nervous system development are DHA and omega-3 fatty acids. During pregnancy, you and your baby need 300 mg of DHA a day, or 500 mg of an omega-3 supplement of EPA and DHA. (The EPA and DHA requirement for women who are not pregnant is 220 mg a day.)

Food Sources: Eat three ounces per day of cold-water fish, such as sockeye salmon (the richest source), herring, or sardines.

1 NOURISHING THE LIFE WITHIN

Hens fed an omega-3 enriched diet lay eggs that have five times more omega-3 than conventional eggs.

Vegetarian Sources: If you are on a strict vegetarian diet, DHA supplementation is that much more important because your diet is lacking in fish, a source rich in DHA. In this case, be sure to take a fish-free DHA supplement. Algae is high in DHA. (It is where the fish get their DHA from!) Algae grown in mercury-free steel tanks is available in capsules.

Fish Oil Supplement: Read the Label

Look for pure fish oil derived from healthy fish in clean water and quickly processed and packaged under strict conditions. The label should say it is molecularly distilled and free of contaminants, mercury, and pesticides. Buy your fish oil at a health food store so you know it is fresh and pure, and avoid cheap generic brands. One reason fish oil is cheaper at large retail stores is because it may have passed its shelf life and is starting to become rancid. Do not buy "flavored" fish oil, as flavoring is used to cover up the taste and smell of rancid oil.[9] Fresh fish oil supplements do not taste fishy.

DHA for You and Your Baby after the Birth

When you breastfeed, your baby continues to get DHA from your milk. Studies show that children whose mothers took a DHA supplement during pregnancy, compared with those whose mothers did not, scored higher on intelligence tests at four years of age.[11] Babies whose mothers had high blood levels of DHA at delivery had longer attention spans into their second year of life. During the first six months of life, the attention spans of these infants was two months more advanced than those whose mothers had lower DHA levels.[12] In addition, mothers who take DHA supplements during pregnancy tend to have a reduced risk of postpartum depression.[13]

Mercury-Free Womb

The developing nervous system of unborn babies is more vulnerable to mercury than the adult nervous system. While your health may not suffer from eating moderate amounts of fish or shellfish, your developing child's thinking, memory, attention span, and motor skills may be impaired through exposure to mercury in the womb. Not all fish contains mercury. This is why you should buy mercury-free fish and fish oil supplements.[10]

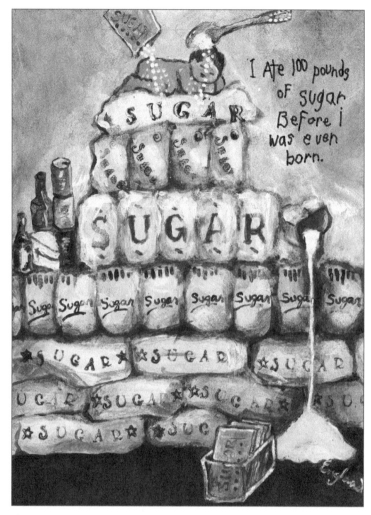

The average American eats 150 to 180 pounds of sugar a year. Read labels: sugar, in one form or another (dextrose, sucrose, fructose, corn syrup, or corn sugar), is in just about every packaged food. According to one source, "Most infant formulas have a sugar equivalent of a full can of Coca-Cola, and that amounts to metabolic poisoning of all infants taking the formula."[14]

Another Sweet Lesson in Nutrition History

The average annual sugar consumption was 4 pounds per person between 1700 and 1800; 19 pounds from 1800 to 1900; and is now 156 pounds—that's thirty-one 5-pound bags![16, 17]

PROBIOTICS DECREASE THE INCIDENCE OF GESTATIONAL DIABETES

Western diets high in sugar, processed grains, unhealthy fats, meat, antibiotics, and calories have decreased or eliminated certain intestinal flora, causing a bacterial imbalance that may contribute to diabetes.[15] Probiotics, good bacteria that restore and maintain a healthy balance in the gut by reducing the growth of harmful bacteria, reduce the risk of gestational diabetes and reduce the risk of the mother and baby developing diabetes later in life.[18]

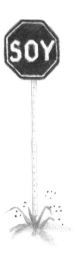

What about Soy Foods and Formula?

Although you may think of soy products such as tofu, soy-based meat substitutes, and soy-based cheeses as health foods, they are not healthy foods for your developing fetus or infant. This is because soy foods contain plant estrogen in the form of isoflavones, which act as hormone disruptors during fetal development.[19]

There is growing concern that ingesting excessive amounts of soy estrogen, especially in the first trimester, may contribute to low birth weight, malformation of a baby's sex organs, poor thyroid function, and may alter the timing of puberty and fertility in boys and girls later in life.[20] And yet, it is nearly impossible to avoid soy altogether as soy products, in one form or another, are in many processed and packaged food in supermarkets and health food stores. Read labels and be mindful of your soy consumption.

Fermented Soy Is Okay

Fermented soy products—for example, soy sauce, miso, natto, and tempeh—are okay to eat.

Breast milk is the ideal food for infants. But if formula is needed, soy-based formula is not preferable to cow's milk formula. The adult body can handle some soy, but daily intake of soy formula may be toxic to young children. An infant who consumes soy-based formula gets 20 times more phytoestrogens than an infant consuming non-soy formula, and her serum soy level is 1,000 mg, which is 13,000 to 22,000 times higher than the estrogen level in a pregnant woman's body and 3,000 times higher than her estrogen level during ovulation.[21] The plant estrogen in soy formula is equivalent to five birth control pills a day.[22] A baby's endocrine system can't metabolize this much estrogen. It is speculated that there is an association between soy in foods and formula[23] and an increase in premature puberty among girls and delayed puberty among boys in the United States.

Reduce the Wait, Eat a Date

In recent studies, eating six dates a day in the last four weeks of pregnancy significantly enhanced labor in the following ways:

- Labor was spontaneous in 96 percent of women who consumed dates versus 79 percent in the control group, and their labors were shorter, too.

- Membranes remained intact in 83 percent of women who consumed dates versus 60 percent in the control group.

- There was more advanced cervical dilation upon admission (3.5 cm) among women who ate dates versus those who did not (2.0 cm).

- There were significantly fewer labor inductions and augmentations among women who ate dates (28 percent) versus those who did not (47 percent).[24]

- There was reduced bleeding postpartum among women who ate dates (see chapter 40).[25]

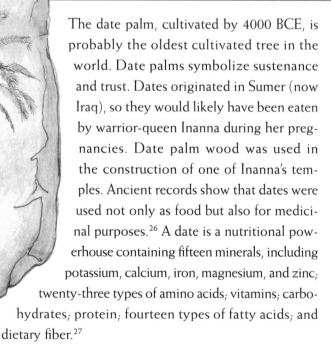

The date palm, cultivated by 4000 BCE, is probably the oldest cultivated tree in the world. Date palms symbolize sustenance and trust. Dates originated in Sumer (now Iraq), so they would likely have been eaten by warrior-queen Inanna during her pregnancies. Date palm wood was used in the construction of one of Inanna's temples. Ancient records show that dates were used not only as food but also for medicinal purposes.[26] A date is a nutritional powerhouse containing fifteen minerals, including potassium, calcium, iron, magnesium, and zinc; twenty-three types of amino acids; vitamins; carbohydrates; protein; fourteen types of fatty acids; and dietary fiber.[27]

A good diet can help prevent many complications

- Anemia
- Preterm birth
- Undernourished baby and placenta
- Intrauterine growth restriction (IUGR)
- HELLP syndrome* and pre-eclampsia (high blood pressure)
- Fetal distress in labor
- Low birth weight
- Postpartum hemorrhage
- Learning disabilities
- Fetal programming for adult-onset type 2 diabetes, coronary heart disease, hypertension, and obesity

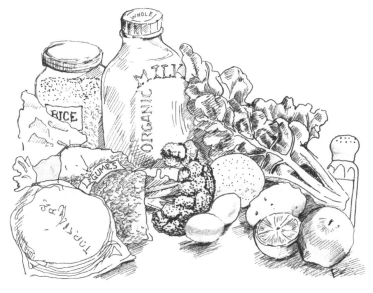

Eat Whole Foods

Replace packaged foods with whole foods. Dollar for dollar, you get more nutrition when you buy whole, unprocessed foods and cook them yourself.

It's up to you

It takes only a few minutes at the end of each day to compare what you have eaten with recommendations listed in the Pregnancy Diet for Healthy Mom and Baby.

Bon appétit!

Pregnancy Diet for Healthy Mom and Baby
Daily minimum: 70 g. protein a day

Food Groups	Meat 'n' Taters	Vegetarian/Vegan
Dairy	**4 servings a day:** 8 g. protein per serving 1 c. whole milk or yogurt; 1/4 c. cottage cheese; 1 oz. hard cheese (1 square inch)	**4 servings a day:** 8 g. protein per serving 1 c. whole milk or yogurt (Greek yogurt is highest in protein); 1 oz. hard cheese (1 square inch). Note: Almond and rice milk have 1 g. protein per 8 oz.
Eggs	2 eggs (DHA fortified): 7 g. protein each	2 eggs (DHA fortified): 7 g. protein each
Protein	**2 servings a day** (in addition to dairy and eggs) 12 3 oz. servings of (organic/grass-fed when possible) meat, liver, free-range poultry, mercury-free fish: wild salmon, catfish, canned light tuna, or sardines. Substitute 1 serving of meat with any 2 servings on right =>	**4 servings a day** (in addition to dairy and eggs) **6–8 servings for vegans** (50 g. protein) ½ c. cooked lentils or beans (pinto, aduki, etc.); ¼ c. almonds, peanuts, sunflower seeds; 2 Tbsp. peanut or almond butter; 1 c. cooked quinoa; ½ c. green peas or black-eyed peas; 2 oz. tempeh; 2 Tbsp. pumpkin seeds (pepitas). *No tofu/soy
Whole Grains	**5–6 servings a day** 10–20 g. protein 1½ slices of whole grain bread; ½ c. rice, millet, bulgur; 1 corn tortilla; ⅓ bagel; 1 pancake/waffle; ½ c. granola or hot cereal/oatmeal; ½ c. noodles/pasta	**5–6 servings a day** 10–20 g. protein 1½ slices of whole grain bread; ½ c. rice, millet, bulgur; 1 corn tortilla; ⅓ bagel; 1 pancake/waffle; ½ c. granola or hot cereal/oatmeal; ½ c. noodles/pasta
Vitamin C Fruits & Vegetables	**1–2 servings a day** 1 orange, kiwi; ½ grapefruit; ½ c. orange juice; ¾ c. strawberries; ⅓ papaya; 1 tomato; 1 c. cantaloupe or cauliflower (steamed); ½ c. broccoli; ½ c. bell pepper; ⅔ c. Brussels sprouts	**1–2 servings a day** 1 orange, kiwi; ½ grapefruit; ½ c. orange juice; ¾ c. strawberries; ⅓ papaya; 1 tomato; 1 c. cantaloupe or cauliflower (steamed); ½ c. broccoli; ½ c. bell pepper; ⅔ c. Brussels sprouts
Dark Leafy Green Vegetables	**1–2 servings a day** ½ c. broccoli greens (kale, spinach, arugula, romaine, etc.) ½ c. cooked or 3 c. raw salad/smoothies	**1–2 servings a day** ½ c. broccoli greens (kale, spinach, arugula, romaine, etc.) ½ c. cooked or 3 c. raw salad/smoothies
Vitamin A Fruits & Vegetables	**1 serving a day** ½ c. sweet potato, winter squash, pumpkin; ¼ c. carrots (juice, cooked, raw); ¼ c. spinach or kale (cooked); 3 apricots; 1 c. red peppers	**1 serving a day** ½ c. sweet potato, winter squash, pumpkin; ¼ c. carrots (juice, cooked, raw); ¼ c. spinach or kale (cooked); 3 apricots; 1 c. red peppers
Healthy Fats	**3 servings a day** 1 Tbsp. butter, mayonnaise, or coconut (olive, nut) oil; ¼ c. avocado; 1 Tbsp. peanut butter	**3 servings a day** 1 Tbsp. butter, mayonnaise, or coconut (olive, nut) oil; ¼ c. avocado; 1 Tbsp. peanut butter

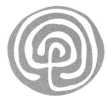

INCUBATION RITUALS

As your baby gestates in a warm cave of muted sound and seclusion, find time alone to gestate motherhood. Set a time once a week to retreat from the noise in the world and the noise in your mind to tune in to the larger rhythms of life.

One of your Tasks of Prenatal Preparation is to learn to hear your inner voice. In his book *The Middle Passage*, James Hollis asserts that "we will never hear that inner voice unless we risk solitude."[1] Give yourself the gift of a daily or weekly ritual of solitude to escape the busy, noisy world and abide in the heart, in silence. Use your ritual of retreat to do what you long to do but tell yourself you don't have time for, such as walking in silence in nature or a botanical garden fully sensing the scents, shapes, and subtle colors of petals and leaves; reading and contemplating poetry or a spiritual book (not a book on birth); taking a leisurely bath by candlelight, followed by a nap; making something for your baby; or sinking your hands into the earth by gardening or sculpting.

MAKE A MOTHER AND BABY ALTAR

Making a mother and baby altar is a ritual of preparation that connects you with the sacred and honors your transition to motherhood.

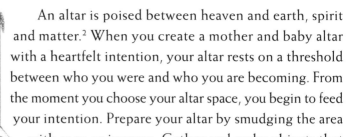

An altar is poised between heaven and earth, spirit and matter.[2] When you create a mother and baby altar with a heartfelt intention, your altar rests on a threshold between who you were and who you are becoming. From the moment you choose your altar space, you begin to feed your intention. Prepare your altar by smudging the area with sage or incense. Gather and make objects that symbolize your intention: healing, opening in labor, transitioning into parenting, protection, gratitude, strength, awakening, or whatever else is calling to you.

After your altar is set up, have a dedication ceremony. During your childbearing year your altar will likely change. Objects will get moved around, or you may remove some and add others to reflect your evolving focus and feelings about pregnancy and motherhood. Your Warrior Bundle (see pages 166–167), open or closed, can be part of your altar. Move the object representing whatever is important to your inner work to the center. Keep your mother and baby altar alive. Adorn it with fresh flowers, fruit, candles, or a bowl of clear water. Keep it clean; tending your altar is a form of prayer and declares your intention. The more you nurture it and meditate near it, the more life it will bring forth for you.

CONNECTING WITH YOUR ANCESTORS AND WOMEN MADE WISE THROUGH EXPERIENCE

There is a wisdom that only women experienced in birth can pass down to you. The medicalization of birth has left four generations of women spiritually and psychologically wounded. But no matter what women experienced in birth all mothers know something other people do not know. Unfortunately, many women underestimate or devalue their experience and knowledge concerning birth. Or they may not realize that their deepest understanding is what people are really interested in. So if you want more than a medical report you have to ask the right questions.

Describe the character of a wise woman sharing her understanding of birth with you. If a wise woman is not available

to you, create a detailed mental picture of a grandmother, re-
membered or imagined; give her a name; describe her in your
journal; then ask her:

- What is your strongest memory giving birth?

- What helped you most when you gave birth?

- What was your spiritual experience of giving birth?

- What did you know after giving birth that you didn't
  know before?

- What was your first thought when you saw your
  baby?

- If you could do it over again, what would you do the
  same?

- Is there anything you would do differently?

- What do you wish you had known beforehand?

KEEP A PREGNANCY DREAM JOURNAL

Some women have vivid dreams in pregnancy that inform or
guide them. Keep a dream journal and pen by your bed so
you can jot down dreams and imagery, or make sketches right
after you awake from dreams.

ANCIENT PREGNANCY AND BIRTH ART

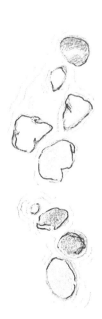

Prehistoric peoples' awe at the mystery of pregnancy and birth
is reflected in the exquisite form and power found in their art.
One of the most beautiful representations of the Goddess of
Lausell (ca. 19,000 BCE) is carved on a limestone slab at the
entrance to a rock shelter in Dordogne, France. She holds in
her raised right hand a bison horn with thirteen notches,
which may represent lunar months. Her left hand points to
her vulva or rests on her swollen, pregnant belly. Traces of red
ochre, the color of menstruation and birth, are still visible on
her body.[3]

The most common representations of the Goddess were
sightless, headless, or with her head inclined toward the middle of her body. The icons are typically rounded vessels with a

gigantic belly and breasts. Her arms are only suggested; huge thighs taper to thin lower legs, with no feet or feet too fragile and small to have survived intact.[4] These Great Mothers still exude a quiet power and exemplify the ancient perception of pregnant women as big and strong. Anthropologists Monica Sjöö and Barbara Mor remind us that two to three million years of human survival can be attributed to women's physical strength, noting that "the human race couldn't have survived…if women had been as physically weak and mentally dependent during those hard ages as we are supposed to be today."[5]

⊚

MAKE A BIRTH POWER SCULPTURE

I am being formed by the clay. I am reconnecting with the earth, and with the other basic elements, too—air, water, fire—and life itself. Every gesture leaves its trail in the clay. Every fingerprint, a message. My breath fills the cavity. My touch curves the wall of a bowl. And inwardly, I am being formed by the outward practice.

—MARJORY ZOET BANKSON

Begin by quietly holding a small lump of clay in your hands. Notice your breathing. Listen to your thoughts as they come and go. When your mind becomes quiet, begin working the clay until all the air bubbles are out and it is malleable. As you knead the clay, continue to pay close attention to your outward breath. If the clay seems a bit dry, dip your fingers into a small bowl of water or vinegar to moisten it, but avoid getting the clay too wet as this will weaken your sculpture. Sinking your fingers into moist, malleable earth takes you to a deeper, unconscious, earthy kind of knowing. Make a power sculpture that connects you to the unbroken chain of mothers, to your source of power, courage, and strength. It might be an animal that reminds you of easy birthing or good mothering.

"I like picturing connections in my head. I am making my connection with clay. Clay turns me on and it turns me in. It seems clearer and clearer that I was drawn to clay by its plasticity. For it is plasticity I seek in my life. To be able to move into new and deeper forms…In which I make the connection between the life I'm living and the objects I'm forming."

—PAULUS BERENSOHN[6]

If your sculpture could talk, what would it say to you?
Did it surprise you?

If you want to save your sculpture, set it aside to dry for a week, covering it lightly with plastic so it will dry slowly and evenly. At this stage, sculptures are called greenware. Firing your sculpture in a kiln, for a nominal charge, will make the piece resistant to breaking. If you want color or a smooth shiny finish, glaze your piece and have it fired a second time.

I have watched women in labor hold, squeeze, rub, or gaze at their birth sculptures, recalling the empowering awareness they experienced while making them. When your child is grown, you can pass down the sculpture that helped you bring her into the world. Not only is this another thread connecting the generations, but it also begins your child's preparation for her rite of passage into parenthood.

Part 4

Tasks of Preparation

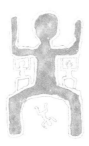

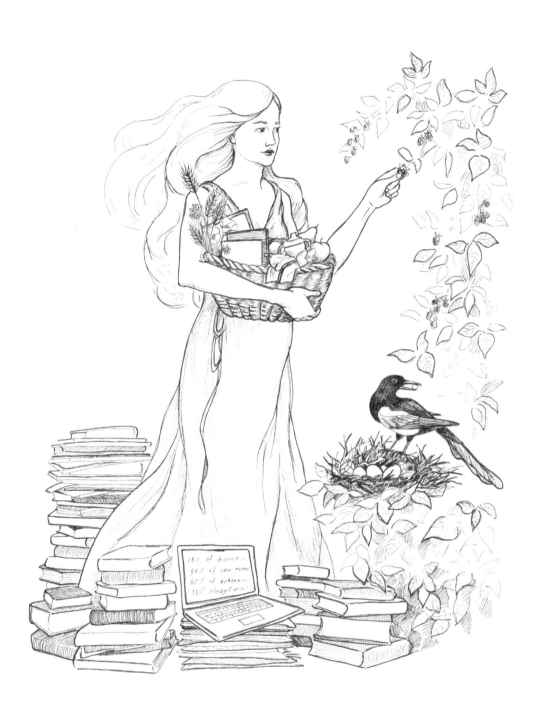

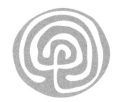

THE GATHERER

The child you are carrying into the world brings out the Gatherer in you. Pregnancy is the season to gather. Gathering is a Task of Preparation in anticipation of a long winter and uncertainty.

There was a time when we knew so little about the science and management of pregnancy and birth that there was practically no information to gather. But today, to be a discerning, decision-making patient and a savvy mother ensuring the well-being of her child, pregnancy is a time for gathering timeless and current information.

Questions arise: What size gathering basket? How much information is enough? How much is too much or too little? Anxiety about being taken advantage of fuels a feverish gathering of every scrap, study, and opinion. A modern woman who believes she is best informed by her own beliefs and intuition may, in the end, regret her innocence and trust. Then again, there is wisdom in knowing that more is not necessarily better.

The Gatherer Is:

> Active in every child, busily collecting shells,
>> sparkly stones, fallen nests, words, numbers, and songs;
>
> Picking berries of knowledge; squirreling away information,
>> opinions, and trivia;
>
> Stockpiling terminology, strategies, and maps, collecting
>> prenatal vitamins and baby clothes—
>
> Filling her basket until it is overflowing.

She gathered the seven *mehda* for her upcoming
    descent into Laborland
And took them into her hands.
With the *mehda* in her possession, she prepared
    herself:
She placed on her head a crown of expectations
    and seven books on birth;
She blow-dried and braided her hair;
She tied her blessing bead necklace around her neck,
Packed up the birth ball, aromatherapy oils, and
    camera;
She daubed her eyes with waterproof mascara,
Bound the maternity bra, inscribed "Come, Baby,
    Come," around her chest,
And took her insurance forms and birth plan in
    her hand.
Then she slipped the hospital ID band over her
    wrist
And wrapped the hospital gown (or labor T-shirt)
    around her body.

WHAT TO DO WITH YOUR BASKET?

It is natural to become attached to the things we have collected in our baskets. People seldom change their most deeply held convictions. To do so takes a powerful experience— such as pregnancy, birth, and parenting—and an openness and willingness to risk altering our worldview.

To better understand this challenge, imagine a baby being given a big basket to collect knowledge, stories, rules, beliefs, jokes, judgments, assumptions, and expectations about how the world works and how to be loved, belong, and feel safe. At the moment she is born, her basket is already partially filled with family and world stories, philosophies, customs, and beliefs. Throughout childhood, anyone can throw stories into her open basket. Over time, the child will add her own stories, rules about life, and beliefs about what it means to be a lovable, worthy, and responsible human. Everything in her basket will affect her preparation for birth and motherhood. Therefore, by the time this child grows up and hears the call to motherhood her basket is overflowing with a thousand beliefs about birthplace, birth attendants, books, classes, and other important items. Beliefs that are borrowed or contradictory will cause confusion; and to the extent that assumptions and expectations remain hidden, ignored or fixed, she will be limited by them, especially while they are driving her decisions, fears, and wishes.

SORTING THROUGH YOUR BASKET

After hearing the call to motherhood, you will need to sort through your basket, paying special attention to everything you tell yourself about who you are as a pregnant woman, a laboring woman, and a mother. In fact, an essential Task of Preparation is to examine the stories you tell yourself and the stories others tell you about yourself.

Every so often you have to empty out your pockets or your purse to see what is in there. The same is true with your basket of beliefs. You put some of the contents back, throw the rest out, and then continue collecting. Before making decisions and plans such as where to give birth, who will be with you, and how you will deal with pain and unpredictability, once again rummage through your basket to see what you've collected, then discard what is no longer needed, helpful, or true for you.

Among the Native people of the Southwest, baskets were made for gathering, storytelling, and ceremony. The art of designing and making baskets has been passed down from mother to daughter for hundreds of years. The design woven into a traditional Navajo basket always appears broken in some way, allowing a pathway from center to periphery. In ceremonies, this gap is oriented to the east and referred to as "the way out." It represents the Navajo people's exit from one world and emergence into the next, as well as the ever-forward progression of individual human thought.[1]

LEAVING "HOME"

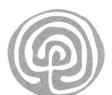

13

A change of heart must precede leaving "home"—that is, leaving behind familiar routines, ways of thinking, and relationships to embark on a great journey. When you answer the Call, not only do you change but so do your relationships (with friends, co-workers, and even your parents), temporarily or permanently, in ways you didn't expect. It might be tempting to try to keep things the same or preserve a familiar dynamic in relationships, even if it means forfeiting an opportunity for

Inanna abandoned her seven temples to descend into the underworld. Temples represent thought patterns that house our points of view, past stories, future ambitions, and all that is trusted and treasured. Abandoning our temples is a necessary first step on the Warrior's journey. In cutting her ties to places, responsibilities, routines, and relationships, Inanna shows her intention to attend fully to her initiation.

personal growth. What you don't know yet—but need to accept anyway—is that you will meet new friends, mentors, and allies whose presence and caring will be crucial to completing your journey.

Coming to terms with the necessary changes can lead to confusion or disconnection, and as a result you may feel neglected or abandoned. If you accept your Call, then pack, walk out of your comfort zone, and lock the door behind you. When others don't agree with you, it doesn't mean they don't support you.

Take your first step in a new direction and head toward a path called Uncertainty.

PRENATAL TASK OF PREPARATION

Strengthen autonomy ◎ Find your voice ◎ Be authentic

For a Warrior, leaving home is not an impulsive or rebellious act. It is a courageous act and another mindful Task of Preparation. Name the "temples" you are ready to leave behind to descend into Laborland, such as the following.

I am abandoning my:

In early pregnancy she abandoned partying for a new life

In mid-pregnancy she abandoned her maiden figure for a new life

In late pregnancy she abandoned bladder control for a new life

In labor she abandoned her modesty for a new life

In labor she abandoned her birth plan for a new life

In postpartum she abandoned her nights of sleep for a new life

In motherhood she abandoned hollow ambitions for a new life.

Temple of Spontaneity or Procrastination
Temple of My Family History
Temple of Fear, Doubt, or Shame
Temple of Approval-Seeking
Temple of Not Enough Time
Temple of My Career
Temple of Perfection
Temple of a Clean and Orderly House

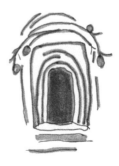

Circular Breathing

The ancient Taoist meditation known as circular breathing was written about in the I Ching five thousand years ago. It was developed while contemplating the mystery of the human fetus growing beneath its mother's navel, absorbing nutrients from her and "breathing" through its own navel. It is not surprising that the sages came to think of the navel as the starting point for the dynamic circulation of our primordial life energy, also called "chi."

There are two kinds of chi energy: yin and yang. Yin is "cold"; yang is "hot." In the womb, the baby's yin and yang energies are balanced and unified, creating a flow of lukewarm chi.[1] According to Taoist teachings, by the time we reach adulthood chi energy divides: the hot yang energy rises to the upper part of the body, and the cold yin energy settles in the lower abdomen and legs. Taoists believe this split in energy causes physical fatigue and mental imbalance.

What is chi?
Where does it come from?

Chi is primordial life force. From the moment the sperm cell penetrates the egg, the human is continuously infused with chi.

In his book *Awaken Healing Energy through the Tao*, Mantak Chia describes the ancient practice of circular breathing (also known as "rejuvenation breathing," "ovarian breathing," and the "microcosmic circuit"). Drawing on the generative power of chi, this breathing meditation rejuvenates hope, calms the mind, and increases your ability to concentrate. Rejuvenation breathing is beneficial every day throughout pregnancy, and whenever you feel exhausted in labor or unable to focus during contractions.[2] This breathing meditation works best when you sit or stand tall with your eyes closed or slightly open, softly gazing downward.

Breathing in

Imagine, as you breathe in, that you are pulling life-giving energy up from your tailbone to the crown of your head. Follow your breath upward, along the inner curves of your spine (one inch inside your body). Notice the brief pause between your inhalation and exhalation while focusing your attention on the crown of your head.

Breathing out

Follow your exhalation from the crown of your head downward through the front of your body, finishing just above your pubic bone. Imagine this life-giving breath rejuvenating every cell, organ, and muscle in your body, your womb, and your baby. Picture your baby being showered in red-, purple-, and gold-colored light.

Filling and spilling your cup of chi

Imagine a little cup sitting behind your pubic bone; picture it filling with your exhalation. With your next deep inhalation, watch the cup tip back and spill chi across your perineum. Breathe out easily.

Listen to the audio recording to learn how your birth partner can enhance Circular Breathing in labor with touch.

Repeat this cycle

You can practice continuous Circular Breathing as a meditation for 20 minutes and as a pain-coping practice using 60-second "ice contractions."* Then you will be experiencing the relaxation, focus, and ancient power of Circular Breathing.

Birth Attendants

14

Doctor ◎ Midwife ◎ Nurse ◎ Doula

Choosing a birth attendant is a significant mile-marker in the life of every modern pregnant woman. There are many factors to consider, so take time to think over your options.

Depending on where you live, your financial re-sources, insurance coverage, politics, and other considerations, you may not have the privilege of choosing your birth atten-dant. In some communities, just finding a birth attendant has become increasingly difficult. In addition to insurance plans that limit free choice, at least half of the states in this country (especially in rural and underserved areas) are short of obste-tricians, family practice doctors, and midwives, requiring some pregnant women to drive an hour or more to get care with few options. In many countries, birth attendants are assigned, not chosen by women, unless they can pay for private-practice care.

If you are birthing at a hospital, you may be able to choose a prenatal caregiver, but it is unlikely that the doctor or nurse-midwife you develop a relationship with during prenatal appoint-ments will be the one who attends your labor. Since private practice is nearly a thing of the past, it is very likely you will enroll in a big practice where patient care is shared among as many as twenty doctors, nurse-midwives, physician assistants, and other care providers. It is not possible to completely agree with the philosophies of—or even meet with—everyone in such a large practice. If you're considering an all-physician practice, take note: one study found that among healthy women who received joint care from a physician and nurse-midwife 81 percent birthed vaginally, compared with only 63 percent who received care from an all-physician group. And there were fewer operative deliveries and less use of epidural anesthesia.[1]

Keep in mind that when you are in labor it is likely that the birth attendant on call will be busy caring for other patients. Also, your postpartum care will probably be with someone who was not at your birth and who may be a complete stranger. These uncertainties motivate some women to consider home birth or hire a doula who will be with them during the whole process.

Interviewing Birth Attendants

In any relationship we are obliged to ask,
"What am I expecting of this person which I ought to do myself?"

—James Hollis

"I found out I was pregnant in the college campus clinic. The first question they asked me was who would be my doctor. I didn't know! They handed me a list with about five hundred names on it, but I still didn't know who to choose. I wanted a home birth, but, I reasoned, why pay three grand for a home birth when I could co-pay 10 percent or less on the plan? At the time, it seemed like it was all the same anyway. Now I know maternity health care is a profit-making commodity."

—Tara

The first visit with a potential birth attendant is an interview to find out how your maps align—or don't. This is your chance to learn about their standard practices, their attitudes regarding prenatal and labor management, their communication style, and their expectations of you. Much like the early stages of dating, during the first prenatal appointments with a birth attendant many women gloss over concerns or ignore important questions to avoid risking conflict. As a result, hard but important questions are often postponed until late in pregnancy, when switching attendants is nearly impossible. Discussing your preferences and concerns with your birth attendant *before* a relationship has developed may actually be easier.

When you meet with a birth attendant for the first time, you should both be fully dressed. You are not on equal footing if you are only wearing a flimsy paper gown. The physical exam can wait until the second visit when you are not a complete stranger and, more importantly, have already chosen this practitioner to attend you in labor.

What happens in your first visits with doctors, midwives, and doulas is a preview of what will likely happen in other prenatal visits—and in labor. Here are some things to keep in mind while interviewing birth attendants to see if they will guide you through labor safely and respectfully:

- Go to every appointment with someone (a partner, relative, or friend) with whom you can later compare notes and talk over impressions.

- Pay attention to your gut feelings about competence, philosophy, and mutual respect; your instincts can play an important role in successfully choosing birth attendants.

- You want to be a member of the birth team, not on the sidelines. Are your values being taken into consideration? Are decisions being made *for* you or *with* you? Do you have shared dialogues about how you will work together rather than simply being instructed in standard practices?

- Notice how the birth attendant speaks with you. For instance, does the birth attendant call you by your name or instead call you "Sweetie," "Mom," or "Honey"—terms some women find condescending.

- Be aware of any pressure you feel from the prospective birth attendant to make decisions or another appointment. Go home and sleep on it.

- If something doesn't feel right, resist the temptation to dismiss your feelings. Track any clues and your gut feelings *before* making any decisions.

If you ask questions in a way that suggests the answer you want, then you might get the answer you want to hear but not the truth. For example, if you say, "I don't want an episiotomy. Do you perform routine episiotomy?" you won't know if the answer you get is the one that makes the sale or the one that describes the doctor's philosophy of practice.

Instead, ask open-ended questions, such as, "How many of your patients require episiotomy?" or "How will you help me avoid tearing or having an episiotomy?" Notice whether the caregiver's response is ambiguous or evasive, as in, "I only do that when it is necessary."

Be discerning rather than easily reassured. Clarify their answer with another question, such as, "How often do you find this necessary?"

Second Thoughts?

If during later appointments you realize that the birth attendant you chose may not be a good fit for you, there are still things you can do:

1. Make an effort to understand the birth attendant's perspective (even when you don't agree with it) and attempt to communicate yours. Engage in a dialogue to see where this takes you.

2. Don't assume that you are "stuck" with your original selection even if it's late in your pregnancy. Ask around for references. Choose another birth attendant or change birth locations if you can.

A Shortage of Time

Some couples assume that their obstetric care will be relationship-based and personal but then discover that prenatal appointments are so brief there is no time for developing a relationship, or even having a conversation. Many birth attendants in the system are physically, mentally, and emotionally exhausted, with little time for getting to know their patients. One doctor mourned that "spending time with patients is now considered 'alternative' [medicine]."[2]

If you are expecting your doctor or nurse-midwife to be the one helping you through labor, you might be surprised to find out that she may only visit you briefly in labor, and may not be seen again until it's time to "catch" your baby. More often it will be the nurse who has ongoing contact with you, mostly to monitor your labor progress, check your blood pressure and baby's heart rate, and so forth.

> "The employer gave us monthly color-coded charts that compared us with our peers in terms of speed and number of patients seen.... The pressure to see as many patients as possible is driven by high overhead. There was no time to slow down, no time to think, no time to care."
>
> —Dr. Pamela Wible[3]

Labor Nurses

A caring labor nurse can offer more than clinical care and be highly skilled in labor support. Get off to a good start with your labor nurse: learn her name; acknowledge her vast experience in labor patterns and ways of supporting women in labor; ask for her advice or help to achieve your goals, including suggestions to help you through labor and pushing. The nurse's personality, her attitudes about pain, her communication skills, and her capacity to provide encouragement will all influence your confidence and decisions.

A hospital's cesarean rate is typically attributed to the attending doctors and hospital policies, however, sometimes a nurse's attitude is key. Through most of labor, a doctor's only view of a woman's labor is through the nurse's eyes and reports, often by phone. So her experience, attitude, and ability to negotiate with the doctor on your behalf—for example, to continue laboring under certain circumstances—can be central to decreasing your need for drugs or cesarean surgery.[4] Your labor nurse may end up being your greatest ally.

If the nurse randomly assigned to you when you are admitted, or newly assigned at the beginning of a new shift, isn't a good fit, you or your partner can ask the charge nurse to assign someone whose attitude and personality are a better match with yours. It is more important to feel comfortable with your nurse than be concerned about hurting the nurse's feelings. This kind of request is common.

HOME BIRTH MIDWIVES

A home birth midwife may be difficult to find, depending on where you live. Licensing and regulation of midwives varies from state to state; only twenty-seven states license certified professional midwives (CPMs). Most certified nurse-midwives practice in hospitals.

One of the responsibilities you entrust to a home birth midwife is sound assessment skills so they can distinguish between a healthy low-risk pregnancy and labor and one that would be better managed by a doctor or nurse-midwife in a hospital. You are entrusting her to know when to consult, order tests, and how to accurately interpret them to ensure your well-being.

In a birth story circle, several home birth mothers talked about how they chose their midwives. Their primary motivation to

"Midwife" can mean many things.

Certified Nurse Midwife (CNM):
Trained in an accredited institution,
licensed as a nurse and midwife,
often holds a bachelor's degree, and
is certified by the American College
of Nurse Midwives (ACNM).
CNMs can prescribe a full range of
medications, provide well-woman
care, and work in different settings
(hospital, birth center, and home).

Direct-Entry Midwife (DEM):
Practices midwifery without a
nursing background, having
obtained training through self-study,
apprenticeship, or a midwifery
school. DEMs can be licensed
or certified, or practice without
certification or license.

*Certified Professional Midwife
(CPM):* Has apprenticed or attended
formal training and meets the
practice standards of the North
American Registry of Midwives
(NARM).

Certified Midwife: A new credential
from ACNM that does not require
a nursing degree but holds the
applicant to the same standards
as those of a CNM.

Licensed or Registered Midwife:
Licensure offered in some states for
DEMs, as well as for professional
midwifery regulations and
standards of care.

Lay Midwife: Not certified or
licensed; trained through self-study
or apprenticeship.

have a home birth was to avoid getting "sucked into"
an intervention in the hospital. Jane said it did not
occur to her to ask about her midwife's education
or experience; at the time, she thought a midwife's
level of friendliness was the most important quality
to get her through labor. So she chose the nicest
midwife she interviewed, only to realize later that
her midwife was inexperienced and that experience
and skill are as important as personality.

Patti chose her midwife because they were in
the same spiritual community and because the midwife quoted studies confirming her beliefs that birth
in the hospital had worse outcomes as a result of
interventions. "At the time," Patti recalled, "I
naïvely thought her anti-medical attitudes were going
to protect me from interventions. In labor, when I
was in trouble and wanted to be transferred she
would not transfer me for hours until the situation
became more urgent. And then she would not go
into the hospital with me."

Another woman in the birth story circle, Ava,
said she wished she had had a list of questions to help
her choose her midwife, and to know when going
to a doctor or hospital was the right thing to do.
Following are suggestions of things to consider when
selecting a midwife.

Ask Around

Get recommendations for a competent and experienced midwife from home birth mothers and
birth professionals in your community. Home birth–
friendly doctors and nurses can be valuable sources
of referrals as well. You may also be able to find online reviews from former clients who had home births
in your community. Whenever possible, find out
specifically what worked and what didn't. Unfortunately, even states that license midwives do not

provide the public with information about their experience or complaints brought against them. Therefore, it's best to speak with mothers themselves.

Conduct Interviews

When interviewing a prospective midwife, ask about:

- Her training, experience, and licensure.

- Her reasons for going into midwifery.

- What aspects of the work she loves the most.

- Her attitudes about collaboration with other birth professionals, hospital birth, and the use of medical technology—to determine if she is distrustful of local providers or has a balanced point of view.

- Her reasons for ordering or declining tests and what tests she routinely orders.

- Her rate of transfer to a hospital. (If it is very low, especially if she is proud of it, be wary since delaying or avoiding a needed transfer may cause a minor situation to become more serious, putting you or your baby at risk.)

- Her fee reimbursement by insurance or Medicaid in case of transfer.

- Her criteria for transfer to a physician's care or the hospital during pregnancy or labor. What about preterm, breech, twins, and postdates (past 41 completed weeks)?

- Her transfer protocols. Which hospital you would go to and how you would get there—by car or ambulance? How does the midwife describe her relationship with hospital staff? How would her care and relationship with you change in the event of a transfer? Would she stay at the hospital with you, and if so, for how long? Would she continue care postpartum? How would she care for and support you in case of a cesarean?

Some states have set standards of safe care for home birth midwives; some midwives follow them, others do not. Become familiar with the standards of care for home birth midwives in your state.

DOULAS

While birth attendants focus on physical assessment and well-being in labor, many overlook emotional needs. Consequently, many parents invite a friend or relative, or hire a doula—a trained birth companion—to provide emotional and practical support during pregnancy, birth, and postpartum. A doula may soothe and reassure you, make suggestions for position changes and coping with pain, remind you to ask questions, help your partner support you, or even support your partner by allowing him to take a break to eat or nap. A good doula should be non-judgmental and prioritize being in relationship with you rather than focusing solely on birth choices and outcomes. Some doulas with special training can help you with breastfeeding. Although you might think of doulas as being essential in a hospital setting, they provide valuable support at home births, too.

The benefits of having a trained birth companion cannot be overstated. Research shows that women assisted by a doula tend to have fewer medical interventions and cesareans, as well as shorter labors and higher satisfaction with their births.[5] However, a doula cannot ensure that you will have a positive natural birth; she cannot guarantee that you will avoid a cesarean, epidural, or other medical procedure. Instead, think of a doula as someone who can help you access your inner and outer resources, offer useful suggestions along the way, and be emotionally supportive when you encounter an unexpected twist in your Laborinth.

Doulas come with a wide variety of life and birth experiences, philosophies, and personalities. When interviewing them, be mindful of what is pulling you toward or away from a particular doula. It is important to find someone who shares your concerns. Also realize that choosing a doula who is adamantly pro-natural birth—even if that echoes your beliefs—may have a downside. You may think she will better protect you from unnecessary interventions, but pessimistic attitudes can interfere with building a respectful working relationship with nurses and birth attendants. And if medical support does become part of your birth, you don't want to fear feeling judged by your doula.

Labor support is hard work and often involves long hours. Neither you nor your doula should have an expectation that she will be a superwoman. It is unrealistic to expect a doula to be present continuously, from the beginning to the end of a long labor, and still provide good support. Exhaustion makes it harder to be objective, supportive, positive, and solution-focused. Make sure your doula has a back-up partner, and if possible, meet the back-up doula in advance. When your doula is taking care of herself, she is better able to take care of you.

Even if you hire the most fabulous doula in the world, you will still need to cope with pain, ask questions in order to make good decisions, and deal with unwished-for surprises. Doula care, no matter how excellent, does not take the place of quality childbirth education. Learning about the physiology of birth, practicing coping and labor positions with your partner, and connecting with other expectant couples are just some of the benefits of good childbirth classes.

Asking your partner to be your sole guide through labor is like asking your partner to lead the way on a climb of Mount Everest. Your partner may be smart and trustworthy, and you love this person, but in the Himalayas you'll both be better off with a Sherpa.

Find a BIRTHING FROM WITHIN Mentor and Doula

www.BirthingFromWithin.com

We train and certify Childbirth Mentors (educators) and Birth Doulas around the world.

One final word: Don't abandon yourself

On a long journey, after turning the wheel over to another driver it's easy to fall asleep in the car and let the driver take responsibility for getting you home safely. Many women realize later that in relegating too much responsibility to others, they abandoned themselves: not tuning in to their bodies, not acting on their urges to change positions, not following their intuition, and not asking for clarification, more time, more support, or whatever they needed. By assuming that all her needs will be intuited and met by others, a woman risks becoming passive and later judging herself harshly. A Birth Warrior views birth attendants as valuable consultants who are doing their best. She understands that no matter how much they know, they are still human and fallible. So she stays alert on the jour-

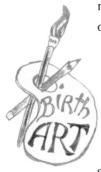

ney and, even more importantly, does her best to walk the path of the heart.

BIRTH IN OUR CULTURE

For millennia, humans have been recording their lives, including childbirth, in drawings on cave walls, clay tablets, and in sculptures. In the 1970s, before launching the Pioneer and Voyager spacecraft, NASA prepared time capsules with sound recordings and images that portrayed the diversity of life and culture on Earth, so that if future humans or extraterrestrials found the spacecraft they would have some idea about the people who created them.

Imagine that you are invited to contribute to such a time capsule. Make a drawing that shows how humans give birth; our birthplaces; and our contemporary, mainstream birth customs, objects, and beliefs. This image may not represent your own birth expectations or values, but it captures birth in our culture.

15

BIRTHPLACE

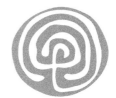

Pregnancy and birth are at once intuitive, instinctive, and cultural. A woman will prepare her "nest" for birthing according to the style of her culture in the same way that a particular species of bird will build its nest.

At a time when the philosophy and customs of birth in our culture are undergoing tremendous transformations, women often agonize over the decision of where to give birth. Weighing the pros and cons of home birth, a birth center, or one hospital over another can leave some feeling caught between a rock and a hard place. If this decision is not determined by your insurance or health conditions, take time to choose the place that you feel is right.

Consider and explore birthplace options in your community. Call on your Huntress to look within at your attitudes and feelings about birthplaces. Where do you imagine building your labor "nest"? Where do you imagine you will feel most "at home" in labor? What draws you to this place?

Every day women are giving birth in unbelievable places: at home; in hot tubs, birthing centers, hospitals; on birthing balls, birthing chairs, operating tables; in cars, birth huts, checkpoints, refugee camps, even in a tree.

On a March morning in Mozambique in the year 2000, when the Limpopo River overflowed, a very pregnant Sophia Pedro saw her home and all her belongings washed away. She strapped one of her children to her back and carried the other above swirling dirty water toward one of the three big trees outside her village. Once there, they climbed as high as they could and clung to the branches, waiting for help. For two days they had nothing to eat or drink but drops of rain. Nor did they sleep, for fear of falling down and drowning. At dawn on the third day Sophia went into labor and gave birth. Soon after, a helicopter rescued the courageous mother, her newborn daughter Rositha, and her family. "The birth was over quite quickly," Sophia explained. "It is a painful experience anyway, and in the tree it was dreadful. There was blood everywhere—a terrible mess. But nothing can take away from the joy of seeing a new life enter the world." Rositha was wrapped in the clothes Sophia had been wearing.

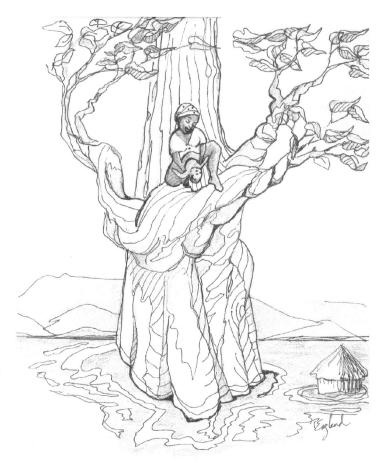

For some women, this place is in a hospital stocked with technology; for others it is in the privacy and comfort of their own home surrounded by family. Keep in mind that even if you envision giving birth in a particular place, your insurance company, an eager baby, or other circumstances determine another place for you. Don't give up if your insurance does not cover your first choice. Call your representative; it is rare but possible that your options could be expanded. And your call will inform the agency that they are not covering consumer choices.

Some women hope that simply "trusting birth" and bringing a positive attitude to any birth environment will create a positive experience. However, in trying to think positively, many women ignore subtle but important signals about not feeling genuinely positive about something, or of not feeling completely safe, heard, or respected. Ignoring these signals limits the depth of your preparation and experience. The ambience and messages of your prenatal care and birthplace can affect your confidence and, to some degree, your body's readiness to labor.

Hospital

What facility has a 7 percent cesarean rate?

The Zuni Indian Hospital near Ramah, New Mexico[1]

Contrary to research findings, our culture generally assumes that the more medicalized and technologically managed labor is the safer it is. Therefore, it is often assumed that hospital birth is the most safe and responsible thing to do—for all births, even normal ones that do not require medical support. This is why 99 percent of all births in the United States take place in hospitals, even though there is no evidence that hospitals make a birth safer for healthy mothers and babies.

Economics also plays a role in promoting the hospital choice. Even when parents want to choose an out-of-hospital birth attended by a midwife, they may not be able afford her services. Some insurance companies do not offer full, or any, coverage for midwifery care provided in home or birth center settings, thereby forcing women to "choose" an approved provider, usually a doctor, in a hospital setting.

Hospital birth is for women who:

- Want to birth in a hospital for whatever reason

- Are birthing before 37 weeks or after 42 weeks

- Have a high-risk condition, such as pre-eclampsia, twins, or breech

- Have chronic medical problems, such as high blood pressure or diabetes

- Have a poor diet, poor weight gain, or smoke

- Desire access to pain medication
- Planned a home birth but require medical support

EARLY TASK OF PREPARATION
Take a tour of labor and delivery

Don't wait until you are in labor to visit the labor and delivery unit in your hospital for the first time. The strange new environment, noises, and smells may be overwhelming and distracting in labor, a time when you need to be as calm and internally focused as possible. Most women take a tour in the third trimester; however, the risk in waiting to see the hospital until late pregnancy is that if you then realize that the place where you've planned to birth is not right for you, you may have fewer options for change.

Take a tour of the labor and delivery unit in your first trimester to learn about its routines and philosophy of care; do this even if you are planning to birth at home. Talking to your tour guide will help you make a mental map of how you will be steered once you arrive at the hospital—from triage to admission, to a labor room, to the postpartum floor and nursery, and finally to discharge from the hospital. Additional advantages to being aware of the facility's procedures and rules are that you will discover which requests you can make to best care for yourself and your newborn, and your worries may be relieved sooner if the environment is less clinical or hostile than you had imagined.

Labor at home as long as you can

If you are healthy and believe that the privacy of your own home will make labor easier for you, but you are not planning to give birth at home, consider staying at home until labor is active. You may want to hire a midwife or doula to offer intermittent support in early labor and to help you decide when to go to the hospital.

"A !Kung mother takes great pride in self-sufficiency in birth. As soon as her contractions become strong, the mother goes out in the veld (grasslands). She collects soft grass and piles it into a mound to make a soft landing for her baby. When pushing, she squats over that mound.

"During her first labor, her mother and other older women assist her. If the first birth goes well, she will give birth to subsequent babies alone. If labor begins at night, she will not wake her sleeping husband as she slips out the door and goes to the veld. !Kung mothers have a keen sense of competence and independence. In the morning, the !Kung mother, glowing with pride, returns home with her newly born child."[2]

Being in the comfort of your own home in early labor has many advantages. At home you can eat and drink whatever and whenever you like. While the trend is slowly changing, most hospitals do not allow laboring women to eat or drink anything other than ice chips and clear liquids. In the privacy of your own home you can also move about freely, take a walk outside, and experiment with the waves of contractions to find your way of coping.

Freestanding Birth Center

Birth centers not affiliated with a hospital can offer a natural approach to labor, birth, and newborn care in a homelike setting. This option is for healthy mothers who wish to birth outside the hospital but not in their own home, and who seek care from professionally certified or licensed midwives (CNMs or LMs). The length of stay is usually shorter and the cost less than a hospital birth. When labor is not normal, mothers are transferred to the nearest hospital. One study showed that out of over 15,500 women who planned to birth at a birth center, 84 percent did; an amazing 93 percent of them had a spontaneous vaginal birth and only 6 percent had a cesarean birth.[4]

Home Birth

There was a time when everyone, regardless of their health status, birthed at home simply doing the best they could. While the majority of births were normal, some women prayed for relief, many of whom would have chosen medical support had it been available. In the last century, science and litigation have changed our values, expectations, and choices. Today, home birth is still an excellent choice for many, although it is not for every woman.

Home birth is for women who are healthy before and during pregnancy; it is for women whose labors progress normally and whose (unborn) babies are healthy. Home birth is for

Percentage of women giving birth in hospitals in the United States:

1900: 5 percent

1927: 15 percent

1935: 37 percent

1945: 45 percent

1960: 97 percent

2014: 98.3 percent[3]

What midwives bring . . .

The introduction of IV, antibiotics, and sterile gloves in the 1940s did more to reduce maternal and fetal mortality than any other interventions since, including the shift to hospital birth. These supplies are available to, and used by, licensed home birth midwives in addition to the following essential equipment: oxygen, Pitocin for postpartum bleeding (not used during labor or for inductions), fetoscope or Doppler, suctioning equipment, and suture materials (for repairing minor tears).

women who believe that birth is hard work, that they can do it, and that medical support should only be used when necessary. Unfortunately, home birth is also restricted to women or couples who can afford to pay out of pocket for professional midwifery care and lab work.

About 1 percent of mothers in the United States give birth at home.[5] In a study of over 11,000 home births attended by nurse-midwives, the overall transfer rate (including prenatal) was 16 percent, and during labor 8 percent.[6] Other researchers found that 25 percent of first-time mothers who planned to birth at home, and 4 percent to 9 percent of women giving birth again, transferred to the hospital.[7] Most transfers were for nonemergency reasons such as preterm breech, postdates, high blood pressure, prolonged labor, and pain relief.

You are a good candidate for a home birth if you are:

- Healthy and low risk

- Well nourished

- A nonsmoker

- Birthing within thirty minutes of a hospital

- Willing to take an active role in giving birth with minimal intervention

- Prepared to cope with normal labor pain, exhaustion, and hard work

- Carrying a single baby in head-down presentation

- Birthing between 37 weeks and 42 completed weeks of pregnancy

- Insured or able to cover additional costs of midwifery care

Labor is hard work wherever you are. Laboring in the comfort and privacy of home, surrounded by people chosen by you, generally makes focusing and coping easier. When everyone around you believes in you and is cheering you on, it is easier to believe in yourself and to keep going. However, being at home during labor can also mean being "at home" psychologically. Sometimes when a woman has an unrecognized belief that she would be safer in the hospital she might not be able to let go and give birth at home, but as soon as she enters the hospital her baby is born. Having too many people, or the wrong people, at a birth can also cause enough stress and distraction to slow labor down.

Most women and couples choose home birth because it resonates with their philosophy and lifestyle, and because the idea is familiar—they often were born at home or know others were. Choosing to have a home birth involves taking more responsibility through a holistic process of preparation. In addition, developing a trusting relationship with a midwife, or a small group of midwives, increases confidence and decreases stress.

Women who had traumatic hospital births sometimes choose home births for their next babies to avoid encountering problems they experienced previously. Unresolved emotional birth trauma can cause fear and stress in the body. If fear of hospital birth is a starting point for you, in addition to changing the birthplace take steps to heal the trauma and release fear and stress. Ultimately, even when a woman is wary of the routines and high rate of interventions in a hospital her primary motivations for a home birth should come from a deep place of comfort with herself, her body, and birthing at home.

TIMELY TRANSFER

When the hospital is the right place to birth

If you are planning an out-of-hospital birth, transfer to the hospital is probably the last thing you want to think about or plan for. But as a Birth Warrior one of your Tasks of Preparation is to plan for the unexpected and for your safe Return.

Anyone who plans an out-of-hospital birth should be prepared to acknowledge circumstances that make a transfer to the hospital a wise choice. If a couple or their midwife avoid preparing for a transfer and one occurs, it would likely cause additional stress. One preventive would be to take a tour of the hospital in advance; another would be to go over your midwife's transfer protocol.

An experienced and watchful midwife can tell when a labor problem begins developing and arranges for a timely transfer. Most transfers to a hospital are for nonemergency problems that require medical support, such as being overdue, the water breaking without labor starting, prolonged labor without dilation progress, pushing for a long time, or the baby being in breech position. Because most transfers are not emergencies, it is usually possible for the couple to drive to the hospital in their own

A story about birth in our culture

"My second baby was a planned home birth. In early labor, I took a shower while my husband made dinner. Eventually, we called the midwife. The contractions became stronger, and my water broke. The next few contractions were more intense. I reached down and felt his head crowning; just then, I felt the urge to push. Out he came; my husband caught him. I didn't need stitches. When we told our family our baby was born at home, they were baffled that a baby could be born at home without a doctor.

They asked, 'How did the baby get out without a doctor?'

'Did you wear gloves?'

'Who gave the baby a bath?'"

—OLIVIA

These questions reflect how deeply conditioned we have become to believe that it is the doctor, not the mother, who delivers the baby, and that parents are not competent enough to even bathe their own newborn.

Cost of modern birth

The cost of a straightforward, unmedicated vaginal birth in a hospital is between $3,300 and $37,000.[8] With insurance, co-pays can range from $500 to $10,000. If there is an induction, cesarean birth, or the baby goes to the NICU, the price tag goes up and up. The all-inclusive fee for home birth from a licensed midwife ranges from $3,000 to $8,000, which includes prenatal care (an average of twelve hour-long visits), being on call for you, labor and birth (including assistants and all supplies), newborn exam, and postpartum visits. If you are birthing at a birth center, there may be an additional facility fee.

vehicle (sometimes with the midwife in attendance) without needing to run red lights.

A transfer to the hospital does not mean you won't have a vaginal birth or a positive birth experience. In fact, in one study the incidence of epidurals and cesareans was significantly lower among 5,400 home birth transfers than for low-risk women who intended to birth in the hospital— only 4.6 percent had an epidural and only 3.7 percent needed a cesarean.[9]

When the plan changes drastically from birthing at home to birthing in a hospital, it can be disappointing and stressful. However, there is no shame in having to transfer and give birth in a hospital. Rather than think of transfer as a failure, acknowledge that as a Birth Warrior you are doing what needs to be done next, that you are being responsible and responsive to unwished-for circumstances. This takes as much courage and determination—if not more—than birthing at home. It may help to think of a planned home birth as a planned home labor. If the baby is born at home, it is a home birth; if not, then it is a home labor followed by a hospital birth.

IF YOU AND YOUR PARTNER DISAGREE ON THE PLACE OF BIRTH

When one parent wants a home birth but the idea seems crazy to the other, who decides? Optimally, a woman should be able to choose the place in which she feels most safe and least self-conscious. Laboring in an unfamiliar and undesired place can increase her tension and fear, which may physiologically interfere with the progress and outcome of her labor. If her experience of labor or labor management is traumatic for her, she may later resent her partner for not supporting her choice of birthplace or for subjecting her to a labor experience she wanted to avoid.

Too often pregnant women, to avoid conflict, judgment, or

being ostracized, defer to their partners or to pressure from family. Deferring to keep the peace or to save money is not really choosing a birthplace. Worrying about being isolated or judged by those closest to her can diminish a mother's experience of birthing and bonding with her baby.

Choice of birthplace is a women's rights issue. Labor and its medical management happen to women's bodies. Women have the legal and ethical right to autonomy over their bodies and to making decisions that affect their bodies during childbirth.

Even the American Congress of Obstetricians and Gynecologists (ACOG) recognizes this right, stating: A woman has the "moral right to bodily integrity [and] to self-determination regarding sexuality and reproductive capacities."[10]

Even so, the opinions and concerns of people closest to a pregnant woman, including the baby's other parent, must be taken in account. They will be co-parenting for a lifetime, so the way they make important decisions during pregnancy sets the stage for years to come.

Following are a few suggestions for respectful and productive communication if you and your partner don't see eye to eye about the birthplace for your baby. Listen to and acknowledge each other's perspectives and fears. Create a spirit of openness as you investigate all your options. Together, interview several doctors as well as home birth and hospital midwives. Talk to other mothers and fathers about their experiences with the birth attendants or birthplaces you are considering. If finances or insurance are important factors in your birthplace decision, talk about how to budget for any out-of-pocket birth expenses. Even if investigating is hard or takes time, it is crucial to reach a loving consensus about your baby's place of birth. Toward that end, it is important to remember that the terrain of birth is already filled with so many unknown and uncontrollable events that when the mother has a strong voice about where to birth she feels more empowered, confident, and supported.

It's not just the birthplace that makes your birth memorable or powerful. It's you and what you bring to it.

WEAR YOUR BREASTPLATE

A warrior acknowledges that she will be vulnerable in battle, so she goes through great pains to prepare to protect herself. As a Sumerian warrior, Inanna made her own breastplate and knew when to put it on to protect her heart and when to take it off. There are times when you may feel bombarded by others' opinions, fears, and advice. Before each prenatal appointment, and when gathering information before making important decisions, visualize putting on your symbolic breastplate as a ritual of guarding your heart, tuning in to your heart's wisdom, and consequently taking ownership of your health care.

JOURNEY THROUGH A LABOR LANDSCAPE

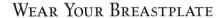

Instead of thinking of labor as a physiological process in your body, imagine labor as a landscape in which every element is a symbolic representation of your physical, emotional, and spiritual journey. Close your eyes. Put yourself in the labor landscape and imagine moving through it. Draw the geographical terrain; it might be wooded forest, desert, mountainous, or a body of water. Notice the season and weather. Who, if anyone, is with you? How do you traverse this landscape—on foot, boat, or the back of an animal? Include as many details as possible while making this internal map.

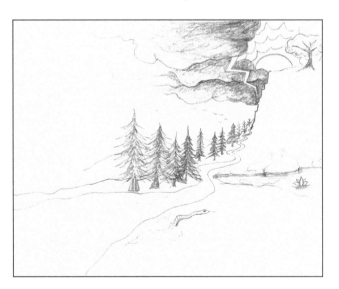

RELAXIN' AND OPENIN' YOUR PELVIS

Turn your attention inward and imagine your baby's journey through the internal landscape of the pelvis. The body follows an ancient map relying on hormones to relax your pelvis in preparation for childbirth, but as a modern woman you also need to bring attention to your posture.

Your whole body—breasts, uterus, abdominal muscles, and joints and ligaments in your pelvis—softens by the end of your first trimester. This is made possible by a hormone called relaxin, produced by your ovaries and placenta. Relaxin softens the cartilage in your joints and relaxes the ligaments that hold your pelvis together, thus allowing for increased mobility of the joints during pregnancy and labor.

YOUR PSOAS MUSCLES IN PREGNANCY AND BIRTH

The psoas (pronounced SOH-az) muscles are a pair of massive, sixteen-inch-long muscles deep in your core that connect your upper body to your legs and allow your legs to swing when you walk. Each psoas wraps around the inside of your pelvic basin, drops down over the hip joints, and attaches to the inside of your thigh bones (figure 16.1). Nerves embedded in the psoas go directly to your reproductive organs. These muscles influence everything from low-back pain to full-body orgasm.[1]

Pauline Scott and Jean Sutton, in their book *Understanding and Teaching Optimal Foetal Positioning*, coined the term "optimal fetal positioning" (OFP) to describe the best position for a baby within the mother's pelvis. They explain many ways in which the woman's posture and movements, in the weeks prior to birth as well as during labor, can help the baby get into a good position, get labor started and progressing well, and even decrease labor pain.

Liz Koch's work has been influential in teaching mothers the importance of optimal maternal position during pregnancy. Having dedicated over thirty years to understanding the psoas muscles, she is a respected international authority, author, and teacher. This section draws from her ideas. For more information, visit her website (CoreAwareness.com) or read her books.

When the psoas are released or lengthened, the tilt of the pelvis increases the size of its opening, making more room for your baby to get into a good position during the final weeks of pregnancy to descend and rotate through your pelvis during labor. Releasing your psoas muscles has other benefits, too, such as enhancing your overall comfort, ease of breathing, and feelings of well-being. Many mothers also notice relief from sciatica and back pain.

On the other hand, when contracted, psoas muscles alter the shape and position of the pelvis, reducing the amount of space for the baby to enter and move through the pelvis. If the psoas muscles are chronically shortened during pregnancy, they may literally hold up a baby before birth.[2, 3]

OPTIMIZING YOUR BABY'S POSITIONING FOR BIRTH

Most birth professionals acknowledge that the way a baby is positioned in its mother's pelvis can dramatically affect the timing, progress, and sensations of labor. However, many doctors only check to see if the baby is head down. It is equally important to note if the baby is posterior (face forward) or otherwise not well situated in the pelvis since in such instances there is an increased likelihood of induction, Pitocin use, epidural, or cesarean. While many factors contribute to the timing, length, and sensations of each woman's labor and birth, and no one can predict or control all of them, there are a few things you can do in pregnancy to make it easier for your baby to move into a better position for birth.

Maintain Optimal Maternal Posture

When you achieve and maintain optimal maternal posture, your psoas instantly release, increasing your energy and providing relief from some of the minor discomforts of pregnancy. Sitting positions that are upright decrease compression of the diaphragm from your growing uterus and allow you to breathe more easily. You may find you "drop down" out of your head and into your belly. It is an important Task of Preparation to learn how to optimally position your body not only for these physiological reasons but also for practicing mindfulness and getting in touch with your intuitive knowing.

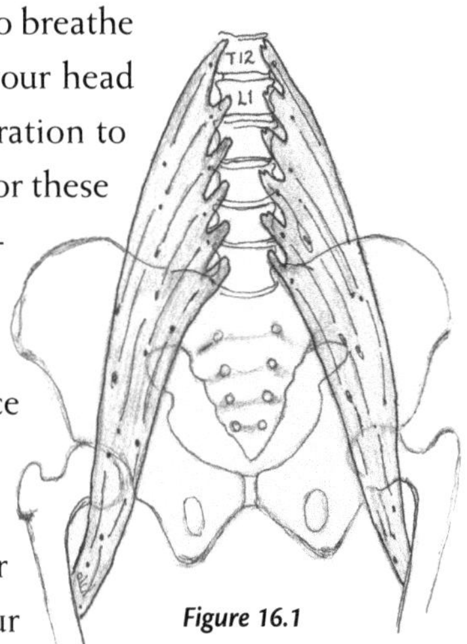

Begin by choosing a chair with a firm surface. Place a Cando wedge, cushion, or zafu (meditation pillow) on the seat to ensure that your hips are higher than your knees (figure 16.2). Then sit down and find your center of gravity by rocking side to side until your weight is evenly distributed, right and left. Now rock slowly, front to back, until you settle on the front curve of your sitting bones (ischial tuberosities)—not resting on the back curve.

Figure 16.1

When sitting with the weight on the front part of your sitting bones, you are "centered" and will feel relaxed and balanced; back and abdominal muscles release because they are not trying to hold you up or compensate for being off-center. When your psoas muscles are relaxed in this position, you can actually feel your pelvis open.

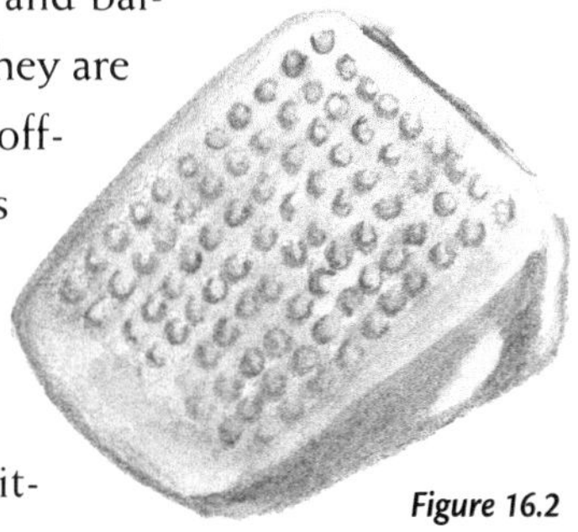

By contrast, when sitting in comfy modern armchairs, sofas, or garden chairs, it is tempting to lean back so that the weight is resting on the back of the sitting bones and on the sacrum (figure 16.3). In this position the pelvis tucks and contracts. Whenever the knees are higher than the hips or the legs are crossed, the flexible joints of the pelvis close and reduce its diameter. This "slouching" position also tips the pelvis and baby backward, causing the psoas muscles to contract to "catch you" as you fall backward. Sitting in these postures occasionally is not a problem. However, most

Figure 16.2

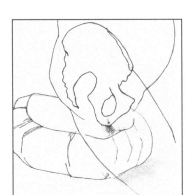

Figure 16.3

Be sure your sit bones settle on the front third, using the wedge or zafu to help you relax into this optimal position.

Gail Tully, a midwife in Minnesota inspired by the work of Scott and Sutton, created Spinning Babies, a training program (with workshops, books, and videos) that increases awareness of the impact on birth of the relationship between the mother's and baby's positions, as well as offers low-tech ways for mothers and their birth attendants to assist in the baby's descent and rotation through the pelvis. Visit her website (SpinningBabies.com) and check out her book, *Belly-Mapping.*

modern women spend a good part of their day driving in bucket seats and sitting slouched in office chairs at desks, in front of computers, or curled up on soft couches.

Be mindful to achieve and maintain optimal maternal posture every chance you get—while eating, driving, working, and while practicing mindfulness and pain coping. Once you experience this comfort, you will not want to be a slouching couch potato anymore.

From your 34th week on, it becomes even more important to focus on being in positions that make space in your pelvis, release the psoas, and help baby move into a good position for birth. In addition to the sitting posture described earlier, many women in late pregnancy find that forward-leaning positions are comfortable and help relieve pressure and pain in the back and pelvis. Try hands-and-knees position, sitting or resting forward on a birth ball, and sitting backwards on a narrow, armless chair and leaning forward over the back of it (padded with a pillow for comfort).

WALK ☉ HIKE ☉ DANCE!

Walking, hiking, and dancing all help to release and lengthen the psoas, increasing the diameter of the pelvis. Take every opportunity you can to move about: Walk to the store. Stroll in a park. Hike in nature. Take the stairs instead of the elevator. Many women find that prenatal yoga emphasizing release of the psoas muscles through "cat-cows" and gentle stretching, benefits their bodies and minds. And remember to dance.

Visualize Opening and Releasing

Imagine that your pelvic bones are sailboats floating on a peaceful lake.
Breathing down through the center of your body...
Pushing each pelvic bone–boat apart... drifting apart.

Breathing in . . . pulls your bones back . . . gliding toward your body . . .
bobbing up and down on gentle waves.
Breathing out ...your pelvic bones drift away ...
Breathing in ...your bones float back ...toward you.
With each releasing breath ...belly, hips, bot-
tom, and thighs melt into the lake ...
Feel your pelvis open ...a little more ...as warmth
and ease diffuse
throughout your body ... allowing you and your baby to enjoy
the good feelings of release ... in the calm, spacious pool.

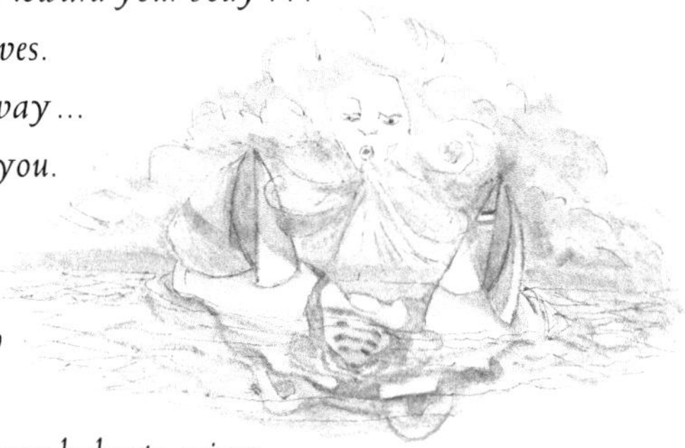

Wear a Pregnancy Belt or "Cradle"

A pregnancy belt or prenatal "cradle" may help decrease movement in your lax sacroiliac joints, thereby reducing inflammation and pain in your lower back, hips, or pelvis. A study found that a belt worn in a high position (figure 16.4) decreased pelvic joint laxity to a significantly greater degree than a belt worn in a low position (figure 16.5).[4] With four points of support, the prenatal "cradle" provides the maximum support and is ideal for women carrying multiples (figure 16.6). A pregnancy girdle offers the least amount of abdominal support.[5] You may also experience relief and support wearing your belt after giving birth.

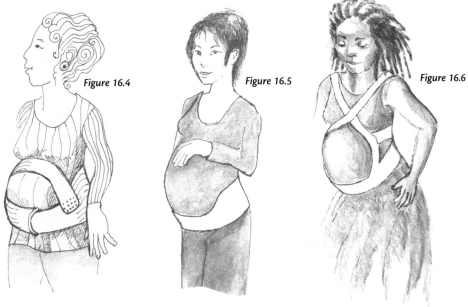

Figure 16.4

Figure 16.5

Figure 16.6

Calming an irritable uterus

Some women experience frequent but painless uterine tightening in the third trimester, brought on by normal activity, exercise, or orgasm; this has been dubbed "irritable uterus." It is also associated with dehydration, being out of shape, or subsequent pregnancies. It is not predictive of preterm labor; the cervix does not change or dilate with an irritable uterus. Many women find that wearing a pregnancy belt or cradle makes their uterus much less "irritable." Drink plenty of fluids. And don't worry.

FIVE CULTURAL CHANGES THAT HAVE NEGATIVELY IMPACTED WOMEN'S POSTURES AND BIRTHS

The human pelvis has not changed dramatically in the last thousand years. Our great-grandmothers' lifestyles included having optimal maternal posture without having to think about it. The chairs they sat in were firm and upright, and they didn't sit in them for long. Their many daily tasks kept them active—and their pelvises rocking—as they cared for the garden, animals, and household. But since 1960 many changes occurred in our culture that altered the mobility of women and their pelvises in pregnancy and in birth. This subsequently impacted the position of their babies, leading to longer and more difficult labors, increased use of Pitocin, and higher cesarean rates. Here are five cultural changes that have negatively impacted women's postures and births:

1. The arrival of television in almost every home meant that to be comfortable while watching for hours, "couch potatoes" needed cushy places to sit. Furniture makers now create lines of sofas that force us to slouch, sit on our sacrums, or recline with our knees higher than our hips.

2. The use of bucket seats in cars, with their hollow for the bottom, causes our weight to resting on the back curve of the sitting bones and sacrum.

3. Computers and excessive desk work contribute to poor posture. Many pregnant women now spend hours sitting in front of computers, often in chairs that foster slouching positions and strain the psoas muscles.

4. The electronic fetal monitor, introduced in the mid-1960s, immobilizes women in labor. This decreases the opportunities for the pelvis to change shape, making it harder for the baby to find his way through.

5. Loss of the "confinement" tradition decreased the amount of rest women have late in pregnancy. The term "estimated date of confinement" (still recorded on many prenatal charts as EDC, now meaning "due date") originally referred to the time when a woman near delivery was expected to withdraw from daily routines, responsibilities, and relationships, to rest during the last weeks of her pregnancy. A few weeks of reflection and separation from the world might have served a woman physiologically as well and increased the likelihood that she would have an easier birth. Today, however, economic pressure and social values have many women working up to the day they go into labor. So at a time when instinct calls a woman to withdraw from the busy world—to sleep more, walk in nature, or make a cozy "nest"—instead her mind and body are firing on all cylinders. While working up to her due date may allow her more time to be with her newborn later (at least in the United States, where paid maternity leave is nearly nonexistent), this cultural expectation could be taking a toll on the bodies and minds of pregnant women.

The standardized map of pregnancy and birth has perhaps unwittingly traded an attunement to nature and trust in grand-

It's easy to make a bucket seat flat by placing a foam or inflatable wedge or folded towel in the hollow. This will raise your hips slightly, making you instantly feel more comfortable because your knees will drop slightly, allowing your psoas and back muscles to release.

Tips for improving your posture at the computer

- Position the monitor at eye level so you are not straining your neck and spine.

- Breathe deeply as you work to keep your psoas "juicy."

- Drink four ounces of water every hour.

- Get up and eat elsewhere.

- Every hour walk around, do a few stretches, or go outside for some fresh air. Walking up and down stairs is an excellent way to stretch and balance the pelvis.

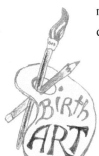

mothers' wisdom and traditions for an expectation that if labor doesn't start or gets stuck technology and surgery will fix it.

WATERCOLOR THE ENERGY IN YOUR BODY

Have your paper, watercolor paints, jar of water, and brushes ready before you begin this meditation. You can do it in silence or while listening to native flute or meditation music.

Lie down and close your eyes. Take a few minutes to practice Breath Awareness. Then imagine the energy in your body as liquid, moving watercolors. Imagine your inhalation picking up a color from a palette.

Watch the watercolor carried on your exhalation, tinting the inside of your body. Witness each colored exhalation moving dreamily, slowly...sometimes in a rush of color, sometimes changing colors. Allow several paint-dipped exhalations to follow the energies in your womb, placenta, amniotic water, and baby.

After the meditation, draw an outline of your body. Inside, create a watercolor painting based on the energy flow within.

MAPS THROUGH LABOR PAIN

17

Because the inner and outer landscapes of labor are varied and uncharted for each woman, there is no one map through labor pain. Navigating your personal course through pain can be best achieved the more you explore your attitudes and beliefs about labor pain, discover how the birth environment can influence your experience, and find practical ways to prepare for your journey.

I n addition to thinking about the baby on the way, most pregnant women wonder how they will cope with labor pain or how they can avoid it. It is essential to our survival to avoid or eliminate pain that is life threatening. Yet pain in a normal labor doesn't need to be eliminated; it is one of the healthy sensations that alerts women to the fact that labor has started, that it is progressing, and that it can offer guidelines on how to move and when to push.

Women who worry the "right amount" about pain are often those best prepared for the intensity of labor. Worrying activates the inner Huntress, initiating a search for resources, both inner and outer, while there is still time to become skillful and confident in mindfulness practices. By contrast, women who are overconfident or have a casual wait-and-see attitude, or are planning on an epidural, do not prepare well for coping with labor pain and are likely to be in for a surprise. Regardless of their optimistic hopes and plans, the unexpected can happen—labor may be harder and more intense than imagined or the epidural is delayed, doesn't work, or there isn't time to get it.

Taking time to explore the work and intensity of birth is an essential Task of Preparation for every pregnant woman regardless of her plans. Preparing for birth requires making plans for both external and internal challenges. The physical sensations of labor have been described in many ways, anything from "rushes" to "waves," sharp pains, or pressure. But it is not just the physical sensations of dilation and pushing that you will have to cope with; it is also the intensity of labor, which can encompass exhaustion from the hard work and lack of sleep; fear about unexpected twists and about adjusting to medical technology; and dealing with other physical sensations such as nausea, vomiting, shaking, and back pain. Your preparation should therefore include plans for dealing with the many internal challenges of birth, including coming to terms with uncertainty and anxiety about the unknowns: not knowing how long labor will take, if you will be able to cope as planned, and how your partner and birth attendants will support you emotionally.

OUR PAIN STORIES

Pain myths are like viruses;
they get passed around and are hard to get rid of.

Labor pain, like all pain, is experienced in the brain yet shaped by a range of external factors—including, in this case, the physical and social environment of the and the people in it. Our perceptions of pain in birth are also colored by stories and myths about pain in birth, as exemplified in the flowing anecdotes.

Grantly Dick-Read, a colonial doctor from Britain visited the Tulkarm region of Kenya in the 1930s. While there, he observed a woman giving birth in a "quiet and dignified" manner. Dick-Read did not speak the language of the local people, so he could not ask the woman about her inner experience. Instead, he drew his own conclusions and began telling this story:

> The primitive [woman] knows that she will have little trouble when her child is born. Natural birth is all that she looks for; there are no fears in her mind; no midwives spoiling the natural process; she has no knowledge of the tragedies of sepsis, infection, and hemorrhage. To have conceived is her joy; the ultimate result of her conception is her ambition. Eventually, and probably whilst even yet at her work, labor commences . . . There is unquestionably a sense of satisfaction when she feels the first symptoms and receives the impatiently awaited indications that her child is about to arrive . . . [She] isolates herself, and, in a thicket, quietly and undisturbed she patiently waits.[1]

Inspired by his assumptions about women's experiences of birth, both primitive and modern, Dick-Read wrote *Childbirth without Fear*, in which he put forth his oversimplified thesis: labor pain is caused by fear, anxiety, and ignorance, and if these are eliminated childbirth would be painless, dignified, and joyful. Dick-Read's theory is still alive and well today among certain groups. And many women who try to follow this premise later wonder where they went wrong because, in spite of their efforts to stay on course, they did not arrive at the pain-free promised land. The assumption that a woman's subjective experience of labor pain is due solely to fear or her state of relaxation is simplistic, leads to judgment, and is not even true.

In fact, fifty years after the publication of *Childbirth without Fear*, a woman anthropologist also witnessed someone giving birth in the Tulkarm region of Kenya. But because the anthropologist could speak Tulkarm she was able to ask the woman if her labor had hurt. The woman answered that the pain had been great. When asked why she did not say so in labor, she answered, "This is not the custom of my people."[2]

Right before the baby was born there was more pain than I could think of, but then I saw the baby and there was a happiness more than I could think of.

—A TONGAN WOMAN WITH THREE CHILDREN

As these anecdotes indicate, there is nothing absolute or universal about the perception and meaning of pain. In addition to attitudes, other important factors influence how a woman responds to labor pain: the labor environment, length of labor, personal resolve and hardiness, and the attitudes and skills of support people. Internal factors have a strong impact as well, such as size and position of the baby, the physical health of mother and baby, the mother's age, and whether it is her first birth. Equally significant is the fact that women in labor are deeply conditioned by their past experience with pain and cultural messages about pain. As one researcher reports, "the women in labor rooms in Oslo do not shout out, not because they are not in pain, but because it is not the custom of their people. Women in Naples shout loudly in labor, not because they are in more pain than the Norwegians, but because those around them would be worried if they did not shout."[3]

Sort through Your Basket of Beliefs and Assumptions

Sorting what went into your basket is an interesting Task of Preparation. This heart-opening exercise will give you more self-compassion and free you up to embrace pain and various ways of coping you may have initially thought impossible.

Begin by noticing where you are now. Acknowledge that the family and culture you were born into handed you a basket of attitudes and assumptions about pain in general and childbirth pain in particular.

Next, take an inventory of all of your beliefs about pain in childbirth. In response to the following questions write down, as fast as you can, all your assumptions and fears about labor pain and how you should react to it. Don't censor yourself or slow down, even if your thoughts are contradictory.

- What is okay to do when you are in pain?

- What are others supposed to do when you are in pain?

- What judgments do you have about women who use pain medications and those who don't?

- What kind of pain medication is acceptable for you?

After completing your inventory, reflect on what you wrote, considering the following questions.

- What surprised you?

- What is the emotional tone of your writing?

- Do you notice any patterns or conflicting ideas?

- Which beliefs or expectations work for you and which do not?

- Which of your current attitudes about pain in labor would you like to change?

Enhancing Pain-Coping Confidence

Lyn vividly recalls working to resolve emotional trauma from her first birth. When asked about her expectations for her upcoming second birth, Lyn tried to bury her fears, saying she was confident it would be easier. She did not want to believe it would be or could be as intense as her first labor. When challenged with, "But what if it is as bad or worse this time? What would you do then?" Lyn replied, with a nervous laugh, "Oh, it just couldn't be!"

These questions compelled Lyn to look more deeply into her fears with the purpose of preparing to meet any challenge. In doing so, she realized she could cope with another long, hard labor. Lyn's second labor, while much faster, was just as intense as her first. Yet because her preparation had included seeing herself coping with even more pain during this labor she had been able to do it.

Scaling Pain

Even if you have never experienced labor, you may have a picture in your mind of being in labor. As a means of preparation, invite your Huntress to explore this image. On a scale of 0 to 100, with 0 being no pain and 100 being the most intense pain you can imagine, how intense do you anticipate active labor will be?

- At this number, see what you are doing to cope. Then name one more thing you can do to help yourself get through contractions.

- Suppose that to get your baby out the number has to be another five or ten points higher. Imagine what you would have to do now to keep going that you didn't have to do at the lower number. Women in our classes often give answers such as "Ask for more help"; "Rock and moan"; or "Swear."

Overcoming Pain Shame

Consider the following:

- Is there anything you are telling yourself that you should not or cannot do in order to "do it right" or be proud later?

- Imagine yourself doing it. How does it feel? How might it help?

- To whom would this response be unacceptable? Is your belief influenced by someone important to you?

- If you acted this way in labor, what do you think it would imply about you?

- What would you say to another woman who coped with pain in this way?

Finding Your Baseline Response to Pain

To get the most out of the pain-coping practices in this book, it helps to find your baseline response to pain. You can start doing this by experiencing an unpleasant sensation and noticing what happens in your mind and body.

Get a bowl of ice, a towel, and a timer. Close your hand around an ice cube for 60 seconds, or hold an ice cube against your wrist. Focus on feeling the cold, burning, aching sensation of the ice. Allow yourself to complain or whine. Try not to distract yourself, even if you know how. When the time is up, put down the ice. Immediately notice what you were telling yourself, your habitual response or strategy, or how you looked for a way out. As you learn various mindfulness practices, watch your ability to concentrate increase and your suffering decrease.

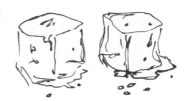

THE DIFFERENCE BETWEEN PAIN AND SUFFERING

Pain is experienced in the body, while suffering arises from the mind. Suffering is more than simply experiencing unwanted or unpleasant physical sensations. We suffer when we fixate on negative stories about what is happening to us. In labor, thinking about the past or worrying about the future, as well as judging the pain itself or our response to it, creates suffering. As humans, our greatest gift—and downfall—is our ability to respond to our current experience by creating internal stories. Suffering, a narrative thread that is wrapped around the pain, quickly leads to doubt, fear, habitual responses, and avoidance. Such ongoing negative mental chatter is what needs to be addressed and changed.

Although nothing can simulate the rhythm, fatigue, and hard work of labor, holding ice during 60-second "ice contractions" can help you investigate your responses to pain. When you use ice contractions regularly to practice the pain-coping exercises in this book, it can help build your confidence and stamina.

Pain may be an inevitable part of childbirth
but much can be done to ease suffering.

MINDFULNESS AS SOLUTION

We suffer when we are in our "monkey mind"—a Buddhist phrase referring to the constant mental activity that occurs when the unfocused mind is jumping and swinging from one thought to another. The solution is to quiet the mind. But how can this be done amidst the intensity of labor? One way is to get in the habit of quieting your mind every day while focusing on breathing, thus invoking mindfulness so that when labor begins you can perform this familiar activity. Mindfulness promotes curiosity and courage that allows you to "enter" sensations rather than feel you must avoid them, ignore them, judge them, or eliminate them. When you move into the sensations, or with them, and focus on your breath or steady your mind, even in states of intense pain or fatigue you can find islands of deep peace and stillness.

There is a common misunderstanding that if you are doing a mindfulness practice "right" you will be relaxed and not feel the "ice contractions" or the uncomfortable sensations of labor. But since the body is designed to register changes in temperature, pressure, cervical dilation, and so forth you may continue to notice sensations, including pain, during mindfulness practice. The real question is not whether you feel physical sensations but whether you *suffer.*

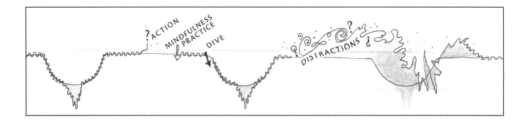

Entering a Contraction in Mindfulness

In my classes, I illustrate a series of contractions to help mothers and their birth companions be mindful in labor. In the first image, pictured above, the even squiggly line represents breathing, focus, and mindfulness. The "leak" shown in the middle of this contraction is where it reaches its peak intensity and, for about five seconds, most women float, or just breathe, then resume their pain-coping or mindfulness practice. A woman who does not know to expect this brief lapse in concentration may, upon losing her concentration, tell herself she is not doing it "right" and feel discouraged.

The label "? action" appearing between the first and second contractions, marks a good time for birth companions to ask a question or for the laboring woman to change positions, have a drink, or go to the bathroom—without disrupting her concentration.

The downward arrow labeled "mindfulness practice" reminds the birth companions and woman to redirect their attention inward and return to their mindfulness practice for about 15 to 30 seconds before the expected start of the next contraction.

The arrow labeled "dive" at the beginning of the next contraction indicates the importance of continuing the mindfulness practice as the contraction builds, which is much easier than lapsing and suddenly returning to it when the contraction begins.

The squiggly line through the third contraction shows how a mother who is distracted by chatter at the start of this or any other contraction can become so overtaken by its intensity that she forgets to engage in her pain-coping or mindfulness practice until the contraction relaxes. If this happens occasionally, it is no problem; however, with repeated occurrences it can undermine her pain-coping confidence.

KNOW THY BODY
The physical story of giving birth

Nature's blueprint for women giving birth includes pain, and this pain is part of labor's amazing hormonal biofeedback loop that keeps labor on track.

Women often wonder how the pain of labor was endured before epidurals. First, when women knew there were no other options, they (and everyone around them) expected they would get through it. But they didn't do it alone, and neither will you. The amazing thing is that nature prepares women's bodies and minds for this intense, inescapable event. When the brain perceives pain, especially with stress, endorphins are released. Endorphins are chemical compounds secreted by the brain and adrenal glands; they produce pain-relief ten times more potent than morphine and provide the euphoric and optimistic "runner's high" needed in the marathon called labor, which usually lasts longer than a typical five-hour running marathon.

As the cervix opens and the baby descends, stretch receptors in the dilating cervix, pelvic floor muscles, and the vagina signal the brain to release more oxytocin. This, in turn, fuels closer and stronger contractions, which further increases dilation and finally the urge to push. As dilation and pain increase, more endorphins are released to help you cope. Elevated endorphins also cause a shift in thinking, from being rational to being more instinctual and in a dreamlike state that meshes well with the task of birthing. Additionally, the pain and pressure sensations of labor guide you in changing positions to help get your baby out.

While there are a number of labor scenarios in which the use of pain medications is wise and compassionate (see chapter 36), in an ordinary progressing labor there is a downside to eliminating pain. When pain is relieved through IV narcotics or an epidural, the biofeedback loop is interrupted. Without pain, the message to produce endorphins and oxytocin is reduced or eliminated. Without oxytocin, labor and dilation slow down or stop. This is why, after an epidural is started, most women receive synthetic oxytocin (Pitocin) by IV to keep the uterus contracting. Having an epidural also means being confined to bed and hooked up to IVs and a fetal monitor.

Investigating the Sensations of Labor

Most women describe cervical dilation during uterine contractions as a sharp sensation just above the pubic bone. Some women also feel pressure or sensations in the groin or back and sometimes in their thighs. The baby's presenting part, usually the head, pressing against a full bladder (in the front) or sacrum (in the back) can increase the intensity. Pain in labor does not come from contracting uterine muscles; you should not feel pain in the upper part of the uterus during labor.

Some women do not feel significant pain in labor. When I was a midwife, a woman told me during a prenatal visit that she was noticing an intermittent "stitch" on one side. Imagine our surprise when I checked her and discovered she was dilated 8 centimeters! But stories like this are not typical, especially for a first birth, and unfortunately, a painless labor is not something that can be manifested by setting an intention, being strong, relaxing, or breathing correctly.

Women have widely different experiences with pain in labor—and with orgasm. In her book *Vagina*, Naomi Wolf describes the complexity and variety of women's pelvic nerve network and how this impacts women's sexual pleasure. While the nerve network of the male pelvic region is about the same for each man, every woman's pelvis nerve map is unique; there are no two women exactly alike. Wolf explains that the most concentrated nerve bundle in women is focused in one of three areas, depending on the woman: inside the vagina, around the clitoris and labia, or through the perineal and anal area.[4]

Could it be that different women experience more pain or intensity in labor because of individual biological variation? Could this explain why some women describe pushing as incredibly painful, while a few others have orgasms (0.3 percent in one study[5])? Perhaps our inborn physiological map has as much of an impact on the experience of labor pain as the birth environment, affirmations, and other planned preparations. The knowledge that the map of nerves within each woman's body is unique and cannot be controlled can take the shame or pride out of our personal experiences of the sensations of labor and birth and our responses to them.

A Softer Memory of Birth

Endorphins have a dramatic impact on how we remember our births. Having given birth with and without drugs, I was fascinated by how drugs affected my memory.

Late into my first labor I was given an epidural in preparation for giving birth by cesarean. The endorphin haze lifted suddenly, as if a curtain had been raised. I became acutely aware of my surroundings; everything around me was in sharp focus again. My memories are still distinct: the clock on the wall, time passing, sterile blue drapes, glaring lights, medical conversations, and the clanging of instruments. Years later, the fear and loneliness associated with those moments remain vivid.

By contrast, memories of my second birth, in which I had no drugs, are more like viewing an impressionistic painting through a veil. Endorphins are nature's gift to us, keeping us "out of our mind" in labor and leaving us with softer memories of birth.

After an epidural, external events seize the foreground of awareness. Without the endorphin haze, memories are shaped and stored in a way that makes them more vivid when retrieved. Part of the trauma of certain labors where pain medication is used is that the woman's experience and memory are clearer.

Kick-Starting Your Endorphins

Exercising and being physical during pregnancy is a healthful way to get into the spirit of being in your body in labor. During pregnancy, try to get thirty minutes of moderate exercise three times a week. You don't need to join a gym or run a marathon; just take a brisk walk, ride a stationary bike, stretch with yoga, swim, or dance or listen to music. Working up a sweat prenatally helps increase your pain threshold. One study showed that pregnant women who exercised three times a week for thirty minutes maintained higher endorphin levels during labor and reported less pain than women who were sedentary during pregnancy.[6] So get your endorphins flowing.

THE POWER OF THE BIRTHPLACE

To understand how the birth environment influences our responses to labor pain, some background in brain wiring may be helpful. The primitive part of the brain (the brain stem)—the part we have in common with other mammals—controls instinctive behavior and regulates automatic responses in the body. The more developed new brain, the part we use to think and plan, can inhibit instinctive, primal activities such as sex and birth.

When the physical environment is clinical, filled with strangers, and requires frequent decision-making, the new brain is engaged, which makes it harder for a woman to turn inward and tune in to her natural rhythms—essential elements of coping with pain and the unknown. A woman can connect more readily with her primitive brain processes and natural coping responses during birth by reducing verbal and visual stimulation in her environment.

Focus on providing privacy, warmth, dim light, water for drinking and bathing, freedom of movement, and a respectful relationship with people attending the birth.

Your ability to cope with the intensity of labor pain may be less influenced by your sensations and more influenced by your birthing environment (the room, temperature, and the attitudes and behavior of those around you). Although your birthing environment is not always within your control—for example, women birthing in a hospital can automatically become part of that "terrain"—do whatever is possible to create a supportive external landscape for your internal landscape, your emotional well-being.

> "Traditionally, above the head of a Zulu woman of South Africa is a hole in the roof of her hut, where, at night, the stars shine through. She tries to focus on this sky; that is why Zulu women say that in labour they are 'counting the stars with the pain.'"
>
> —Caroll Dunham[7]

It's Not Really about the "Pain"

The perception of pain is influenced by expectations, imagination, attitudes, and how you and others talk about it.[8,9]

Hearing horror stories that emphasize the pain and suffering of labor can reinforce fear and dread in pregnant women. Expectations profoundly influence behavior and pain perception,[10] especially when the birth stories are not accompanied by information about how the women coped.

The word *pain* evokes many associations, varying widely from person to person and culture to culture. Many of the women I work with find the word descriptive but neutral, not likely to invoke feelings of dread or fear. Some women prefer using other words to describe the sensations of labor. But eliminating the word *pain* from a pregnant woman's vocabulary and assuming an "out of sight, out of mind" attitude could inadvertently cause her to miss an opportunity to explore her assumptions and cultivate a new mindset.

What we tell ourselves and imagine matters because it focuses our attention on a particular goal. Shifting our awareness away from what we fear toward what we desire can therefore help us achieve goals. Where we put our attention is a form of self-hypnosis. Considering the numerous accounts of people who, using hypnosis, were able to have surgery or give birth without fear or anesthesia, self-hypnosis can be a valuable tool, especially when the attention is focused on "doing" something rather than simply wishing for some outcome. For example, repeatedly visualizing your body opening, or seeing yourself engaging your heart, body, and mind in the process of birthing and coping, is different from repeating positive affirmations or verbalizing only what you want, such as saying, "I will have an uncomplicated, joyous, and pleasurable birth." Repeating such desired intentions can be a tempting "shortcut" to avoid thinking about something scary or to override a habitual pattern of focusing on negative images and thoughts, but consider the risk of putting all your eggs in the "magical" basket: if your hoped-for outcome does not occur, then who is to blame?

More important and effective than repeating a desired intention is awakening your inner Huntress and Birth Warrior. All of Birthing From Within's pain-coping practices and visualizations in this book are designed to help you focus your attention and imagination and to increase your receptivity to a solution-focused mindset.

Mindfulness Practices

Mindfulness practices help focus your attention and eliminate negative mental chatter that leads to emotional suffering. Mindfulness is simply a new routine for the mind to get into.

There are three givens about labor: it's hard work; it hurts a lot; and you can do it! That's the bottom line. All the rest you learn about it is icing on the cake.

—SUZANNE STALLS

Practice Pain Coping

Readers and parents who take our Birthing From Within classes tell us that the best way to learn pain-coping and mindfulness practices is not just to read about them or try them once but to practice them repeatedly in the weeks and months leading up to the birth. Using "ice contractions" to deepen your focus, enhance your resilience, and quiet your mind is an empowering ritual of preparation. Daily meditation lowers stress hormones. As a result, an attitude of mindfulness is gradually absorbed by your subconscious so that later, in labor, when your conscious mind is swept away by the intensity and exhaustion, the habit of mindfulness will be there for you to tap in to.

The intensity of labor is such that no one technique, mantra, or method can promise a pain-free or calm labor. For this reason, Birthing From Within does not advocate "planning" to birth with or without drugs no matter what is happening. In fact, we encourage parents, as Birth Warriors, to commit to doing what needs to be done in the moment. Cultivate this helpful habit by meeting each moment in pregnancy as it arises.

Labyrinth as a Pain-Coping Tool

When I was in active labor, I traced my clay labyrinth over and over while I was in the tub. It kept me calm and helped me concentrate. And now my labyrinth holds special memories for me.

—MICHELE

For centuries people have used the labyrinth as a tool for meditation and problem solving. Walking or tracing a labyrinth balances the activity between the right and left hemispheres of the brain and slows down brain waves, turning the attention inward and inducing a feeling of calmness and well-being.

When we are alert, thinking, and conversing, our brain waves are faster; when they slow down, we worry less about comfort, modesty, or looking good. As a woman shifts from being in the world to being in Laborland, she experiences a wordless, mindless, and egoless immersion—even surrender—into the work of labor.

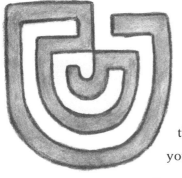

A childbirth yantra in the classic labyrinth form, with the opening at the top, from Rajasthan or Gujurat ca. 1750. To fully appreciate this labyrinth, meditate on it, moving your eyes through it.

To deepen your mindfulness practice of Breath Awareness, hold an ice cube in one hand while tracing a clay labyrinth with the other. Alternatively you could hang your hand-drawn Laborinth on the wall and trace it with your eyes. Doing two things at once takes concentration and helps train your mind to focus in labor.

Practice through seven consecutive 60-second "ice contractions." Give yourself a minute or two of rest between contractions, switching hands each time.

Have your labyrinth drawing or a clay labyrinth ready to use. Before picking up the ice (as well as during rest periods between ice contractions), quiet your mind, focusing on your breathing. This allows you to begin tracing the labyrinth as the contraction starts so you stay in the flow. If you are distracted when the contraction begins, both during practice and in labor, you may not be able to catch up before the contraction peaks.

For more about labyrinths and how to draw your own, see chapter 2.

For this practice, you will need:

- A drawing of a labyrinth or a glazed clay labyrinth
- A bowl of ice cubes and a towel
- Someone to time your "ice contractions" (or a timer set for 1-minute increments)

If you are using the clay laborinth, when the ice contraction begins bring your full attention to your outward breath as you glide your finger along the labyrinth's pathway. It might feel as though your exhalation is propelling you through the labyrinth. When you breathe in, your movement through the labyrinth may continue, slow down, or even stop. There are no rigid rules; do whatever works for you. After you master this practice while holding an ice cube, deepen your concentration by instead immersing your hand in a bowl of ice.

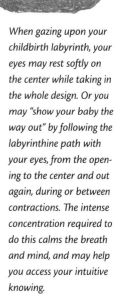

If you are using your labyrinth drawing, hang it so the center is at eye level. Make sure the drawing has fairly even pathways and is large enough to see at a distance without straining.

Midwives in northwest India instruct laboring women to gaze upon their hanging labyrinths by letting their eyes rest softly on the center while taking in the whole design. Mothers can "show their babies the way out" by following the labyrinthine path with their eyes, from the opening to the center and out again (either during or between contractions). The intense concentration required to do this calms the breath and mind, and may help a mother access her intuitive knowing. If she gets lost during a contraction, it doesn't matter; she just picks a point and keeps going.

Remember to take your Laborinth to your birth!

When gazing upon your childbirth labyrinth, your eyes may rest softly on the center while taking in the whole design. Or you may "show your baby the way out" by following the labyrinthine path with your eyes, from the opening to the center and out again, during or between contractions. The intense concentration required to do this calms the breath and mind, and may help you access your intuitive knowing.

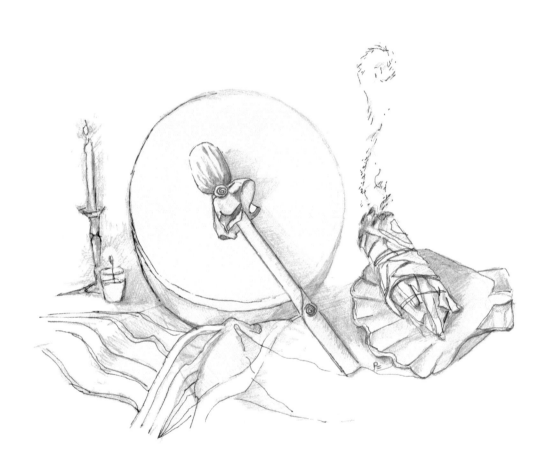

Ceremony and Celebration

Ceremony is at once empty and full. When a potter shapes a clay vessel, it is the empty space within that holds what we want; ceremony carves out a place for us to act out our heart's intention.

Every pregnant woman deserves and needs to be celebrated, to feel loved and special. A birth ceremony is not optional or frivolous; it is a necessity, so mark your prenatal map of preparation with a star for "ceremony." As you prepare for your rite of passage, step out of your busy life and commit to a time and place to be honored by those close to you. A birth ceremony allows you to get in tune with the sacred, renewing relationships with yourself, your baby, your "village," and the archetype of the Great Mother.

The Traditional Baby Shower

Baby showers bring family and community together before a birth; yet these social gatherings are a remnant of more meaningful rituals originally designed to help women prepare for the self-transformation that occurs during birth. Showers are usually baby-focused and materialistic, with an emphasis on presents and games, mirroring the general cultural shift away from honoring the mother and her experience.

One woman, Renata, tells how such an atmosphere at a baby shower made her feel alienated and depressed because it lacked a connection with her transformation to Mother. Like many modern women, Renata yearned for other mothers to recognize and guide her spiritual transition into motherhood. In a birth art session, she made a pastel drawing entitled *Being Pregnant* (figure 19.1) that beautifully depicts a mother's metamorphosis from Maiden to Mother. Yet as she reflected on her recent baby shower she revealed how disappointing it was for her:

> Everybody was generous and happy, but afterward I was terribly depressed. There was a huge pile of baby presents, but not one woman recognized me as a mother. If a baby shower is supposed to get the mother ready, it should be something different. It's not just about babies. There was nothing that connected me with other women—yet mothers know something that other people don't, and they should tell us.

With an eye toward celebrating motherhood as a right of passage, let's explore some deeper ways of honoring the pregnant woman.

Figure 19.1

It looks like an oven, a cave, or an horno (type of oven used by Pueblo Indians to make bread). You go in there alone . . . give birth in there . . . . It's more like an incubation of motherhood than birth. On the other side, you join all the women who have ever done it.

—RENATA

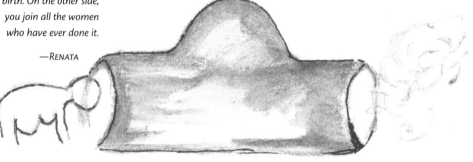

MOTHER BLESSING CEREMONY

All ceremonies symbolically destroy one world to create a new one.
A Mother Blessing Ceremony acknowledges the woman's new status
as mother and helps her say good-bye to the life she is leaving behind.

When friends and family gather for a Mother Blessing Ceremony with a collective intention to honor the pregnant woman as she prepares for birth and motherhood, the mood and experience are very different from those of a baby shower. Many women decide to have both events, choosing to invite only specific people to their Mother Blessing Ceremony. Such a ceremony may be large or small, women-only or not—whatever feels most supportive and meaningful to the mother-to-be.

While each person comes to the ceremony in support and celebration of the pregnant woman or the couple, they also partake in personal preparation, learning, and healing. Therefore, it is helpful to spell out the expectations and purpose of the Mother Blessing Ceremony to all participants in advance. The following suggestions, gleaned from my experiences in leading such ceremonies for mothers and couples, have been culled to help guide you in creating your own wonderful Mother Blessing.

Choosing a Ceremony Leader

A Mother Blessing Ceremony needs a leader to organize and prepare the mother and the guests, carry the vision, build momentum, and maintain cohesiveness. With a timid leader or no leader at all, the ceremony could quickly lose focus. When the boundaries and agreements are not clear and there are "too many cooks in the kitchen," distraction can turn everyone's attention outward instead of inward. Because we don't usually have village elders or storytellers to call on to lead birth ceremonies, it is a good idea to ask someone you trust to help prepare and lead your ceremony. Or perhaps someone will volunteer to plan the event for you. (Every village elder has to begin somewhere!)

Not just anyone can lead a Mother Blessing Ceremony. Choose someone who:

- Knows how to organize and mobilize a group

- Is contemplative, self-aware, and open to the life of spirit

- Has experience participating in or leading ceremonies

Planning the Details

Working with your ceremony leader and a few friends, plan how you want your event to unfold: the time of day, how long the event will last, its location, and so forth. Blending ideas from different people will make for a richer event.

- Choose a theme, structure, flow, and intention.

- Select music and decorations.

- Make a menu (or plan a potluck) for feasting.

- Create a guest list and invitations with information about what to expect, how to prepare, and what to bring (a bead, a blessing, food to share, and so forth).

See the rest of this chapter for more ideas.

Preparing the Mind and Heart

When a Japanese tea master pays attention to every detail associated with preparing and serving tea, he is acting out the intention of a life lived in mindfulness. In a tea ceremony, the attention given to preparing tea is as important as drinking it. Before entering a Japanese tea house, it is customary for guests to walk through the garden to separate themselves from the busy world and to become centered in the moment. Then they rinse their hands in a stone basin under running water, symbolically washing away the outside world.

An important part of preparing for a Mother Blessing Ceremony is to plan personal rituals that will engage the mother's mind and heart. You might make a Warrior Bundle (pages 166–167) and bring it to the Mother Blessing Ceremony, perhaps opening it and sharing it at the event. Other ways to prepare are to take a special bath of renewal before going to the ceremony or to wear special clothing to it.

In Native American culture, ceremonial smudging of the ritual space and the group clears the air and purifies the hearts and minds of those who have gathered. The aromatic smoke from sage, pine, and sweetgrass connects us to spirit and helps us on our spiritual journey. Sage banishes negative energy; sweetgrass calls forth good energy. Other ways to create a ceremonial mood are by lighting candles and incense, using aromatherapy oils, decorating with flowers, face painting, playing music, or drumming.

Opening the Ceremony

Once everyone has arrived, the group enters the circle together, stepping into a world of possibilities, perceptions, and feelings. When you enter ceremonial space, time slows down and the world stops. The heart's gate opens to receptivity, wisdom, and far-seeingness. Observing and participating in a series of shared blessings, actions, and processes entrains everyone who has gathered, strengthening intentions, deepening emotional bonds, and building momentum. Being energized by a loving and supportive group may help each participant suddenly see possibilities they could not see before, opening the way to a new direction.

A Few Ideas for the Ceremony

- Share poetry, prayers, songs, and blessings.

- Give the mother a fragrant, soothing herbal footbath. Float flower petals in the water. Gently dry, massage, and oil the mother's feet.

- Make a blessing bracelet or necklace with beads brought by guests for the mother to wear as a reminder of the support of her circle.

- Bring or make prayer flags and string them together.

"In the warm, womblike waters of the bath, I reconnect with my own potential for change, and my perspective shifts from fixed to fluid. Troubles seem to wash away, and I emerge renewed."

—EILEEN LONDON AND BELINDA RECIO[1]

Incense

"When our ancestors first observed that smoke rises, it came to symbolize the union of heaven and earth, and spirit and matter. As a result, smoke became the vehicle for communication with the spirit world, capable of carrying our prayers to heaven. Burning aromatics is also an ancient way of gaining access to the spirit of plants. . . . Many cultures have long believed that the wisdom and energy in a plant can be released by burning it."

—EILEEN LONDON AND BELINDA RECIO[2]

- Invite a belly dancer to lead a group dance. Belly dancing was originally a birth dance performed by women for a laboring woman, to show her how to move the baby down.

- Create a candle ritual. The oldest way of bringing light to darkness in ceremonial space is through candles. There are many ways to create candle rituals within your ceremony. Each guest can bring a candle or be given one at the ceremony. From a candle burning on an altar, each person can light their candle and offer a silent prayer. Guests can walk a candlelit labyrinth as a group meditation on birth.

- Candles can be blessed and taken home by guests, who will later will be called when the mother goes into labor. Lighting the candle will remind them to send positive energy to the laboring couple and their birth team. Give introductions using the guests' maternal lineage. For example, each person could say, "I am the daughter of [name of mother] and the granddaughter of [name of maternal grandmother] and great-granddaughter of [name of maternal great-grandmother]," as far back as she knows.

- Tell mythic stories to inspire group learning and sharing. Perhaps you can invite someone who can could tell a mythic story about an ancient heroic journey that would entertain and inspire.

- Discourage guests from dishing out medical birth stories in great detail. Instead, recount one moment of a birth journey that was memorable, humbling, loving, or enlightening. From these brief sharings, mothers are gifting something personal to the woman who is about to become part of the lineage of mothers.

- Paint the mother's belly with henna (*mehndi*) or make her a flower crown.

- Document the ceremony for the mother. Line up a photographer (a friend or professional). Have a "scribe" make note of the special things people say, the meaning of the beads, songs, and other things the mother will want to remember.

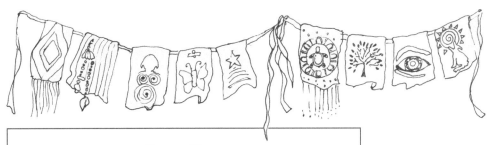

Prayer Flags

For my sixtieth birthday, Birthing From Within Mentors from around the world sent handmade red prayer flags decorated with images symbolizing their prayers and blessings for me. The 170 flags—each one uniquely embroidered, painted, beaded, or quilted—were strung together. They grace my teaching space, showering me with blessings and friendships every day.

Prayer flags can shower the mother and baby with blessings before and during labor. It is easy to transport the flags and hang them in the birthplace during labor. Colorful, handmade prayer flags not only brighten the birthing room but also create focal points for the mother and remind her of the love and support of her community. During her Return, and for a long time to come, these prayer flags continue to send blessings.

Some Mother Blessing Ceremony hosts include flag making as part of the ceremony; others provide the materials and instructions in advance so guests can bring their prayer flags ready made. In this instance, invitations to a Mother Blessing Ceremony could include these simple instructions:

• Cut a paper or cotton cloth rectangle to your preferred dimensions—5 x 8 inches to 9 x 12 inches works well. (Specify the color if there is a color theme.) Fold the top over and glue or sew a seam, leaving an

---

inch-wide sleeve at the top through which a cord or ribbon can pass for stringing the flags together.

- Design a simple drawing or symbol to represent your blessing or prayer.

- Avoid using words like *trust, relax,* or *open.* Instead, be more creative: come up with a symbol, animal, or image to represent your blessing or wish for the mother and baby. Pictures are ambiguous and allow the viewer to contemplate a meaning for them, whereas words or affirmations send a direct message that might not be meaningful or helpful in a given moment.

- Embroider, appliqué, quilt, bead, or paint your design on the flag. (If using fabric paint, keep the fabric taut by tacking the flag to a board.)

- Sign your prayer flag on the back so the mother will always remember you.

Closing the Ceremony

Ending the ceremony in a memorable way that mirrors the opening of the ceremony creates a satisfying sense of symmetry. For example, people can enter the ceremonial space in a clockwise direction and exit in a counterclockwise direction. Or candles can be lit to open the ceremony and blown out to close it. A Mother Blessing Ceremony can be so moving that, after it is over, all participants—not just the mother—return to their lives changed. Postpone socializing, feasting, and gift-giving until after everyone has left the ceremonial space.

The Ceremonial Feast

Celebration is a kind of food we all need in our lives . . .
Each individual brings a special recipe or offering
So that together we make a great feast.

—CORITA KENT AND JAN STEWARD

A ceremony can work up an appetite. So after the ceremony is closed, it's time for a nourishing and bountiful feast to feed the guests, the emerging parents, and the baby everyone is waiting to meet. Put someone in charge of coordinating a potluck or catering, setting the table, and cleaning up.

Make, Bake, and Decorate a Birthin' Mama Cake

Parents get a kick out of specially baked and decorated "birthin' mama" cakes. It's fun to assemble and frost a cake shaped into a birthin' mama in advance, then let everyone decorate it using small tubes of frosting and a variety of small edible treats, such as candy, nuts, and raisins. You can also serve it as a "birth-day" cake with candles. Bread shaped into a birthin' mama can be baked and served with hummus, cream cheese, or peanut butter. Birthin' mama pizzas are fun as well.

BIRTH PARTY

Pregnant women deserve a party to
celebrate what their bodies have done and are about to do.

If a ceremony is too formal for you or your circle, a Birth Party may be a better choice for celebrating the upcoming birth. A Birth Party can be enjoyable as either a surprise or a planned event. You may want it arranged for you so you can be treated as the guest of honor. Or you might prefer to organize your own event and invite friends to come. The event could be just for you or for you and your partner; and it could be for family or your workplace peers, for women only or co-ed.

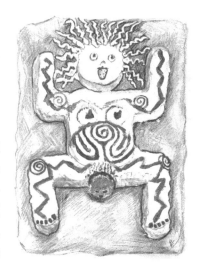

Anything can happen at a Birth Party:

- Beading of necklaces
- Party favors
- Pedicure
- Body painting
- Dancing
- Potluck or a special catered meal
- "Meal train": everyone brings a delicious homemade frozen dish to nourish the new parents after birth, or everyone signs up to bring a meal
- Presents for baby and mother

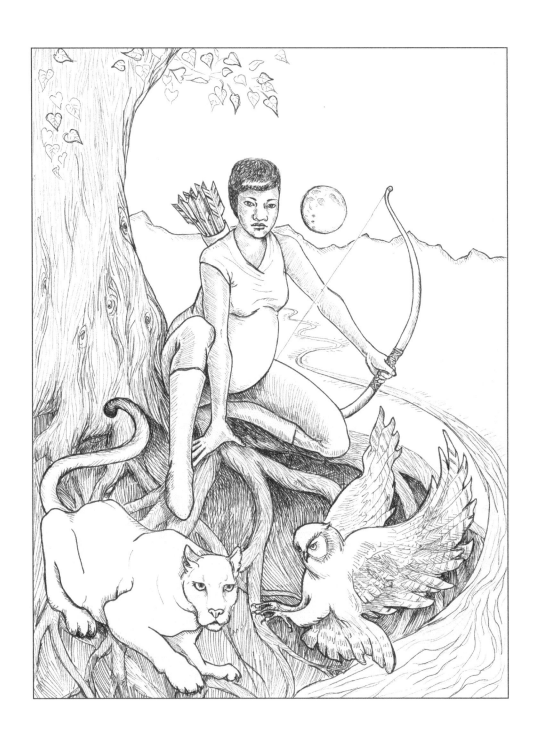

THE HUNTRESS

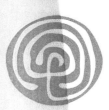

Depending on what you hunger for, you will either gather or hunt. The archetypal Gatherer looks outward, collecting information, research, and the opinions of others. In contrast, the archetypal Huntress looks within, tracking habitual patterns of thinking when seeking change, self-knowledge, and personal freedom.

Gathering external information is an essential Task of Preparation, reinforced by the standardized birth map (see chapter 12); however, for some it can become a time-consuming preoccupation leading to a hoarding of nuts of research and opinion berries in the pursuit of "getting it right." Another part of you, the Huntress, is not satisfied solely by such nuts and berries and is hungry for an internal search for self-knowledge. The Huntress is not hunting something "out there" but instead watching the "habit mind," the ways of thinking that keep you stuck in routines. When you are following this path, you take time for reflection, explore personal motivations and beliefs, access your unconscious mind through art and dreams, and discover new solutions and ideas within.

The Huntress is not awake or active in a child who is still being "fed" by adults, be it food for the body or "food" for deciding what to think and do. As long as the child is comfortable, secure, and being fed by others, she is not "hungry," so there is no Call to go hunting.

To learn how to hunt, the novice Huntress requires the guidance of an experienced hunter. Imagine a hungry, ambitious youth going into the woods with a bow and arrow, eagerly tromping around looking for game; if he doesn't know the habits of his prey, he is likely to scare it off or not know where to look. In the same way, "hungry" pregnant and postpartum women benefit from the wisdom and skills of a mentor, someone who is well-versed in the art of the search for self-knowledge. Consequently, an essential Task of Preparation is finding a mentor who is introspective and familiar with the ancient map of birth, such as a Birthing From Within Childbirth Mentor.

The Huntress

Questions of the Huntress

What is keeping me from following my intuition or taking action?

What do I really need to know?

How do I know to want or avoid _____?

Why is someone else's opinion so important to me?

What am I telling myself it would mean about me, if I chose or did _____?

How would doing _____ be a solution or a problem for me?

Knows what she is hungry for;
    nothing deters her hunt.
Senses and listens to everything
    with her whole body, alert, observing.
Notices small changes early,
    a broken twig, a change of heart.
Patiently tracks her mind, follows her instincts,
    and is willing to change directions.
She is drawn toward beauty,
    aligning her energy with Spirit.

HUNTING GROUND

A Huntress is attentive to everything in her environment. She neither makes up a story to explain away what she senses nor assumes that she already knows what it means. Instead, she registers her observations and listens. During pregnancy a Huntress is tuned in to the shifting landscapes of her body, mind, and emotions, and she is patient enough to stalk, without judging, small changes in herself and in her surroundings.

An ordinary person seeks comfort within the boundaries of

what she already knows. Upon approaching a threshold to the unknown, she may equate the unfamiliar or unexpected with danger, which could lead to complaining, feeling confused, deferring to others, panicking, or retreating to familiar ground. Not so for the Huntress. The Huntress is alert and aware, listening to her intuition and ready to take action at any moment. When she comes to the threshold of the unknown, she is eager to cross it because she knows wisdom and greater perspective lie on the other side. When you are the Huntress, you trust your instincts. When sensing something is not quite right, whether it is with a person, your body, or in the birthplace, you closely examine the situation, changing direction if necessary.

The Huntress speaks her mind firmly and does not strive to be polite or "nice." Conversely, the Nice Girl or Good Patient archetypes—the parts of you that have been taught to be seen and not heard and to dismiss your emotions or concerns—may cause you to passively wait for someone else to act.

Keeping Your Huntress Alert

When your Huntress is alert, instead of passively listening to opinions, rushing to make decisions, or reacting impulsively, you stalk what you are hearing or telling yourself, as well as subtle messages from your body—during prenatal visits, childbirth classes, while reading about birth, or when hearing birth stories. For example, while taking a hospital tour, some first-time parents are in awe of the aesthetics of the birthing room, or how the bed breaks down, or how nice the nurse is; they are only gathering details and forming opinions or strategies. They tell each other: "The ____ freaked me out" or "I loved the _____." But a Huntress notices the feeling in her body when learning about protocol and touring the rooms; she is curious about why she feels safe or guarded or disappointed. Rather than just accept or ignore her initial responses of satisfaction or fear, she looks within, asking herself: "Where

Faux Hunting

Don't fool yourself. Know the difference between pretending you are "fine" versus actually doing change work. One clue: truly tracking to its source a belief or story that is keeping you stuck in habitual behavior requires discipline, effort, and patience.

Sustenance for Your Huntress

- Your heart's question
- Your first birth story
- A Birth Tiger Safari
- Non-focused awareness
- Meditation

does this feeling come from? What do I need to know or do next?" Hunting takes practice and hunger for self-awareness. Always be on the lookout for tasty morsels that sharpen your senses and keep your inner Huntress alert and active.

Non-Focused Awareness

Japanese Samurai call quiet mind "mushin" (pronounced MOO-shin). This is a mind that, like a still pool of water, reflects the immediate surroundings without distortion, an observing mind with no plan, no preference, no fear or wanting. We call this this mindfulness practice, which is particularly suited for pregnancy and birth, Non-Focused Awareness.

In our busy world, without training and devotion to daily practice we don't know how to achieve or sustain *mushin*. But Japanese Samurai warriors practiced achieving and sustaining *mushin* as part of their preparation for battle, giving them unwavering mental focus to perform without fear, without being distracted, and without thinking or judging. Being acutely present, aware of everything yet not distracted by anything, was a matter of life and death.

Mushin is like a sword cutting through distractions.

Although it is not likely you will encounter a sword-wielding warrior during your childbearing year, you still have to prepare for a kind of battle: to be in quiet mind amid the modern distractions of traffic, the Internet and social media, opinions and advice, being overscheduled, and multitasking. In this practice you are observing what you are seeing, hearing, and touching—without interpreting the sensation; labeling anything as "positive," "negative," "annoying," or "soothing"; or telling yourself a story about what it means.

Resisting an unwanted situation, or whining, judging, or complaining about it, is exhausting, counterproductive, and weakens resolve. Non-Focused Awareness (NFA) provides a more helpful response to changing conditions during labor.

The Huntress knows that you can't always control your environment but you can change the story you are telling yourself in the moment. Everything arising in your birthplace is a part of the birth, whether chosen or wanted—or not. When you are a Huntress, you are ready to harness the power of whatever is in your surroundings, including the unexpected, to aid your journey instead of feeling hindered by such potential obstacles.

> "I planned a homebirth so that I could birth in a relaxed and familiar environment. Yet on the day I went into labor there was road work right outside: jackhammers, people shouting, trucks coming and going. I was angry and felt powerless. How dare they ruin my birth!"
>
> — ELLIE

Practicing Non-Focused Awareness

Practicing Non-Focused Awareness during pregnancy helps you prepare for labor. Practicing it in labor helps you maintain mental focus during contractions, deepen rest between contractions, and utilize distractions to enhance concentration and quiet mind.

In your practice of Non-Focused Awareness, you are equally aware of all sensations—light and shadow, sounds, the words spoken, touch, the soles of your feet on the floor—but do not focus attention on any one sensory experience. And you are in touch with how all these sensations are not fixed but are appearing and disappearing. You may also notice nausea, exhaustion, thirst, shaking, and contractions appearing and disappearing.

Expanding your awareness without judgment or preference means that you do not become fixated on one sensation. So instead of trying to avoid a particular sensation,

Download live teaching of NFA

Listen to the audio teaching and guided practice. Practice NFA daily as you go about your ordinary activities. Challenge yourself to a longer session with "ice-contractions" at least once a week. At first you may be able to maintain a "mind like still water" only briefly, but with practice you will enjoy longer and longer periods of quiet mind.

such as pain or exhaustion, or assessing your experience as positive or negative, you experience any given moment in its wholeness.

In labor, resisting what is and wishing it were different can take energy and focus away from the task of birthing your baby—one that will require every bit of attention and energy you can summon. Non-Focused Awareness is a tried and true practice for increasing stamina and a positive outlook in labor.

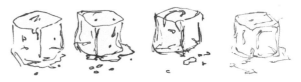

Seeing

Hearing

Touching

Breathing

Although a calm birth environment is preferable, when practicing Non-Focused Awareness you don't need a specific environment; in fact, distractions around you can help deepen your mental focus. If in labor something is annoying or distracting you, when you get through a contraction you can be assertive and instruct, "Turn off the lights" or "Stop talking," and with the next breath continue with your practice of Non-Focused Awareness.

The more you practice Non-Focused Awareness before labor, the more likely it is that you will be able to practice it when you are in Laborland. Practicing it daily during pregnancy will also help you, in general, cope with physical discomforts, unwanted advice, and other distractions.

ⓢ

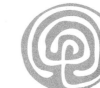

Worry Is the Work of Pregancy

Many new mothers are surprised that they didn't feel prepared for birth; they express deep regret that they didn't acknowledge or listen to feelings of doubt or fear during pregnancy, instead dismissing them with positivity, denial, or obsessive information-gathering. Yet worry is part and parcel of experiencing a rite of passage. Worry is a kind of curiosity, wondering about what might happen and how you could respond. Worry can help you use your imagination and creativity to awaken hidden sources of courage and power within you.

Years ago, Dr. Lewis Mehl Madrona made a lasting impression on me when he said, "Worry is the work of pregnancy." Women all over the world have always worried about labor pain, the health of their baby, and dying in labor. Modern women have new things to worry about: whether a doctor or midwife they trust will be on call when they are in labor; if they will be given balanced information; if they will be separated from their baby; losing control; if they'll feel coerced into interventions or cesarean if their labor takes too long; and so forth. Couples worry about the cost of health care and changes in their income, relationships, and child care.

Especially during a first pregnancy, it is normal for women to worry about both big and little things. However, many mothers try to sidestep worrying, wanting to remain hopeful and trusting. Not everyone thinks that worry is an essential or normal part of pregnancy. Some people believe that talking about worries will make them happen. They tell pregnant women, "Don't worry; just trust birth. Your body is made to give birth. Women are strong!" Such advice is commonly given even when intervention rates are soaring. Wanting to appear relaxed, confident, trusting, and motivated to birth normally, some pregnant women try to follow this advice by ignoring their worries or by trying to convince themselves that if they trust enough all will turn out well. This strategy, however, offers little motivation to prepare to cope with all kinds of labor experiences.

Both the impulses to worry about birth and to try to gloss over concerns are common, and when they are present at the same time an inner conflict of opposing beliefs, both of which have an element of truth, cause women to feel stuck and indecisive. The task of the innocent under-worrier is to "get real" and face the immense changes that an initiation through birth will bring. The task of the over-worrier is to explore her concerns realistically and find ways to calm her mind and nervous system.

"Worry is a way to pretend that you have knowledge or control over what you don't—and it surprises me, even in myself, how much we prefer ugly scenarios to the pure unknown. Perhaps fantasy is what you fill up maps with rather than saying that they too contain the unknown."

—REBECCA SOLNIT[1]

When a woman focuses on the worst possible outcome, she either worries obsessively, to the point of gathering excessive amounts of information, or is immobilized by fear or dread. In either case, she may become dependent on others or technology to avert or manage the problem. The problem is not worry but rather the absence of a solution-focused outlook that includes a plan for what she can do to cope with the unwished for situation should it actually happen.

Worrying is not a sign of weakness,
nor does it weaken resolve.

A BIRTH WARRIOR WORRIES EFFECTIVELY

A Birth Warrior who prepares to face the unknown naturally worries, but worries effectively. When worry is accepted as an essential Task of Preparation, images of not coping can be transformed into images of taking action. To understand how this occurs, first acknowledge that the outcome you worry about could actually happen. Then imagine one small thing you could do to help yourself cope if it did happen. In the long run, doing that one small thing may serve you better than doing nothing, hoping it won't happen, or expecting someone else to save you or fix it.

Each Guatemalan worry doll takes on a worry of its own.

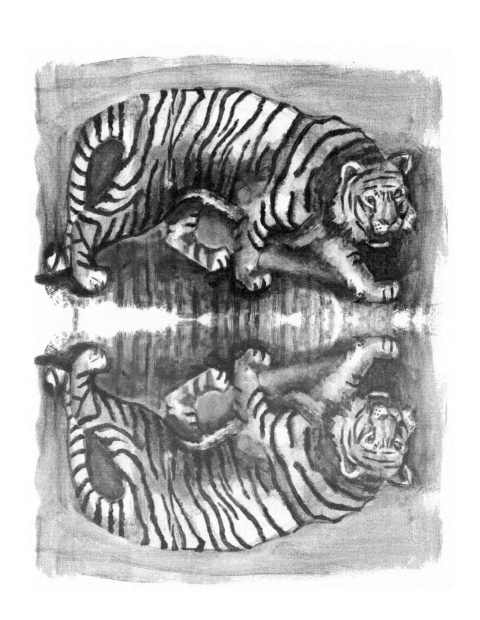

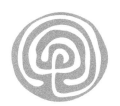

Birth Tiger Safari

Many ancient maps depict dragons and other strange creatures; one contains the phrase "Hic sunt dracones" ("Here be dragons"). Dragons represented the unknown, a territory not yet traveled. A true adventurer might wonder about such uncharted territory, make an effort to find out what surprises lie ahead, and plan ways to prepare for them. You may already be seeing wild beasts hiding in the corners of your map of birth and in your mind. One of Birthing From Within's most loved processes—Birth Tiger Safari—guides you to examine and change your perception of and relationship to things you are hoping to avoid.

In myths, dreams, and art, animals convey both universal and personal meanings. The tigress represents the fierce huntress, protective mother, courage, and nobility. Coming face-to-face with any tiger, whether it's a Bengal tiger or a metaphorical Birth Tiger, is something we instinctively try to avoid. Moving beyond avoidance and fear takes courage and effort, qualities that your Huntress has in spades.

Examples of Birth Tigers

A really long labor

Being transferred to a hospital from a home birth

Laboring so fast I birth at home

Episiotomy

Laboring while my partner is out of town

Being too tired to cope or finish

Being separated from my baby

Induction

Cesarean

Not being listened to or respected

Losing control of my plan

What Is a Birth Tiger?

A Birth Tiger represents any unwanted event, situation, or medical intervention you would like to avoid. These often begin as "kittens"—fleeting concerns—which then grow into bigger worries that anxiously pace back and forth in your mind, distracting you from peace of mind during pregnancy.

In the same way that bears inhabit some national parks, Birth Tigers inhabit the modern prenatal inner landscape. Knowing that you can't predict or control what a bear might do, you can try to avoid an encounter by staying in your car or passing up national parks altogether. Or you can learn what to do to increase your likelihood of survival should a bear cross your path; then, when you arrive at the park, get out of your car and enjoy a hike and the beautiful views. An essential Task of Pregnancy is learning and planning constructive responses to your Birth Tiger.

What's *Your* Birth Tiger?

Is there a topic, intervention, or outcome that you:

Hope won't happen? Try hard not to think about? Research obsessively? Intentionally avoid reading about? Try to control?

If so, that is your Birth Tiger.

Two Ways Birth Tigers Are Problematic

Physiological Stress

Since the brain cannot distinguish between real and imagined images of danger,[1] a vivid mental picture of something threatening your well-being triggers a neurohormonal response. Within milliseconds of perceiving an actual or imagined threat, the brain and autonomic nervous system turn on a survival mechanism that is forty thousand years old, engaging an intricate hormonal symphony of thirty stress hormones that produce

1,400 different physiological and biochemical changes in the body.[2] This brief physiological reaction—called the fight, flight, or freeze response—makes you feel alert, aggressive, strong, and able to take action, including potentially performing super-human feats. It is a healthy stress response designed to be short-term, allowing stress hormones to return to baseline levels once the threat has passed.

However, in a pregnant woman elevated stress hormones can't return to baseline when a Birth Tiger is continually pacing back and forth in her mind and she cannot envision a solution or see herself coping with the imagined event. When stress hormones remain high for long periods of time, her appetite, self-care, ability to sleep, and overall health and well-being are negatively affected. In a state of dread, hypervigilance, and self-protection, the pregnant woman is guarded and tense at a time she should be preparing to open and release.

Psychological Stress

Imagine a Birth Tiger pacing back and forth in your mind as you search for ways to avoid or control it. What you truly fear or are trying to avoid is not so much the event itself but rather the personal meaning you give it. A Birth Tiger has power over you because of the negative beliefs that you link to it. Your confidence, peace of mind, decision-making ability, and sense of well-being are directly influenced by the beliefs that you and others hold about various birth-related scenarios. For this reason, it is important to acknowledge, explore, and change what you are telling yourself *about yourself*. A sense of relief and genuine positivity follows from envisioning a broader range of possibilities.

There are two (mutually exclusive) strategies for dealing with Birth Tigers: ignoring them or going on a Birth Tiger Safari

WHY PEOPLE DON'T FACE THEIR BIRTH TIGERS

There are lots of reasons pregnant women and those around them ignore birth-related fears or worries. Some people believe that talking or reading about the situation they hope won't happen will plant a seed in their mind and that the power of the mind is so strong their thoughts will create the reality; on the other hand, people who set aside their concerns instead of addressing them create a reality of powerlessness, inhibiting their ability to respond in helpful ways. For still other people, admitting to a concern or fear about an imagined situation is a sign of weakness or lack of trust or faith, so they minimize their concern and wear a mask of bravery.

For most individuals, dismissing a concern is a way to suppress feelings of fear, powerlessness, shame, or uncertainty associated with an imagined situation. It is uncomfortable—even painful—to imagine not knowing what to do, feeling like a failure, or being judged. So the response is to try to not think about it, or think positively. But this does not make us more powerful or less afraid of a Birth Tiger. Moreover, trying to deny or avoid a Birth Tiger does not bypass the stress response but instead gives the Birth Tiger more power over you. In the presence of a wild tiger, nobody would pretend that there was no tiger or utilize a "think positive" strategy and forge ahead with their plan. So Birth Warriors look forward to going on a Birth Tiger Safari to tame their fears.

Birth Tiger Safari

1. Start by identifying your Birth Tiger—one situation related to pregnancy, birth, or the first week postpartum that you are hoping won't happen. The situation could be one that poses a potential threat to your own or your baby's physical well-being or survival, or it could be one that threatens your self-esteem or your sense of worthiness or belonging. To name your Birth Tiger, tune in to sensations in your body, sinking feelings, stress responses, or strategies of avoidance. Be specific.

2. Invoke your Huntress to track your Birth Tiger. Since this Birth Tiger is in your imagination, begin noticing your thoughts, visions, and feelings when you consider this unwanted possibility: Are you afraid, immobilized, helpless, freaking out, resistant, or trying to find ways to avoid it?

3. Next, get in touch with how it would be a problem for you if this unwanted situation happens: What negative self-belief is linked to the imagined scenario? What are telling yourself it would mean about you, such as believing you are weak, powerless, unworthy, a failure, or a bad mother?

4. Now imagine entering the scene as a Birth Warrior who doesn't judge herself or others because such a scenario is happening but instead abides in her heart and responds one moment at a time. (Keep in mind that Birth Warriors are not magicians who can instantly make the problem vanish.) Keep the undesired event in mind, but pay attention to what changes when your Birth Warrior takes over. Notice how differently you feel in your body, breath, and posture when the Birth Warrior responds.

5. Be aware of how the story you are telling yourself about yourself has changed. What more helpful, true, or positive self-belief can you hold when you imagine coping with this unwanted situation? For example, "Even when _____ is happening, I am doing my best" or "I am a good mother" or "I am present to myself and my baby" or "I have an inner strength."

6. Journal about what changed, how you now see yourself coping in this situation, and what your new more positive self-belief is. Capture your new knowing in a drawing or painting to further impress the positive image on your mind and heart.

An Ambush of Tigers

A tiger in the wild is a solitary animal. For a Birth Tiger Safari to be effective in changing your outlook, you will therefore need to select one particular "tiger." A man-made environment, on the other hand, may force tigers into a group, called an "ambush." Worrying about having a cesarean is equivalent to dealing with an ambush of metaphorical Birth Tigers—a group of unwished-for moments such as hearing that you need a cesarean, being strapped to the operating table, and having your baby taken away. For a Birth Tiger Safari to be effective in dealing with fears of a cesarean, just one of those unwished-for moments must be chosen at a time.

> ### What Birth Warriors have done:
>
> "I asked for a second opinion."
>
> "I focused on my breath for a minute."
>
> "I imagined my baby inside me, safe and sound."
>
> "I looked into my husband's eyes, knowing I was loved."
>
> "I asked for an epidural."
>
> "I got up and changed positions."
>
> "When I felt exhausted, I lay down on my side, closed my eyes, and just rested for a few minutes."
>
> "I reminded myself that I could push just five more times."
>
> "I told my mom to leave the birth room."
>
> "I shut myself in the bathroom, alone."
>
> "I noticed my jaw was clenched and tried to release it."

HUNTING SELF-LOVE

To fully embrace all possible outcomes, you must first truly embrace yourself.

The Birth Tiger Safari is not another birth plan. The rigors of labor can overwhelm even the most prepared and confident parents. The exhaustion, pain, and ongoing uncertainty mean that nothing about birth is predictable. Be gentle with yourself; do not use the solutions imagined in your Birth Tiger Safari against yourself should you later find yourself not able to respond in exactly the way you hoped or imagined. Letting go of attachment to specific ideas or solutions (no matter how rational they may seem now) is an ongoing task of the Birth Warrior. Commit to simply doing your best in each moment.

STALKING A BIRTH TIGER IN LABORLAND

In the modern birthplace, when imagination and emotions are at play we may be tempted to take drastic measures to ensure safety even before we know for certain whether a Birth Tiger is real or imagined. This is partly because imagining and fearing a Birth Tiger can instantly produce a rush of adrenaline, neutralizing the effect of oxytocin, the hormone that stimulates uterine contractions. Without regular surges of oxytocin, labor contractions would slow down or stop, not resuming until the real or imagined tiger was gone.

A story about someone who reported seeing a white tiger in a field in Southampton, England, illustrates how people can react to an imagined tiger as they would a real one. Officers were sent to the scene; a helicopter with thermal imaging cameras circled above; a nearby cricket game was stopped; and golfers were told to go indoors. Contingency plans were put in place to close the motorway while animal experts at the zoo prepared to send a team with tranquilizer darts to overcome the tiger. Meanwhile, in the field, police stalked the tiger, which was sitting very still. Just then a gust of wind rolled the tiger over. It was merely a life-size stuffed toy tiger.[3] In the face of uncertainty, the police had to respond as if it were a real tiger. Similarly parents and birth attendants may, in the face of uncertainty during pregnancy or birth, overreact when perhaps watchful waiting would be wiser.

If you like, download and listen to the guided Birth Tiger Safari visualization.

So remember: before raising the alarm, take time to stalk your Birth Tiger. First, use all your senses and resources to determine whether it is real or imagined. If there is no urgent need to act, wait and see what happens. Maybe a timely "gust of wind" will tell what you need to do next.

HOW TO TAME A LABOR TIGER

Sometimes watchful waiting is not the appropriate response. If fear is magnified, it can become a problem in labor when the mother is overwhelmed by exhaustion and pain, a series of unexpected events, or an intervention that she was not prepared for or does not understand. When she is fearful or freaking out, true courage and creativity can make all the difference. Here are some ideas for taking action:

- Turn out the lights, enforce privacy, and keep the mother warm.

- Take time to regroup and refocus.

- Guide her compassionately through the Gates of Doubt and Holy Terror.

- Slow things down when she feels pressured or the situation seems urgent. A one-minute explanation about what is happening, or what needs to happen next, can be extremely calming, especially if the mother is very worried about her baby or prone to catastrophic thinking.

As a child, my son Lucien heard me lead the Birth Tiger Safari process many times. He drew this image when he was about nine years old.

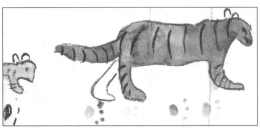

A word to the wise: Don't misuse the tiger metaphor or simplify the complex physiology of fear by presuming that all fear will stop a labor in its tracks, by blaming the mother for having a Birth Tiger, or by making a rule to always act or always wait. Tigers—fear and uncertainty—are integral to the inner landscape of a rite of passage. It is a natural and spiritual part of birth for the mother to cross thresholds of the Gates of Doubt and Holy Terror; it is neither a failure nor something that always needs to be fixed.

Drawing on Your Animal Nature

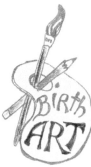

What qualities do you want to develop and embody as a mother? As a Huntress? Which animal or animals come to mind? Choose one that brings those qualities alive in you. Drawing or sculpting the animal helps you imagine and embody the qualities you want to develop. This image can be part of your Warrior Bundle or altar.

You might need to research animals as mothers—perhaps watching videos of mother animals with their offspring on YouTube—to learn about their unique qualities and habits. For example, elephants have the longest pregnancy (twenty-two months). Crocodiles are surprisingly gentle as they carry their young in their mouths. Gorillas carry their babies on their backs, nurse for three to four years, and share their nest for six years.[4]

Some Animals That May Invoke Desired Qualities in You

Nocturnal: Big cat (lioness, tiger, jaguar, cougar), owl

Courage, protectiveness: Big cat, bear

Endurance: Horse, polar bear

Perseverance, hard work: Llama, ant, salmon

Strength, communication: Elephant

Social, herd- or pack-like: Horse, buffalo, otter, wolf, elephant

Far-seeing: Bird of prey

Deep-hearing: Owl, whale

Instinctive: Wolf

Trickster: Coyote

Playful, joyous: Otter, dolphin

Team player: Bee, ant

Determination, groundedness: Turtle

Deep-diving: Dolphin, sea turtle

Nurturing, maternal: Gorilla, cheetah

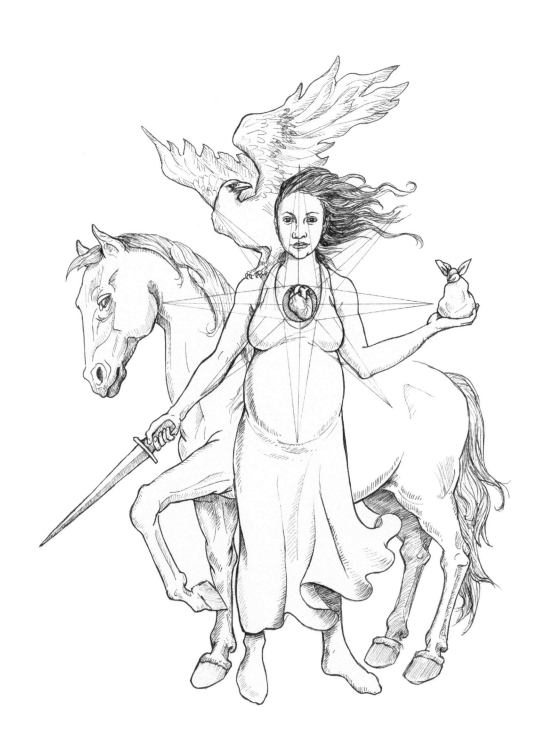

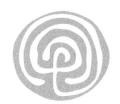

THE BIRTH WARRIOR

No one is born a warrior. A warrior begins her journey as an ordinary person in search of knowledge, clarity, power, pride, or a certain kind of experience.

Some people assume that a Birth Warrior is a woman who shows no fear, experiences no pain, or is victorious in achieving the birth of her dreams. Nothing could be further from the truth: a Birth Warrior does not have to be exceptionally brave, experience no pain, or have an ecstatic or perfect birth. The following is an introduction to qualities of the Birth Warrior so you recognize her when you meet her within.

When you wholeheartedly do what needs to be done without being attached to any particular outcome, including gaining approval, you are the Birth Warrior. When encountering surprises in labor, you continue to do your best without judging the situation or yourself for being in it, even if you don't know quite how to proceed. Doing your best means understanding that your responses are based on a thousand factors (known and unknown). Everything you have lived and learned flows into each moment. It also means taking into consideration that illness, pain, fear, and other people will affect how you respond, and that this is unpredictable and changes from moment to moment.

When arriving at the threshold to the unknown, fear or habits make it tempting to retreat to familiar territory or stick to a plan to avoid terra incognita. When facing uncertainty, it takes courage, support, and creativity to step up and be a Birth Warrior.

Of all the expressions of the Warrior archetype, abiding in self-love and self-respect during your preparation, in the midst of hardship, and on your Return is the most important. In contrast to Hollywood's image of a warrior being a lone crusader, a true archetypal Warrior strives for interdependence; this means that she is self-reliant but can ask others for help, and does not abandon herself while hoping others will show up to support her. Because of our conditioning to be self-critical and to seek approval from others, doing this requires discipline and mental focus.

When you embody the Birth Warrior, you are:

War or Peace?

The word *war* as part of the word *warrior* dates back to ancient times when a warrior led a disciplined life of self-mastery and adhered to a way of being in the world that was beyond what ordinary people could manage. By the same token, today's spiritual warrior does not seek war or conflict.

In beginner's mind, perceiving the familiar as unfamiliar and unknown.[1]

Awake and receptive, gathering information from within and all around you.

Far-seeing, neither focusing on the problem nor being attached to any one possibility or solution.

Decisive and deliberate, knowing every act counts; not overthinking a decision.

Spontaneous, wholeheartedly doing what needs to be done, and nothing extra.[2]

THE BATTLEFIELD

The battlefield becomes the sacred space in which the initiate is tested and where she can prove herself and achieve transformation.

It is not possible for a Warrior to reign calmly on her throne during an initiation, maintaining perfect composure, peace of mind, and confidence. Because birth is a rite of passage, there has to be a struggle between the childlike parts of you and the emerging, more mature parts of you; this struggle is a spiritual battle that calls you to get down and dirty, plunging into doubt, fear, and pain.

Even when, on the surface, the battle seems to be in the birthplace, you must realize that it is an internal battle. The battlefield is where the Child and the Warrior meet within your own mind as you accept the ongoing challenge to transcend your habitual patterns of thought and behavior, such as being passive, not speaking up, pleasing others, or rebelling. The Warrior within you does not fight just to be right or to get her way; nor does she retreat from conflict such as with rigid protocols or her partner wanting a different birthplace. The Birth Warrior requires you to be utterly present in the moment, to choose self-love over self-judgment, to decide rather than defer, and to respond to what is versus clinging to what could have been. Your battle may be learning to surrender without ever giving up.

BIRTH WARRIOR TASKS

You invoke and strengthen the Warrior through any practice that trains your mind to focus, your eyes to see, and your body to be responsive. Here are five ways to prepare to give birth as a Warrior.

1. Practice self-love.

    Be gentle with yourself. This means not judging yourself. When you notice you are being hard on yourself, take a moment to listen to the inner critic telling you that you aren't good enough and that you should try harder or be different in some way. Cultivate a compassionate response to your inner critic. Loving and accepting yourself means that you can look in the mirror daily and say, "I'm good enough, I'm smart enough, and doggone it, I like me!"[3]

2. Do your best.

    In any given moment, do your best. Do what needs to be done next wholeheartedly, without attachment to outcome and without seeking approval. When second-guessing yourself: stop. When matching expectations against reality: stop. Instead of regretting "not doing it right," embrace the you who now knows.

3. Practice *not* doing.

Choose a routine that has become habitual and comfortable rather than necessary, and practice not doing it, without planning to do something else instead. It could be your routine of reading the news, feeding your sweet tooth, or surfing the web. In the emptiness that follows not doing what you ordinarily would do, be receptive to what is happening around you and within you. Notice what you do when you don't know what to do.

4. Be decisive.

If you are not usually decisive, find opportunities in your daily life to strengthen this power so it is more accessible to you in labor and as a mother. Start by making decisions that do not have significant consequences. When something needs to be done, instead of procrastinating make a plan and take action. For example, if you are contemplating taking a childbirth class do research, choose one, and book it. Or if something about your birth partners or birthplace is bothering you, examine the situation and your options then take action, such as communicating your concerns, finding a mutually workable solution, or changing a relationship.

5. Embrace interdependence.

If you tend to be fiercely independent one of your Tasks of Preparation is to cultivate the ability to ask for and accept support from others. If you tend to depend on others for advice or problem-solving, practice being your own counsel.

Make a Birth Warrior Bundle

A Warrior Bundle is not something that can be bought or assembled by someone else and given to you. To make one, you must gather objects that represent characteristics of the Warrior you want to embody now and in labor. When your bundle is open, it becomes an altar for meditation. When you want to keep your bundle under wraps for privacy or to carry it, tie the ends.

Here's what you'll need to gather and do:

The making of a Warrior Bundle is a personal ritual and meditation, so it's best to work in solitude as you gather your objects. Collect or make three to five objects that remind you of Warrior characteristics you want to embody. These can be made from such materials as clay, cloth, or paper. If you buy one ready-made, add something to it to imbue it with your intention and energy; for example, paint it, tie a ribbon around it, or glue a feather or bead on it.

In her visualization to awaken her Birth Warrior, Maggie saw the intensity of labor as a brick wall and herself breaking through it with fierce determination. For her Warrior Bundle, she made a little clay brick to remind her of her determination.

After gathering your symbols, choose a piece of cloth that is large enough to hold them all. The cloth can be any fabric or color; it can be a family heirloom or something new. On the inside surface of the cloth, draw, paint, embroider, quilt, or transfer an iron-on image of a mandala, a labyrinth, or your inner map through birth. With every stitch or step, send a prayer or affirm your determination to do what needs to be done next on your journey as a way of imbuing your bundle with your intentions.

When the cloth is prepared, arrange your chosen symbols on it. Meditate on each symbol. You may want to keep your Warrior Bundle private or share it with special people in your life. Later when you need inspiration, especially in labor, you can meditate as you hold one of the objects in your hand.

A few weeks after your baby is born, in a Return Ceremony of release and gratitude you can bury or burn your Birth Warrior Bundle. Or you may want to save it to give to your child when he is preparing to become a parent.

⑥

THE REWARDS OF EMBRACING
THE UNEXPECTED

Just as Inanna, the warrior queen, makes her descent into the underworld, a woman's descent into Laborland is about embracing the unexpected because what unfolds in labor is rarely what she expected or planned. The Birth Warrior is courageous and does what needs to be done—even when it's something she thought she never would (or could) do. Ultimately, a Birth Warrior knows that she did her best; regardless of how the birth unfolds, she comes out of the labyrinth with a deep sense of empowerment.

The Birth Warrior's quest involves sacrifice and loss of control—the price for personal power and knowledge.

MONKEY TRAP

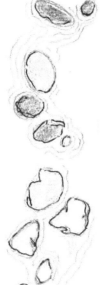

In his book *Fate and Destiny*, Michael Meade describes a monkey trap used in ancient India. Hunters carved a small hole in the bottom of a hollowed-out coconut, just big enough for a monkey's hand to pass through, placed a delicious fruit inside, then pinned the coconut to the ground. When a monkey caught a whiff of the fruit, he would reach inside the coconut to grab it. With his fist wrapped around the coveted prize, the monkey could not pull it back out through the hole. If the monkey would only let go of the fruit he would be free.[4]

It is the nature of the mind to fixate on the first appealing idea or desire, which then becomes the sole idea or desire. Birth attendants can get caught in a monkey trap when they rely on routine protocol. Pregnant women can get trapped by their birth plan.

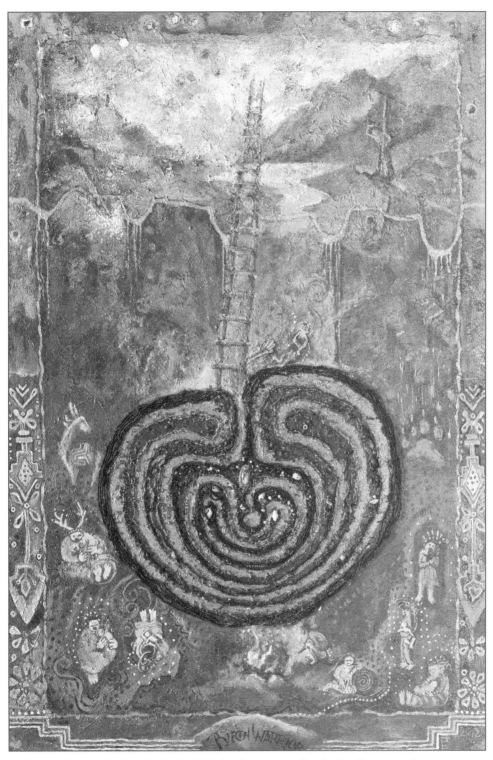

Pam England, Mexican Labyrinth of Birth © 2012, acrylic/mixed media on Masonite.

THE BIRTH PLAN OF A WARRIOR

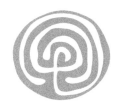

There is a real possibility that birth plans only offer an illusion of control and do not change the course of birth in any real way. Invoke your Birth Warrior to understand what is motivating you to write a birth plan and what is really important to you.

If you are going to write a birth plan, the first step in the process is not researching options, asking others what to do, or filling out a form. The first step is to begin within: if you don't want the frightened or defensive part of you to do this task, consciously invoke your thoughtful Birth Warrior to understand what is motivating you to write a birth plan and what is really important to you. When a woman writes her birth plan with feelings of powerlessness, fear, vulnerability, or distrust, there is a risk that instead of emerging from birth feeling empowered, she may emerge with her deepest fears of being unheard, powerless, alone, and trapped reinforced.

A Birth Warrior knows that she cannot control the attitudes, assumptions, or actions of others with a piece of paper listing her preferences. She knows the importance of building rapport and maintaining relationships with others through direct and respectful communication. When there is a difference of opinion, she does not take it personally. She knows when to stand her ground and when to yield. So if a Birth Warrior writes a birth plan at all, it will not be a wish list of everything she wants. Rather, her birth plan will be firm, concise, matter-of-fact, and polite.

When your Birth Warrior becomes the author of your birth plan, notice how the feelings in your body and the message you are writing change.

⊚

Fifteen or twenty years ago, writing a birth plan was a subversive act. That little piece of paper was symbolic of a couple's determination to have some say in the "management" of their labor and birth.

—KELLI WAY

After a new idea is absorbed into mainstream culture and becomes familiar, it loses some of its original passion and purpose. This may be what is happening to the once thoughtful and time-consuming process of researching and writing a personal birth plan. Today some pregnant women receive a birth preferences form from their birth attendant, while others find standardized birth plan templates online. It has become a routine task that entails very little thought, learning, or personal reflection; simply scroll down the list of choices and check boxes as if ordering from a sushi menu. It's easy to check a box without being aware of what is influencing your choice. Is it your imagination, feelings, intuition, or knowledge?

Out of curiosity, I attempted to enter into "beginner's mind" as if I were a first-time parent filling out a birth plan online. I found hundreds of websites and forms from which to choose, as well as a few apps. Just deciding where to start was stressful. After settling on one, scrolling through and selecting options was simple but tedious. What began as an adventurous act of autonomy ended as an exercise in anxiety. By the time I was ready to click "Print My Birth Plan," my mind was filled with images of all the things I didn't want and strategies for avoiding them. What irony! Later I told a friend, "I took a couple of birth plan tests online today." "Tests?" she asked. Why did I say *tests*? On some level, checking boxes and trying to make all the "right" choices made it feel like I was taking a multiple-choice exam. Women have told me that after completing their online birth plans they felt their work of preparation was done but later discovered they hadn't learned or prepared enough for the possibility of unexpected events.

WHO IS WRITING THE BIRTH PLAN? WHO IS READING IT?

Birth plans typically look about the same. Most women ask for respect, minimal disruption or intervention, and to have a say in their care. The difference that matters most is what motivates each woman to write her birth plan—or opt not to write one.

To understand your motivation for writing a birth plan, ask yourself: Which part of me is writing the birth plan? Is it the "health consumer" collecting information and writing a wish list, hoping to get the right outcome and avoid the wrong one? Is it the "good patient," or the "control freak" part of me that is afraid of not being heard?

One the other hand, if you are not inclined to write a birth plan, perhaps you are a woman who doesn't "plan," or maybe not asking for what you want is a way to avoid getting your hopes up or being disappointed. You may say, "I just want to go with the flow." To understand your motivation for not doing so, ask yourself: Who is *not* writing a birth plan? What is motivating me not to write a plan? Is not setting intentions, goals, or tuning in to what is important to me a manifestation of the Innocent? The Innocent strives to stay positive at all times and trusts that it will all work out. However, this is not a wise course of action when birth in our culture is so complex. Refusal to become aware of your own needs, or to learn about hospital protocols, birth choices, or common complications, will not help you avoid disappointment. In fact, it is more likely to lead to regret and even emotional trauma.

Even if you refrain from actually writing a birth plan, do you carry the desire for perfection in your heart?

Once you discover the source of your motivations to write (or not write) a birth plan, what's next? Explore ways to shift from fear, avoidance, or helplessness in order to compose or formulate your "Warrior's Plan."

TASK OF EARLY PREGNANCY

If you are going to write a birth plan, the best time to do so is in the first half of pregnancy when there is still time to change your birthplace or birth attendants if you want to. Begin by taking tours of local hospitals' labor and post-partum units and nurseries. In learning about hospital protocols, you also learn what is important to you. Ask new parents in your community about what happened to them in the hospital, what surprised them, what they wish someone had told them, and what was helpful or not helpful in navigating the terrain of birth choices. Their responses may help guide you in formulating some questions to ask.

ADVICE FROM LABOR AND DELIVERY NURSES

If you are birthing in a hospital, the first person you meet and give your birth plan to will be a nurse. A long, detailed birth plan is not usually more helpful or convincing than a short one. Since nurses see many birth plans that ask for the same things, the nurse you hand your birth plan to may glance at it without reading every word, and might forget some details. So as you work together through labor, talk directly to your nurse about your needs and desires instead of relying on your written plan to do the talking for you.

Becky, a labor nurse, explains some of the important aspects of a birth plan. "Nurses do not find it helpful when a birth plan states, 'I don't want an epidural' or 'Don't offer pain medication.' What we really want to know is how you have prepared to cope with pain and what we can do to help you. If

"I needed to find out the range of possibilities because I knew that once I was in labor, if something came up I wouldn't be able to say, "Let me google that." It's my personality to research everything, so that's how I used the birth plan to help me prepare. Once I learned what was routine, what was necessary, and what I wanted for myself and my baby, I chose a birthplace and a culture that would not ask me if I wanted an epidural, so this was taken off the table right away."

—TARA

you sincerely want to avoid an epidural, take time during pregnancy to learn various ways to deal with labor pain. Even if we are at your bedside with the best intention to support you, our ability to help you and teach you pain-coping techniques in labor is limited."

Short and sweet birth plans

It's better to use positive language and keep your birth plan short and sweet. Let the staff know about special requests that matter most to you. Also find out what is routine, optional, or no longer practiced at your hospital. Don't create animosity by stating you will refuse practices that won't even be offered (for example, enemas or shaves, which are no longer ordered routinely in the United States). Clearly state what you want and what's important to you, rather than what you don't want. For example, instead of saying, "Don't offer drugs," write, "Follow our lead about pain medications. We will ask about them if we need to."

Here are a few examples of short and sweet birth plans.

Lena and John handed their nurse a card with the following message.

To Everyone:
Thank you for wearing a shirt, shoes, and a smile,
and for supporting us in our effort to have a positive birth.

Written on a scrap of paper and tacked to the door, Audrey's birth plan read:
I plan to bring myself to each and every moment of my labor and birth.
I welcome encouragement and your experienced guidance to help me birth as normally as possible.
I want my baby placed skin to skin on me, wet and wriggly (not swaddled in blankets).
Let us do the breast crawl for the first nursing.

In the first hour after birth, a calm and alert newborn baby lying on his mother's warm belly is able to crawl up to the mother's breast, latch on, and begin nursing without any help. He does not need to be positioned or to have the breast forced into his mouth. The baby's innate survival instincts and reflexes guide him in knowing just what to do.

Watch this endearing little video: http://www.breastcrawl.org/video.shtml.

Bethany worked in the hospital where she was going to birth. Her two-sentence birth plan let her nurses know her special request:

I am in labor and need my privacy.
Co-workers who want to stop in to "visit"
and medical students are not allowed in my room.

CLAY AS A CATALYST FOR EXPLORING ATTACHMENT AND LETTING GO

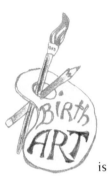

We try to gain control over childbirth by planning and making decisions ahead of time and holding on to whatever makes us feel safe or confident. As a Birth Warrior, your task is to prepare for a birth that has no script, for a journey that always begins with an incomplete map. This requires courage, flexibility, and a capacity for inner awareness. One way to cultivate these qualities is to notice how you are being open and responsive in the moment while making a series of birth sculptures from the same piece of clay.

Begin working the clay in your hands, noticing how forms naturally emerge and sink back into the lump. You may begin without an intentional outcome, then a clear image might surface in your mind, which you can sculpt it into the clay. Or when a shape or symbol in the clay captures your attention, work the clay to bring the image out. It won't necessarily make sense to you or be what you "had in mind." View each of your sculptures as a catalyst for exploring ideas that come up.

Pounding, rolling, smoothing, and coiling a meaningful symbol out of clay is a slow process that requires patience, but it allows you to see aspects of your inner self. As the clay is transformed from a lump into an image, it becomes a kind of soul-portrait.

After five minutes or so, contemplate the shape that has emerged and its symbolic meaning for you. No matter how extraordinary a sculpture is, it only captures the insight of a moment. It is inevitable that perception, understanding, and symbols will change over time. Now fold the sculpture back into a lump, and allow another form to surface. Consider the meaning of this creation then fold it again into a lump of clay.

Be aware of how your mind latches on to a particular sculpture or to the meaning you've given it—either loving it or hating it. Notice when you feel attached to a sculpture and are reluctant to let go of the form you've made. Is there a correlation between your response to creating, smashing, or saving sculptures and what happens with ideas that you capture in a birth plan?

Repeat this process any time during pregnancy when you feel yourself resisting or becoming attached to one idea. With this clay exercise, you can practice being present and creative, letting go, and changing direction, which will serve you well as you compose your birth plan and experience labor.

OPENING IN LABOR

If you are taking a Birthing From Within class, your childbirth mentor may lead you in a visualization about "opening." You can also listen to a recording of this visualization (available as a download at www.sevengatesmedia.com). Even if you don't think you're artistic, boldly draw or paint the image you saw and felt as vividly, and in as much detail, as you saw it during your meditation or visualization. Hang your drawing up; every time you see your image of opening, you are making a positive pathway for your body and mind. Later, display your art in your labor room.

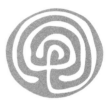

Informed Consent Is a Dialogue

Understanding how most caregivers make recommendations will help you participate more skillfully in gathering information and "incubating" healthcare decisions for yourself and your child. This chapter, drawn from the wisdom of parents, caregivers, and legal professionals, helps you learn about the complexities of engaging in an informed consent dialogue.

For years we gave expectant parents a list of questions to help them ask the "right" questions. However, since the publication of *Birthing From Within* I've heard countless stories from parents who asked the classic questions and still did not feel they were able to give informed consent. Informed consent requires a meaningful dialogue between a mother and those helping and caring for her. Many things interfere with having a true dialogue—among them, feeling paralyzed with information overload, deferring decisions to a doctor or partner, and making hasty decisions out of fear or pressure.

Terms, Definitions, and Rights

Informed Consent: *Your agreement to allow tests, treatments, or procedures after being informed of risks, benefits, and alternatives in dialogue with a birth attendant. Informed consent is more than signing a consent form*

Consider yourself informed if:

- The problem is described in terms you understand.

- A range of best- to worst-case outcomes has been explained.

- You have received a balanced picture of the risks, benefits, and side effects of recommended tests, treatments, and procedures.

- Questions about alternative methods of treatment, including watchful waiting (doing nothing and letting nature take its course before you decide), are answered.

"We [doctors] prefer to do something instead of nothing, and this often means prescribing medications. For the most part, patients encourage this behavior. No one likes to leave the doctor's office empty-handed. The misuse of antibiotics to treat respiratory viruses illustrates this point. . . . Patients want answers and clear-cut solutions, and doctors want to provide them. To admit how much we don't know—how much is out of our control—is frightening for all involved."

—Annie Brewster, MD[4]

for a procedure or surgery. It is being able to have a meaningful dialogue with caregivers before making a decision to sign anything.

You have a legal right, and a responsibility, to be fully informed of risks, benefits, and alternatives before any exam, test, procedure, or treatment is given to you or your baby, whether it is routine or uncommon.[1]

Informed Refusal: Your legal right to decline or postpone any recommended tests, treatments, or procedures after learning of potential risks to you or your baby. By definition, informed consent must also include the right to give "informed refusal."[2]

When in doubt about a decision, you also have a legal right to receive a copy of your medical records and get a second opinion. When you, as an adult patient, decline a recommendation for treatment or surgery, the doctor typically accepts your decision. However, when you, as a pregnant woman, refuse a recommendation for routine testing or cesarean surgery your decision will not always be accepted. Sometimes the conflict or coercion that follows is due to a fundamental confusion about whether the mother or the baby inside her is the patient. Our litigious culture is not clear about who is ultimately responsible for making decisions that may affect the baby's well-being—the mother and father, the doctor, or a judge?[3]

Pre-Admission Consent

For billing or other purposes, you might be asked to fill out pre-admission forms that include a general consent form for treatment. Even after signing a pre-admission consent form, you are legally entitled to receive information about procedures and treatments and to consent to or decline them. This is true for procedures such as fetal monitoring, vaginal exams, IVs, artificial rupturing of the membranes, and episiotomy. Additionally, you have the right to change your mind after you've signed such a form.

Birth Companions, Friends, and Family—Read This:

Even if a pregnant or laboring woman is well informed and usually advocates effectively on her own behalf while under pressure, in labor she may need your help asking questions and considering her options. Here's why:

- In active labor, a mother is capable of hearing information. However, because of the endorphin haze of labor, thinking clearly and formulating or verbalizing questions are often difficult in the brief minutes between contractions.

- Exhaustion, pain, worry, and feeling overwhelmed make it easy for a mother (and father) to give uninformed consent to procedures and drugs in labor.

- Many women later regret having consented to recommendations before asking more questions or thinking or talking about the recommendations.

WHY TRUE INFORMED CONSENT
IS RARELY GIVEN

Even though obtaining informed consent before performing procedures is the law, it is rare for patients to actually have a dialogue leading to true informed consent. This is not because caregivers don't know the law or don't believe in the principle of informed consent. It's because if the process of informed consent were actually followed to the letter, our overburdened clinics and healthcare system couldn't provide it given how time-consuming information gathering and processing can be. Further, there is lively debate within the medical ethics community about whether a woman in labor, especially when exhausted, in pain, or afraid, can ever really give informed consent.[5] In the intense, emotionally-charged world of the birth room, what should happen regarding calm, rational, informed decision-making may not happen. So within the realistic limits of the experience just do the best you can.

WORST-CASE SCENARIO STRATEGY

Nancy Rhoden, author of *Informed Consent in Obstetrics*, observed that birth attendants have two strategies for making clinical decisions: one is "watchful waiting," a low-key plan for when everything is absolutely normal; the other focuses on, and tries to avoid, the worst-case scenario. The latter problem-focused strategy is characterized by birth attendants or parents focusing on the worst possible outcome that could happen—even when it is not actually happening or is unlikely to happen—and then choosing the maximum amount of testing, interventions, drugs, or surgery to deal with potential problems, no matter how small the possible gain. Because uncertainty is common in obstetrics, this strategy is becoming the standard in obstetric practice.[6] When your caregivers are operating according to the worst-case scenario strategy, they might do the following:

- Get tunnel vision and present one management plan (usually the plan that is their typical approach) as the only legitimate one.

- Minimize or fail to mention side effects and consequences of treatment for the mother or baby.

- Appeal to the parents' vulnerable emotional state to sway them to comply.

- Utilize language that triggers vivid imagery of a tragic outcome, thus making the recommendation nearly impossible to question or decline.

- Focus on the worst possible outcome for the baby, typically the possibility of neurological damage or death. (This is often referred to as "playing the dead baby card.")

Worst-Case Tactics

Examples of this worst-case scenario strategy include vague or inaccurate comments such as "Your baby is getting so big we're afraid she won't fit if

Learning to embrace uncertainty is a soulful Task of Preparation necessary for both birth and parenting.

After making a recommendation to induce labor, one way for a caregiver to bypass a meaningful dialogue and gain quick compliance is to play the "dead baby card." A pregnant woman I knew told her doctor she would let him know her decision after talking to her husband. The doctor replied, "That's fine. You go home. Take your time. When you come back, I'll deliver your dead baby." Then he abruptly walked out of the exam room. What do you think she decided?

you aren't induced this week," "Your baby is getting tired," or "We're worried about your baby" (a comment that is especially troubling if delivered while looking at the fetal monitor). Comments like these effectively create images of the worst possible outcome but do not give parents objective, meaningful clinical information with which to make informed decisions. When medical personnel play the "dead baby" card, parents are even less likely to ask questions and employ a rational decision-making process and are more willing to consent to maximum management.

Gathering Information for Decision Making

Not long ago, there was a limited amount of information available to a woman curious about birth; she could go to the library or buy a book or two. Also she had time to think about the material she read and talk about it with a few close friends. By contrast, the current generation of pregnant women is bombarded with a constant stream of (often conflicting) facts, stories, and opinions from social media, blogs, and other online sources. Many women try to arm themselves against unnecessary intervention with more and more information. While a certain amount of information can inspire and guide good decisions, it is easy to reach a point of diminishing returns where too much information actually interferes with good decision making. Information overload can not only cause undue anxiety; it can decrease reflection.

Three Steps to Take before Consenting or Declining

1 Ask yourself: Do I understand what the problem is or am I reacting to fearful imagery? (Don't decide anything yet.)

2. Check assumptions—yours and your birth attendant's—about problems and recommendations. (Don't decide anything yet.)

"I was planning to birth normally. I was a week overdue. They told me the ultrasound found that my amniotic fluid was low and my baby looked like he was enveloped in Saran Wrap. At that moment, I was so scared that I would have agreed to anything they wanted so my baby wouldn't die."
—Molly

While low amniotic fluid can be a concern, frightening images of the baby suffocating in the womb do not inform but instead effectively coerce a pregnant woman's "consent" and cooperation.

How much do you need to know?

Set a limit for your information gathering and then stop. Hoarding excessive information doesn't make you smarter or help you make better decisions; instead, it will make you more anxious and less intuitive.

3. If a decision does not have to be made immediately, wait. When the time comes, decide and give real informed consent.

A review of fifteen studies involving 5,583 women showed no difference between the lengths of labor in women whose water bag remained intact and women whose water was ruptured artificially.[6]

Let's see how this three-step approach plays out in a typical scenario in labor. When Deirdre was in labor, her birth attendant suggested breaking her water to speed up labor, which usually sounds like a good idea to a laboring mother.

1. Deirdre asked, "How is the perceived slow progress of my labor a problem?" The birth attendant said he was concerned that Deirdre and her baby would get tired.

2. Deirdre quickly checked assumptions. She speculated about her caregiver's underlying assumptions. "Maybe he thinks if I labor into the night I will be too tired to push my baby out. Maybe he is worried he'll have to deliver my baby in the middle of the night and he'll be tired. Maybe his positive intention is to shorten labor to help me avoid a long ordeal."

Then she asked, "Do babies get tired in labor?"

"Not tired," the birth attendant explained, "Your baby could go into distress."

"Is my baby in distress now?" Deirdre asked.

"No. Your baby is doing fine. The heartbeat is very strong!" replied the birth attendant.

3. "Then maybe there is no urgent need to speed up labor at the moment. Let me think about your recommendation. I'll let you or the nurse know what I decide. Thank you for coming to see me," Deirdre responded.

It is important to notice that in this dialogue Deirdre questioned what was motivating her birth attendant's assumption that her labor needed to be accelerated and his recommendation to break her water. If she had asked only "What are the risks and benefits of breaking my water?" she would likely have been told there are no risks (which is not always true), but the benefit of breaking water is that it speeds up labor (which is not always true). Those answers suggest (inaccurately) that this "harmless" intervention will speed up labor—and what woman wouldn't agree to that? But by checking assumptions, Deirdre was able to sort out what could happen from what was happening. In doing this, she discovered there was no actual problem and therefore no need to break her water.

A Few Tips

Invite a companion to prenatal appointments

Make it a point to bring someone (your partner, a friend, or a family member) with you to every prenatal and postpartum appointment, however routine, so the two of you can later discuss what was said and what, if anything, was recommended. Also, if you should feel intimidated or space out, your companion might be able to help you continue asking questions while you are still in the office and have ready access to your caregiver's input.

Take pen and paper to prenatal appointments

Write down your questions in advance. During the visit, it may be helpful to have your companion jot down what is said while you concentrate on the questions.

Remember that two (or more) heads are better than one

When facing a difficult decision as a pregnant couple, you don't have to mull it over on your own. Birth attendants often consult with one another, and you can do the same with a friend or relative. When you explore options with another person or small group, you gain a broader perspective by learning from others' experiences. Remember, you are not asking someone else what you should do; rather, you are inviting a shared exploration of problems, assumptions, recommendations, and alternative solutions.

A word to the wise: Be mindful not to have this dialogue with someone who is still in acute birth trauma, since her perspective might be negatively affected by her own still-raw experience and not particularly objective.

Classic Questions to Help You Get Information

For Tests and Procedures

- What will I learn from this test or procedure?

- How accurate is it?

- What are the risks?

- Do the risks outweigh the benefits?

- What could I do differently after getting the results?

- If the results will not change what I can do or the outcome, is there another reason to do the test?

For Treatments, Drugs, and Interventions

Do you understand the problem? If not, ask more questions until you do.

Try these:

- In what way might this treatment, drug, or induction help? How likely is it to help?

- What are the advantages and disadvantages?

- Must this be done now? What might happen if I postpone it for an hour? A week? What if I never do it?

- This may be what you usually recommend, but are there any other approaches to be considered?

- If there are several options, which one might be the least invasive? What is a logical sequence for trying different options?

IF YOU AND YOUR CAREGIVER DISAGREE

Make a genuine effort to build and maintain a constructive relationship with your caregiver. At the same time, be a loyal advocate for yourself and your unborn child. Your relationship with your child will outlast your relationship with your caregiver.

Perhaps the most common question asked by expectant parents is: "How do I know if what is being recommended is necessary?" The answer, which depends on various factors, is vitally important to every parent concerned with birth. If you believe or intuit that a test or procedure is not necessary, or may introduce unnecessary risk to you or your unborn child, exercise your right and responsibility to decline it. Consider getting a second opinion. If circumstances prevent you from getting a second opinion, you might be tempted to avoid conflict and give consent; but try to stay in dialogue with your caregiver and make the best plan together.

If you decline a recommendation, your caregiver may go along with your wishes, suggest watchful waiting, or propose an alternate plan. However, if your caregiver cannot accept your decision you may be asked to sign a form stating you have been informed of risks and benefits and that you release the caregiver and the hospital from liability. Don't be intimidated. This is just a formality in our litigious culture, so sign the form.

Continue observing how the situation is unfolding. Don't get locked in to your decision or attached to being "right" or following your birth plan no matter what. Labor, like life, is perpetually changing. If at any time new developments inform you that what you declined earlier is now the next best thing to do, consent to it.

INCUBATE YOUR DECISION

After you've gathered advice and information for a reasonable amount of time, stop! Stop reading, stop thinking, and stop talking about it. Unless an answer needs to be provided immediately, incubate your decision. You incubate decisions best when you don't try to figure the answer out deliberately but allow your unconscious to sort out

Let the Ants Sort While You Sleep

Symbolically, seeds represent possibilities, choices, resources, and emotions.

In the legend of Eros and Psyche, Psyche is weighed down by the daunting task of sorting a huge pile of seeds. Making decisions is exhausting, and she falls asleep. While she sleeps, ants come to sort the seeds. When she awakes, to her surprise her task is completed.

Symbolically, the ability of ants to work above and below ground could represent our access to conscious and unconscious knowing and the power of allowing our unconscious to work things out while we rest.

what you know and feel and construct a solution or decision. To help your mind rest and your intuition open, turn off the television, your cell phone, and your Internet access for a few hours. Create space and time in solitude by sitting under a tree or by a river. Enjoy a picnic while watching the clouds. Listen to music that opens your heart and moves you emotionally; turn the volume up and dance. Go about your day, allowing the answer to come to you. Whenever possible, sleep on it.

There is no certainty in childbirth. Don't try to make a "perfect" decision or one that has no consequences. You don't have control over that. Instead, make a decision, act on it, and don't look back. In the future, if you learn different information, don't tell yourself you should have decided something else. Know that in the moment, based on everything you—and everyone else—knew at the time, you made the best decision you could.

Enter the Center

When you are in active labor, the intensity draws your attention inward. You may not be able to distract yourself, so go with the flow and learn how to enter the center of the sensation.

Pain is not static, but our ideas about it can be. Once you name a sensation, fix its location, and assign it meaning, you begin responding to that "history" rather than to what is happening in the moment. With training, when you enter the center of pain its magnitude is reduced, making it easier to handle.

Practice Entering the Center for a 60-second "ice contraction." Before the contraction begins, hold the intention to find the center. As soon as the contraction begins, fasten your mind's eye on the center of the sensation. Between one breath and the next, notice how the sensation moves slowly or swiftly in any direction—and keep bringing your attention to the ever-moving center. Stay in quiet mind for 2 to 3 minutes between ice contractions.

You can hold an ice cube or, to get the most out of this practice, immerse your hand in a basin of ice water for 30 seconds then take your hand out and continue practicing Entering the Center for another 30 seconds. This will give you a full minute contraction; the intensity of the ice will peak at 30 seconds (as in labor), after which it will begin to resolve. Since it's impossible to watch a clock with your attention turned inward, have someone time this practice for you, or use a timer.

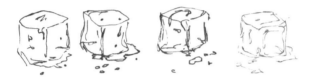

Visualizations for Entering the Center

Be a "hurricane hunter." Hurricane hunters, pilots who fly into the centers of hurricanes, pass through howling winds of 100 or more miles per hour, blinding rain, hail, and a cloud 10 to 15 miles thick before entering the center, where skies are blue and sunny.[7] Many people think it's crazy to risk flying a plane into the eye of a hurricane for weather reconnaissance or other purposes. Similarly, many people think it's crazy to birth through pain. There are other similarities between finding the center of a hurricane and finding the center of pain in labor: both require training to survive flying in "stormy weather"[8] and both require concentration to be able to remain in a calm center for up to twelve "stormy" hours.

To train your mind to concentrate while Entering the Center of pain, using 60-second ice contractions do the following:

Imagine flying a red airplane through the "wall of pain." Feel the wings quiver in the stormy edges before entering the center. Focus your attention on your breath and the cockpit around you to stay in the center. As your plane and labor move forward, keep your eyes fixed on the calm blue center.

No two hurricanes or labors are alike. Therefore, like a hurricane hunter you should be prepared to respond to a variety of situations and unexpected surprises in labor—not just blue skies. Even with all their training and expertise, pilots always feel a bit apprehensive before taking flight and daring to fly into the eye of a hurricane, and so might you as you prepare to cope with labor pain.

Be a martial artist. Martial artists impress us by breaking boards, and sometimes blocks of cement, with their hands. Even a young child can perform this feat. How is it possible? First, the martial artist believes she will succeed. Second, she does not aim to strike the board itself but rather an imaginary target beyond it. Third, she follows through on her strike, utilizing the full force of her speed and intention to go through the board. If a martial artist hesitates at the last second, her hand bounces off the surface of the board and she feels pain. To make this mindset and training relevant to coping in labor:

Imagine a point "on the other side" of the contraction, fix your attention on it, and follow through with each exhalation. When your intention, focus, and follow-through are aligned, you can breathe through contractions rather than pulling back.

"All that I know is I'm breathing.
All I can do is keep breathing.
All we can do is keep breathing."

—INGRID MICHAELSON[9]

Think of your contractions as a rapidly moving river. As you imagine beginning each contraction, envision yourself standing on one shore and looking at a point on the other shore. Then breathe deeply and "swim across the river" toward it.

The Archer and the Arrow

Imagine you are an archer. As each contraction builds momentum, keep your inner eye fiercely focused on your target. Feel your strength and the tension in the bow as you pull back the string. At the peak of the contraction, release the bow-string and become the arrow. Let each long exhalation propel you in straight flight, unimpeded, until the contraction stops and you hit the center of your target.

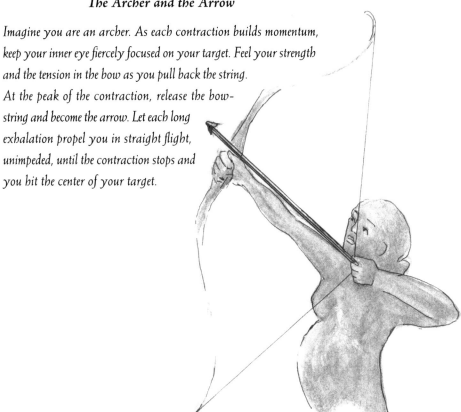

Preparing for Your Return

A Warrior does not leave things to chance. Knowing that the "battle" will require her to give her all to get as far as she can on her own, she must also have the foresight and humility to ask for and receive help when she needs it while she's on her postpartum return.

Inanna, as she prepares for her descent, anticipates that she may be spent and need help to recover and complete the journey intact. As a final step of preparation before going to the underworld, she and Ninshubur, both Warriors, make a pact to ensure Inanna's safe return. Inanna tells Ninshubur:

"I will do everything in my power to return safely on my own. If I do not return in three days and three nights, call on our friends and elders to find me, restore me, and help me get back. Do not leave me in the underworld."

LOOK AHEAD

Take notice of Inanna's wisdom. She didn't wait until she was at the end of her journey in the underworld to figure out how to get "home." The time after your baby is born is almost too late to start wondering what you need and how to get it. When planning ahead, some things you can do are: read part VI of this book to learn about the physical and emotional components of the postpartum period; attend a breastfeeding class or support meeting; hang out with new mothers and babies; and make plans for practical support.

SUMMON YOUR ALLIES

As a new parent, it will be impossible to maintain all your responsibilities and daily habits in addition to recovering from birth, learning to feed and care for your baby, and grabbing sleep and food when you can. It's hard to believe that this new little person will completely turn your world (and time management) upside down, but he will. This isn't a reflection of your competence but rather an essential aspect of becoming a parent, of stepping into an entirely new identity.

ENSURE POSTPARTUM COCOONING

Take time before birth to think about what your daily needs are and will be so you can arrange to have them met later.

- Laundry
- Grocery shopping
- Pet care
- Tidying the house
- Cleaning
- Washing dishes
- Meal preparation
- Breastfeeding support

Mother and baby remain suspended between two worlds for hours, days, even weeks. New mothers and fathers feel their whole world—inside and out—has changed forever, and they need some time to integrate the change. In China, Korea, and among the Hopi of the Southwest, as well as many other traditional cultures, new mothers are secluded for twenty-one to thirty days to ensure a gentle transition into motherhood.[1, 2, 3]

However, modern Western culture tends not to support seclusion for mother and baby. Within minutes of giving birth, a woman is expected to reenter the world. Before she has even had time to connect with her baby, contemplate her experience, or clean up, her birth space is invaded by social media, visitors coming in and out of her room, and nurses going through long lists of questions, instructions, and forms. This is true even late at night, when an exhausted new mother should be resting. Everyone around the woman carries on as usual, because nothing extraordinary happened—*to them*—and because birth is viewed largely as a medical event, not a rite of passage.

So, one of the often overlooked final Tasks of Preparation is to choose a special, nurturing person to ensure that you and baby will have plenty of postpartum cocooning. This will require envisioning what you would like, how to make it happen, and educating your family and circle of friends in advance about the wisdom and ritual of postpartum cocooning so they are on board.

ARRANGE FOR A POSTPARTUM MEAL TRAIN

Eating well often falls to the bottom of the priority list in the first few weeks after birth, with fast food, frozen meals, sandwiches, and cereal becoming the default choices. But excellent nutrition is important for your physical recovery, your emotional well-being, and establishing a good milk supply. People who care about you will want to help, so enlist the aid of your enthusiastic supporters in forming a postpartum meal train to bring you a series of healthy, delicious home-cooked meals. Then before giving birth hand your special nurturing person a list of friends and relatives who agreed to bring you a postpartum meal. Be sure to also provide a list of your food allergies and preferences. Many great online sites and apps streamline meal train organization.

ONE LAST TASK

No amount of knowledge or groundwork can fully prepare you for the wild ride of birth and new motherhood. While you may now feel more confident about and ready for your descent into Laborland and beyond, be humble as you abide in the place of not-knowing. Now is the time to acknowledge what you've learned and done so far. But it also might be the time to do nothing, to let go of control and enjoy the end of your pregnancy without a long to-do list.

Part 5

GATES OF
LABORLAND

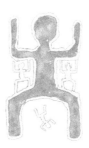

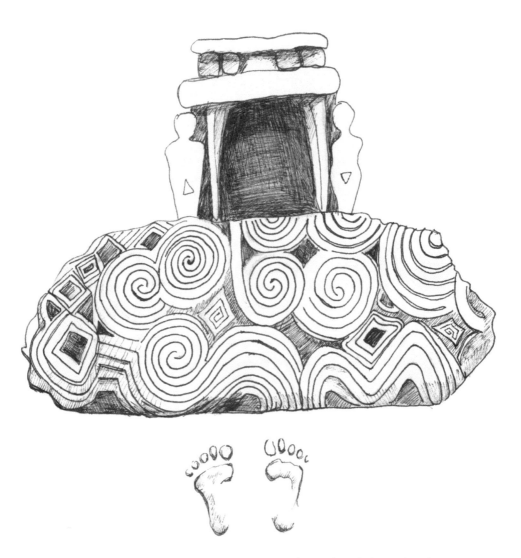

Portal to the Neolithic tomb at Newgrange, with its ornately carved spirals, diamonds, and waves.

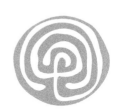

26

CROSSING THE
THRESHOLD

A threshold is a universal symbol of transition and transcendence representing the interface of two worlds, such as the known and the unknown, the mundane and the sacred. In birth, there is a psychic threshold separating the worlds of the Maiden and the Mother.

*T*ypically, a threshold is a place to pause with awareness but not a place to dwell.[1] It marks the point where changes must be made to cross over to a new world. In a symbolic way, crossing a threshold also represents leaving the past, abiding in the present, and entering the future. In birth, a woman crosses the threshold between Maiden and Mother, leaving behind her past identity as Maiden to embrace her new identity as Mother.

To cross this threshold, you may need to become curious about what brought you to it and what motivates you to cross it; to do this, you may need to reach deep down to connect with your body or some forgotten resource within you.

In mythological stories such as "Inanna's Descent," crossing thresholds leads to the underworld, a place where elemental forces are outside the reach of culture and where human control is diminished. In archetypal psychology, the underworld represents the unconscious, or something you have not yet lived, expressed, or realized about yourself. The Descent into the underworld is also the way out—of old patterns and assumptions. Therefore, your journey to the inner world of Laborland allows you to see or do something you were not able to see or do before. While this discovery of something new about yourself can result in a confrontation of sorts, it is also the key to personal growth.

One of the most impressive thresholds of the ancient world is the mega-ton stone portal to the Neolithic tomb at Newgrange in Ireland, ornately carved with spirals, diamonds, and waves. After seeing the stone during a visit to Newgrange, I wrote:

> When I first stood before it, I sensed by its imposing size that this threshold was purposeful; it would have made Neolithic people pause before climbing over it and entering the sacred inner chamber. It was in that moment that I understood the importance of threshold and the purpose of pausing before leaving our ordinary world and entering sacred space.

Like the people of Newgrange, it is important that you, as a Birth Warrior, cross your threshold with awareness. Do not rush or stumble over it. When you realize that you are leaving ordinary life and entering Laborland, take a moment to acknowledge that you are entering a sacred chamber. Connect with women across lands and through all time who have crossed the threshold that is now before you.

A LABOR CEREMONY

Drink Your Laborinth

Plan a threshold ritual to mark your crossing into labor. Draw inspiration from the mothers and midwives in northwest

India who, for hundreds of years, have taken part in this simple ritual at the onset of labor:

Saffron is sprinkled in a shallow dish. After the mother traces a labyrinth in it with her finger, holy water from the Ganges River is poured over it. She then drinks the labyrinth to ensure victory over her fear and the unknown and to symbolically show her baby the way out.[2]

Make this ritual your own. Sprinkle a powdered food, such as cocoa or Emergen-C, in a shallow, flat dish. Trace a labyrinth in it with your finger, then cover it with water, milk, or juice. Finally, drink it as you envision you and your baby finding your way through labor.

Add a Threshold and Footprints to Your Laborinth

You learned how to draw a classic labyrinth in chapter 2. Now you can personalize your map of birth by adding a threshold that holds a special meaning for you. It could be a drawing of a ribbon, a sprinkling of rose petals, a gate, or a butterfly symbolizing transformation. Make a threshold that stretches across the entrance or is tall to invoke the feeling of having to pause or make an effort before crossing it to enter the unknown. You might like to make a guardian to sit by the entrance to your Laborinth, such as a lion, bear, or a gate-keeper (see chapter 29).

In preparation for some journeys, you dress up and put on comfortable shoes or hiking boots to protect your feet and to help you make ground quickly. For journeys of the heart, labyrinthine journeys into the unknown, the underworld, and Laborland, you cannot rush toward your imagined goal. So begin your journey by symbolically taking off your comfortable shoes; walk barefoot, feeling each step of the way.

After you draw your threshold, draw footprints in front of the entrance. Footprints before the threshold remind you that you are standing on the ground of the familiar; they are also a symbol of everything you have experienced in life that brought you to this moment. With every step forward you must move into the unknown, even when you aren't certain where the next step will lead.

Stand quietly resolute and draw energy from Mother Earth before entering your Laborinth. Know that as your birth journey begins—with your waters breaking, your first contraction, or entering the hospital—you cross the threshold between your past life as Maiden and your future life as Mother.

MAPS FOR NAVIGATING LABORLAND

27

Anyone who has probed the inner life, who has sat in silence long enough to experience the stillness of the mind behind its apparent noise, is faced with a mystery. Apart from all the outer attractions of life in the world, there exists at the center of human consciousness something quite satisfying and beautiful in itself, a beauty without features. The mystery is not so much that these two dimensions exist—but that we are suspended between them, as a space in which both worlds meet . . . as if the human being is the meeting point, the threshold between two worlds.

—KABIR HELMINSKI

TWO LABOR MAPS

*I*f you are in an unfamiliar place for the first time, you might rely on a map to show important landmarks and turns. Regarding labor, it could be said there are two very different maps: the modern map based on measurements and medical procedures (the one we understand with our minds, the one birth attendants

Comepass Though LABORLAND

follow) and the ancient map based on inner knowing and intuition. Rather than think that you have to choose between one map or the other, know that you can benefit from the wisdom and guidance of both maps as you traverse the varied terrain of your childbearing year.

Modern Map of Labor

In our culture, the modern map of labor is focused on medical tests and measurements. Routine tests mark milestones; labor progress is assessed by measuring cervical dilation over time. Three more examples of modern labor maps include a cervical dilation chart (figure 27.1), a labor graph (figure 27.2), and charts and tables highlighting the three stages of labor.

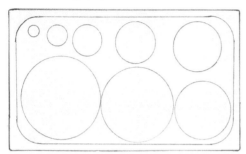

Figure 27.1

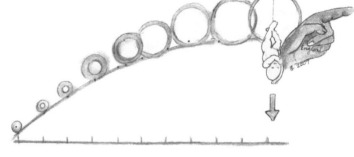

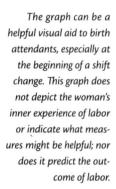

Figure 27.2

The graph can be a helpful visual aid to birth attendants, especially at the beginning of a shift change. This graph does not depict the woman's inner experience of labor or indicate what measures might be helpful; nor does it predict the outcome of labor.

Charts, graphs, and tables make labor seem predictable. For example, the straight lines on a labor graph convey the notion that labor, whether long or short, is linear. If your map only shows you how to get from point A to point B, labor may look deceptively straightforward. But sooner or later, you will come to a twist in your Laborinth that is not shown on the labor graph, one that may be emotional or psychological, causing you to feel doubt or lose faith, even when there is nothing "wrong" with your labor. In addition, the modern map of labor ends with the birth of the baby, with little if any attention given to the woman's postpartum Return. Consequently, even though the modern labor map has value it presents a limited view of a mother's full experience of labor and postpartum. What a woman lives through in her body, mind, and heart cannot be fully expressed through an objective description or a timeline of events.

Ancient Map of Labor

By contrast, the ancient map of labor—the Birth Warrior's map—is based on inner knowing and intuition. In our noisy busy world, it can be difficult to listen to our inner voice and challenging to follow our intuition when evidence-based decision making is viewed as essential for parents and birth professionals alike.

The ancient labyrinth is a perfect symbol for the Birth Warrior's journey through birth; hence, we refer to it as a Laborinth. The labyrinth does not represent medicalized labor but rather a woman's inner experience of labor. Before labor begins, before entering your Laborinth, you are standing on the ground of everything you believe and know. At the start of labor, whether with the first contraction, arrival at the hospital, or your waters breaking, you are crossing a threshold and entering the unknown.

Once you enter a labyrinth, the continuous, winding pathway eventually leads you to the center and out again. In your Laborinth, every moment, every effort brings you closer to giving birth. Yet from time to time, you may feel lost or stuck because, as in a labyrinth, you can't see how far you've come or how close you are to the center. The winding hairpin turns of labor can be disorienting and overwhelming; it's natural to want to give up or look for a way out. But in the Laborinth there are no shortcuts and no stopping. There is only one way to get to the birth of your baby: you must continue putting one foot in front of the other—even when you feel lost or want to quit—until you reach the center of your Laborinth.

Approaching the open, empty space of a labyrinth's center induces a state of receptivity and intuition. Likewise, as labor

When the cervix is not measurably opening or stops dilating at some point in labor, you may believe nothing is happening if you focus only on the modern map of birth, which uses dilation as the main marker of progress. But in fact, not only are contractions dilating the cervix, they are also thinning it, rotating the baby, and squeezing him downward, deeper into the pelvis or against the cervix. The rate of dilation can follow a curve, or, as the Laborinth suggests, it can be very unpredictable. Sometimes there is no dilation for hours, then suddenly labor becomes wildly intense and within a few hours dilation is complete.

progresses you may find yourself in an altered state where you process information differently, turn your attention inward, and let go of control. The physical, mental, and emotional work of journeying through the Laborinth supports you in becoming more in touch with your heart and intuition.

The center of the Laborinth represents the place of birth-death-rebirth: the birth of the child, the death of the Maiden, and your birth as Mother and parent. Being in the center—giving birth—involves dealing with the death of the ego, expectations, and beliefs. Afterward, your journey continues as you make your way out of the labyrinth. The final section of this book will guide you in moving through your postpartum Return.

Preparing for the center—birth—is something you do at each step along the pathway. Each moment of attention to your walk, to your physical body, and emotions slowly quiets your mental chatter; each repetition of the meditation serves to take you deeper into your inner world . . . moving away from your past into the future. There is often a sense of making yourself ready for that which is to come.

—HELEN CURRY

When labor begins, many women apply their mindfulness practices and think, "This is doable"; labor is still what they imagined it would be. Suddenly, at around 6 centimeters dilation the intensity increases beyond what they could have imagined and requires great determination and focus. At first some women are shocked and think they cannot do this, but they rebuild confidence by continuing to do whatever practice is working for them. Finally the baby is born.

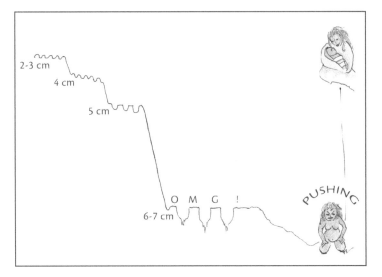

YOU ARE NOW IN LABORLAND

As you read the practical information and suggestions for navigating Laborland, keep in mind that your birth map will be personal and unique. Yet every birth can be a Birth Warrior's journey, no matter how it unfolds.

YOUR AMAZING UTERUS

The uterus is composed of three intertwined layers of muscle that run in every direction. All three layers are coordinated to contract together, making it the strongest muscle in your body (by weight), strong enough to squeeze your baby out into the world. The cervix (opening of the uterus) softens, shortens, thins, and then opens fully to let your baby out.

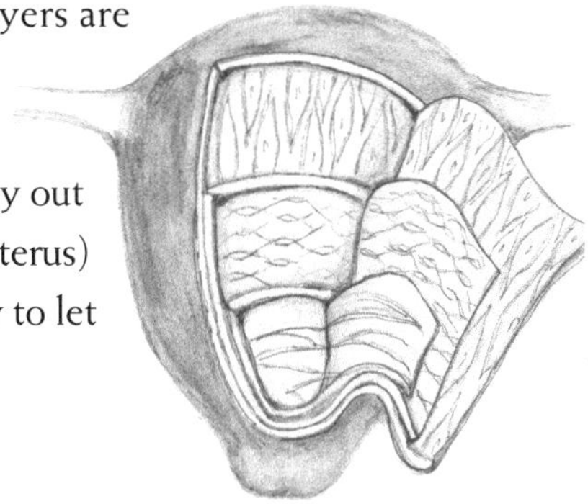

How does the uterus contract?

Stimulated by the hormone oxytocin, uterine contractions move as a wave from the top downward toward the cervix (figure 27.3). The upper segment of the uterus contracts more strongly and for a longer time than the lower segment. Relaxation of the muscle during rest periods between contractions begins at the same time in all parts of the uterus. The riper the cervix is, the more readily it responds to uterine contractions. If labor starts on its own, the cervix is more likely to be ripe.

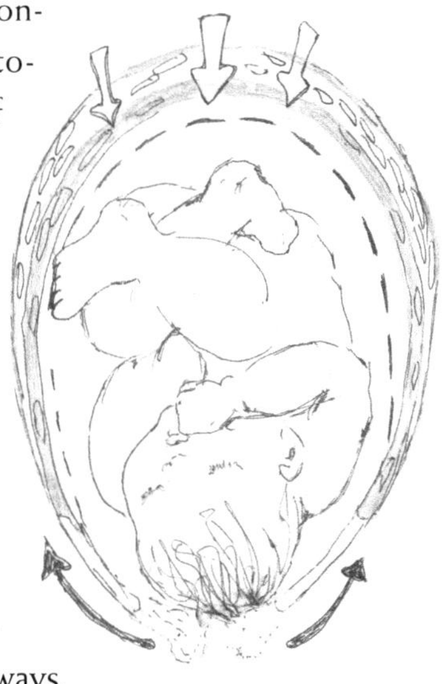

LABOR HORMONES

Labor and birth encompass a vast array of physiological and emotional factors interacting in complex ways. Dozens of hormones—chemical "messengers" in the body—affect the timing, pace, and subjective experience of birth. We'll focus on a few keys ones: oxytocin, beta-endorphin, and stress hormones.

Figure 27.3

Oxytocin

Oxytocin, often called the "love hormone," is connected to a wide range of human experiences, including falling in love, orgasm, anxiety, bonding, breastfeeding, and maternal behaviors. During pregnancy, oxytocin is secreted from the hypothalamus and pituitary in large amounts. As labor progresses, levels peak, bringing about rhythmic uterine contractions of labor, which press the baby's head against the cervix and stimulate stretch receptors in the mother's lower vagina.[1] Oxytocin levels remain high after the baby's birth to ensure birth of the placenta, to sustain uterine contractions to minimize bleeding, and to facilitate breastfeeding and maternal-infant bonding.[2] During breastfeeding, oxytocin is released as the baby sucks, stimulating the milk ejection ("let-down") reflex.

Beta-endorphin

A naturally occurring opiate, beta-endorphin has properties similar to Demerol, morphine, and heroin, and has been shown to work on the same receptors of the brain. Like oxytocin, beta-endorphin is secreted from the pituitary gland, and high levels are present during sex, pregnancy, birth, and breastfeeding. When beta-endorphin is released under conditions of duress and pain, it acts as a painkiller and induces feelings of euphoria. Beta-endorphin levels increase throughout labor,[3] which help you cope with pain; at this point, be more dependent on your birth companion since you have entered an altered state of consciousness.

Stress Hormones

Stress—fight-or-flight—hormones are released in response to fear, anxiety, cold, hunger, or prolonged pain. In labor, high levels of stress hormones can inhibit oxytocin release. This makes sense for mammals birthing in the wild, where the presence of danger would activate the fight-or-flight response, inhibiting labor and diverting blood to the major muscle groups so that the mother can flee to safety.

In the modern birthing climate, the body may perceive excess light and noise, as well as the presence of strangers, as threats and may unnecessarily activate the flight-or-flight response. In humans, high levels of catecholamine* have been associated with longer labor and adverse fetal heart rate patterns, an indication of stress to the baby.[4]

The surge in noradrenaline simultaneously gives the exhausted mother a sudden rush of energy and induces several very strong contractions, both of which are needed to birth the baby.[5] High catecholamine levels at birth "wake up" the baby so he will be wide-eyed and alert at first contact with the mother.[6]

LABOR BEGINS

A few signs that you are getting ready to begin labor include nesting, feeling tired, having diarrhea, having low back pain, feeling crampy, and the baby "dropping" (also called lightening or engagement).

If you have to ask,
"Am I in labor?"
you are probably not.

*When the long-awaited day of labor finally arrives,
you'll always remember crossing this threshold,
although it's never quite what you pictured.*

Ignore the Itty-Bitty Twinges

Back in the day when our grandmothers gave birth, they started counting "hours of labor" not from the first mild contraction but from when they had to stop their tasks of daily life. Counting every itty-bitty twinge will make labor seem really long.

> ### Staving off *Hiesho*
>
> In Japanese, *hiesho* is the diagnosis given to patients who "feel chilly" or complain of sensitivity to air conditioning, poor circulation, or cold feet. One study found that the presence of *hiesho* is associated with premature delivery, premature rupture of membranes, weak labor pains, and prolonged labor, and is most prevalent in women over age thirty-five. A good preventive is to increase circulation by keeping your feet warm in wool socks or soaking your feet in warm water.[7]

RECOGNIZING EARLY AND ACTIVE LABOR

Read the ACOG and SMFM 2014 consensus statement entitled "Safe Prevention of the Primary Cesarean Delivery."[8]

Earthy-Birthy Terms

Bloody show*
Braxton-Hicks contractions*
Mucus plug*
Prodromal labor*

"Early labour is a woman's signal to get settled somewhere safe and to gather her 'women folk' around her."

—RACHEL REED[9]

Identifying early and active labor depends on a number of factors. Early labor refers to the period when contractions are mild, often irregular, and spaced about five or more minutes apart. It can take several hours for these early contractions to thin the cervix before labor becomes "active"; for first births, it may take twenty-four hours or longer. Active labor refers to the part of labor when a woman's cervix is about 6 centimeters dilated, with contractions that are stronger, at regular intervals, and less than five minutes apart; there's no need to time every contraction.

Typically, in active labor a woman can no longer focus on the "outside world" between contractions; her attention is drawn inward; she feels spacey or restless between contractions; and she may begin to spontaneously vocalize and move rhythmically.

Early Labor Project

To labor you don't need to stop living. Although sometimes labor starts like a racehorse bolting out of the gate, usually there is enough time to take care of last-minute business, settle into your birth space, and even do an early labor project.

Rather than watching the clock, telling everyone that labor has started, or timing contractions, doing an early labor project is a good way to keep from thinking too much about the contractions.

In *A Midwife's Story*, Penny Armstrong describes an Amish mother's "labor project."[10] Just as Penny went up the steps to the back porch, the Amish mother, Katie, popped out the back door with a paintbrush in hand. She had just finished putting the final coat of lacquer on a rocking chair when contractions became stronger. "I just wanted so much for it to be done so I could rock the baby in it," Katie explained. The midwife was thinking that Katie couldn't be too far along, but it turned out she was 9 centimeters, and soon her baby was born.

Katie's story inspired me to plan an early labor project of my own: tinseling our Christmas tree. My second child was due a week before Christmas, and we had decorated our tree but left the tinseling for an early labor project since it would require physical movement that could focus my attention and keep me from thinking too much about contractions.

Washing and folding baby clothes

Updating photo albums

Decorating the nursery

Cooking or baking

Making birth art

Gardening

When choosing an early labor project, consider an activity that involves physical movement capable of focusing your attention. It is not essential to complete the activity to perfection. Instead, its function on your labor journey is to help you be present in the moment without concentrating on how difficult it is, how much longer labor will be, or where you are on the modern map of labor.

What You Can Do Now
Visualize Your Cervix Ripening and Opening

Many factors influence who gets sick, who gets well, who goes into labor spontaneously, and who responds favorably to induction. It is impossible to know of or control all the forces at work in birth. However, your inner Birth Warrior can cultivate healthy attitudes and expectations and, most importantly,

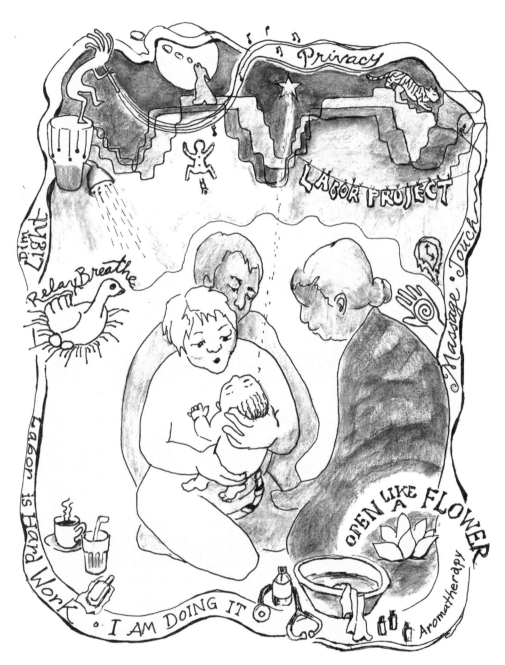

I drew this handout as a visual reminder of what parents could do to help themselves in labor. Make your own drawing—a kind of visual birth plan—to remind you of things you can do to help yourself open in labor.

take action instead of waiting or hoping. As a Birth Warrior, repeatedly and strongly visualizing your body working and opening may help it prepare for a spontaneous, natural labor.

In particular, visualizing your cervix ripening and opening is enormously helpful. This visualization was inspired by the groundbreaking work of Dr. Carl Simonton, a radiation cancer specialist, and his wife, Stephanie Matthews-Simonton, a psychotherapist and counselor, who together developed an effective visualization technique for the treatment of cancer, which is now known as the Simonton Process.[11] The Simontons noticed that cancer patients who were cured had a strong will to live and envisioned getting well, while those who had already resigned themselves to fate did not go into remission or recover.

I adapted the Simonton Process to help you visualize your cervix ripening and opening spontaneously, or during an induction. It is best to experience this outcome while listening to the audio download included with this book.

To help patients imagine wellness, the Simontons showed them what healthy cells look like. Seeing an image of strong, healthy uterine cells might help you build your visualization.

After learning the Simonton meditation and experiencing a visualization, a pregnant woman planning a VBAC drew her new image: *Warrior Uterine Cells*. She experienced a profound shift from feeling her body had failed her to acknowledging how long and hard her uterus worked last time and how it would do so again. With this image came new confidence and hope. Weeks later she had a powerful and normal labor, and she birthed vaginally. (This image is my rendition of her drawing; the warriors' shields are "covered" in golden droplets of oxytocin.)

Welcome to Laborland

Entering Laborland takes you to ultimate surrender. It means dropping social masks. It could mean making noise, being sweaty, pooping, or being physically and mentally naked as you become more in tune with your body and intuition. It means letting go of being "nice" and instead doing what needs to be done to birth your baby. It means being vulnerable and calling on your allies for guidance and support. For someone who "has it all together," doing this—or being made to do this as part of the initiation labor offers—is life changing.

—Shalene

As your labor progresses, hormonal changes in the brain bring about a quiet, internally focused state of mind. Eventually interest in your labor project wanes. In active labor, you might become indifferent to or annoyed by chitchat, and the s p a c e s b e t w e e n your thoughts and words w i d e n. You may become less verbal, and, except when interrupted by contractions, you may be in a trance or light sleep.

Labor works better when you're out of your mind

Other mammals give birth instinctively because they are not thinking about the right way to labor or watching a clock. Being human, you can't stop thinking altogether, but you will get help from elevated endorphins. When your brain perceives pain, endorphins are released. Endorphins cause a shift from being in your rational, thinking mind to being more instinctive and relaxed. They induce a dreamlike state of mind that may help you surrender in Laborland, and also create a hazy, pastel memory of labor.

Out of Control

Many women breathe a sigh of relief when told that they don't have to maintain self-control in labor.

Being natural in labor means doing what comes naturally for you in any given moment. That could mean moaning, groaning, rocking, looking for a way out, asking for help, or white-knuckling. Repressing spontaneous behaviors in labor by trying to follow "rules" and act "properly" would be unnatural.

**If you are afraid of "losing it,"
what are you afraid of "losing"?**

- What does "losing it" in labor mean to you?

- How concerned are you with what other people would think of you if you "lost it" in labor?

- If you completely "lost it" in labor, how would you know? What would you be doing?

- How might "losing it" in labor be helpful to you?

No matter how or where you give birth, you will come to a gate called Out of Control. On this threshold, you might lose control of your lunch, your choice of positions, a calm breathing technique, or your commitment to do or not do something in particular. Whatever it is, embrace it; love yourself unconditionally. The moment will pass—these moments always do. Don't fight it. Don't judge yourself; it only feeds the feeling of not doing it right or of not being worthy.

In Zen, there is a saying: "Fall down seven times, get up eight times."

Places to Go and Things to Do in Laborland

WHEN TO CALL YOUR BIRTH ATTENDANT, DOULA, AND EVERYONE ELSE

Your birth attendant and doula will tell you how and when to reach them, day or night, when you think you have gone into labor. Trying not to bother anyone until you are in active labor (or until daybreak) can lead to increase anxiety and tension, so any time you need answers or support, pick up the phone and call.

Early labor is a good time to build confidence. This can be

done in different ways depending on your personality and circumstances. Check in with yourself about whether spending these early hours alone will help you find your way or whether having someone nearby—your partner or your doula—encouraging you or providing tips will feel supportive and helpful.

Letting family and friends know labor has started can initiate an intrusive, even frenzied "checking-in" on you, despite their best intentions to be supportive. Frequent interruptions throughout labor, including checking social media or having to provide updates, can be distracting enough to cause performance anxiety, interrupt your focus and your connection with your partner, or even disrupt the flow of labor.

> *The timing of when a woman is admitted to the hospital for labor care following spontaneous contraction onset may be among the most important decisions that [she and her] labor attendants make, as it can influence care patterns and birth outcomes.*
>
> —Jeremy L. Neal et al.

Birthing at home is appealing to women because they are typically more at ease in this familiar environment and would prefer not to drive to another location during labor. Even women planning to birth at a hospital want to stay home as long as they safely can. One reason women go to the hospital earlier than is necessary is to feel settled in, to "nest," or to be reassured by experts; sometimes they are sent back home.[12, 13]

Labor at home as long as you can

Until a few years ago, women were told to go to the hospital when contractions were five minutes apart for an hour. Research shows and experienced birth attendants agree, that this is often way too early, especially for a first birth, when early labor may last twelve or more hours. Most women who are admitted too early in labor find the unfamiliar hospital environment stressful, restrictive, and distracting—all of which may increase anxiety and interfere with the ability to cope with even mild contractions, thus undermining a mother's confidence. Arriving at the hospital in active labor (now considered to be 6 centimeters rather than 4 centimeters dilation) decreases the likelihood of receiving Pitocin and pain medication.[14, 15]

One excellent reason to hire a doula is to have more support in early labor, which may enable you to stay home longer. It may be much easier for you to establish coping patterns in early labor in the comfort of your own home. Indeed, one study shows that "first-time mothers who managed to stay home during the latent phase of labor had a sense of power and bodily and mental strength."[16] Yet while being at home in early labor may sound appealing it also raises the questions "How will I know when to go to the hospital?" and "What if I wait too long?"

When to Go to the Hospital

The decision about when to go to the hospital depends on how far you live from the hospital, if you have a special condition that necessitates admission to the hospital in early labor, how comfortable you are with the idea, and how your labor actually unfolds. You may think that timing contractions (or using a smartphone app) is essential to monitoring labor progress, but it doesn't really tell you much. If before calling your birth attendant you want to estimate how frequently contractions are coming, timing three or four in a row is enough to determine the pattern. Don't watch the clock again until the pattern or intensity has really changed.

There are no rules about the perfect time to go to the hospital, but it is usually time to go when:

- You are unable to focus on your labor project between contractions because you feel spacey or restless. If you can still work on your labor project, bake, garden, or sew between contractions, it's not likely you are about to push out your baby.

- Your partner notices that you don't seem like your ordinary self; for instance, you stop talking or socializing between contractions, and your attention is focused inward.

- Contractions get harder and noticeably closer—three to four minutes apart.

- Your intuition tells you to go to the hospital. If your intuition tells you to call your provider or the hospital, even when there seems to be no apparent reason to, act on it rather than overriding your instinct with logic or trying to stick to your preconceived labor plan. Often a mother knows in her heart or gut—even before the experts know—that assistance is needed.

If your water breaks before or during early labor, this rarely constitutes an "emergency," but your birth attendant will recommend whether it is necessary to go to the hospital. If the amniotic fluid is not clear but is instead green or dark, your baby needs to be assessed to make sure he is happy and not stressed.

Arriving at the hospital

Laborland is in some ways a fragile state. Your chances of progressing well after arriving at the hospital improve when customs that preserve the body-mind harmony of labor are observed. Here are a few things to be aware of.

For starters, being admitted to the hospital is not usually a seamless process. Even if you are preregistered at a hospital, when you arrive you will still need to participate in the distracting rituals of triage and admission while coping with contractions. Tasks may include: having blood drawn and an IV started, changing into a hospital gown, starting fetal monitoring, and answering lots of questions about your medical history.

When entering someone else's territory, such as a hospital setting, the primitive (animal) part of the brain produces a surge of adrenalin that facilitates a state of alertness for checking out new terrain and unfamiliar people. Adrenalin neutralizes oxytocin, which can slow labor down for a time. This biological process allows the laboring woman to investigate her environment, interact with new people, and create her birthing "nest." It only becomes a problem if and when the mother feels unsupported, stressed, or unable to settle into her birthing space over a prolonged period of time.

What you can do: After the admission process is complete, focus your attention inward using a mindfulness practice or by listening to music. A gentle massage and a warm cup of broth or tea can be calming. Once you settle into your new environment and become acquainted with the staff, your adrenalin will decrease and oxytocin levels will rise, allowing your labor to reestablish its pattern.

PROTECT YOUR PRIVACY

A woman's mind and body respond as positively to privacy in labor as during lovemaking. When a woman becomes self-conscious or startled by an unexpected distraction during sex or during labor, it takes her away from her body's sensations and into her thinking mind. Frequent distractions and inter-actions with others repeatedly draw a woman's attention out-ward. Having many people present during labor may instill a feeling of self-consciousness or of being "watched." Consequently, it is important to preserve peace of mind and privacy to maintain the internal focus that supports coping in labor.

When a friend or relative assumes they will be with you in labor or witness the birth of your child, it can be awkward and distracting if you don't want that person with you, even if earlier you thought you did. To prevent this situation from happening, prior to labor carefully consider who you want to be at your birth. Also, ask someone who can be tactful and firm to be your "birth bouncer," ensuring your privacy when you need it.

Questions to ponder before labor:

- Who do I want at my birth?

- Am I inviting this person to please them or avoid hurt feelings, or am I inviting them because I am counting on their support?

- In what way does this person support me now? What "gifts" does this person bring me?

- Who can be my birth bouncer when needed?

Years ago a couple passing through Albuquerque came to my birth center and told me about their visit to a rural village in Africa. In the middle of their first night there, they heard a knock on the door of their hut; the woman was summoned. (Her husband was not allowed to come along.) She followed another woman down a path to a round hut at the edge of the village. Upon entering, she realized she had been invited not only to witness the birth of a child but also to be an active participant in spiritually and emotionally supporting the mother's labor.

In the center of the dimly lit hut, a first-time mother labored. Many women from the village, sitting side by side against the wall, had enclosed her in a complete circle. Four women seemed to form an experienced birth team. The team communicated with one another though barely uttering a word. Each team member had a special job to do: midwife, herbalist, a woman who ran errands as needed, and one who led the participants in songs, prayers, and chants to encourage the laboring woman.

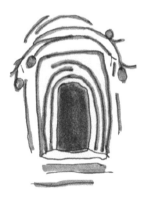

STAY HYDRATED AND NOURISHED

Hydration during labor is important, especially if you want to avoid an IV. In early labor, stay well hydrated: get in the habit of taking a few sips of fluid after each contraction, aiming for 6 to 8 ounces per hour even if you aren't particularly thirsty. Water or ice chips are not sufficient to replace lost minerals, calories, and electrolytes. Instead, choose from:

- Warm tea with honey

- Warm miso or chicken soup, or broth

- Electrolyte-rich drinks (diluted Recharge, Gatorade, or coconut water)

- Vitamin-rich drinks (Emergen-C, fruit juice, Popsicles)

- Homemade "Labor-Ade" (See sidebar for recipe.)

Also be sure to snack when labor starts—even if it is the middle of the night. In early labor, eat a light, nourishing snack every three to four hours, such as cereal, toast, oatmeal, eggs, soup, pudding, or yogurt. This will fortify you before active labor, when you may lose your appetite, at which point it will be time to stop eating solids and try Jell-O, honey, or Popsicles.

An old Italian mother blanched and peeled tomatoes, then simmered and stirred the tomato sauce for hours—slow cooking gave it incredible flavor. She would tend the kids at her feet, get the mail at the door, then return to her pot, stirring slowly. Patience made the sauce. Nowadays we want our tomato sauce—and everything in life—too fast. We open a jar of tomato sauce. When the sauce has warmed for three minutes, we say, "Okay, that's enough. Let's eat." Preparation for labor and being in labor is like making an old Italian tomato sauce—it takes time, stirring, and patience.

—SIGLINDE

Labor "diets" in hospitals

In some hospitals, laboring women are still routinely advised (or ordered) not to eat or drink anything except ice chips or clear liquids after admission.

Homemade "Labor-Ade" Recipe

⅓ c. fresh squeezed lemon juice

⅓ c. honey

¼ tsp. salt

2 crushed calcium/magnesium tablets

4 c. water

Do IVs in labor have risks or benefits?

The importance of hydration in labor is often cited as a benefit of IV therapy in labor. A study of three hundred first-time mothers who received four or eight ounces of intravenous fluids in labor showed that mothers who were well hydrated with eight ounces (250cc) per hour had significantly shorter labors and a tendency toward fewer cesareans.[17] Another study showed that IV hydration decreased vomiting in labor.[18, 19] However, these studies did not look into the delayed consequences of overhydration for mothers or their newborns. During long labors, inductions, or cesarean surgery, women can receive three to six liters of IV fluids within twenty-four hours, which can result in pitting edema from feet to thighs, breast engorgement that lasts for weeks and interferes with breastfeeding, and increased weight loss in the newborn.[20]

**Another Little Lesson in
Obstetric History**
Origin of the NPO Policy

In the 1930s, general anesthesia was commonly used, even for vaginal deliveries, and was not administered by specialists.[21] The widespread policy of restricting a woman's oral intake in labor is an outdated response to a report published in 1946 that referred to an increased risk of aspirating stomach contents into the lungs during general anesthesia.[22] Today, general anesthesia is rarely used in childbirth, but when it is, it is administered much more skillfully than in the 1940s. The World Health Organization and research by a Cochrane Review (2013) recommends that healthcare providers not restrict eating and drinking in labor when no risk factors are present.[23, 24]

In other hospitals, laboring women are allowed to eat and drink unless an epidural is requested, at which point hydration is maintained through an IV and mothers can only have ice chips or sips of clear liquids.

When an IV can help

Eating small regular snacks and staying hydrated on your own decreases the likelihood of needing IV fluids. Sometimes, however, labor has other plans. Nausea can prevent a mother from eating; frequent vomiting can dehydrate her quickly; and a very long labor can deplete even a determined and healthy mother.

In the same way that dehydration, low blood sugar, and diminished electrolytes negatively affect athletes' muscle strength and performance, these conditions can cause the uterine muscle to function poorly during labor. It's easy to solve the problem and quickly rehydrate with an IV. Often well-timed hydration can provide a boost of energy and more effective contractions, allowing the mother to birth without further interventions.

Don't Watch the Clock

"A watched kettle never boils"—or seems like it never boils—because watching and waiting for something to happen can slow down the perception of time. When a laboring mother is watched too closely, she can become self-conscious or anxious. She, or her partner, may worry that labor will take too long and will either inconvenience others by making them wait, or lead to interventions, such as Pitocin or a cesarean. Amy said of her twenty-hour labor, "I was worried after about ten hours that I was moving too slowly, that I was running out of time on the doctor's clock."

Many women are culturally conditioned to avoid inconveniencing others. Countless women, for example, feel anxious about taking too long to orgasm and making their partner wait.

How More Than Three IVs in Labor Changes a Baby's Birth Weight

Two factors are associated with excess weight loss in newborns: mothers who receive more than three IVs in labor and babies who do not nurse well.[25] Babies born vaginally lose 6 percent by seventy-two hours, while cesarean-born infants lose 10 percent.[26] When mothers receive three IVs or more (at rates over 200 cc/hour), their babies are three times more likely to experience excess weight loss at three days compared to babies of mothers who are hydrated at less than 100 cc/hour.[27] This occurs because breastfed newborns normally pee once or twice a day the first two days. However, when mothers are overhydrated in labor so are their babies, which means they pee much more and thus lose more weight in the first seventy-two hours.[28] When babies lose weight, caregivers worry and mistakenly believe that the mother is not making enough milk. As a result, babies of breastfeeding mothers who are, in fact, making enough colostrum or milk are given formula supplementation by bottle.

A Better Solution: Until now, a newborn's birth weight has been used to assess breastfeeding intake and weight loss within the first week of life. However, if you received more than three IVs in labor do not use your baby's birth weight as the baseline for assessing weight change in the first week. Instead, use the twenty-four–hour weight as the baseline—and keep breastfeeding without supplementation unless there is real evidence that your baby is losing weight or getting dehydrated.

This same fear can creep into the labor room; when a woman becomes concerned about what others are thinking, her ability to fully immerse herself in labor can be inhibited. Hospital rooms have a large clock on the wall, facing the labor bed; some women

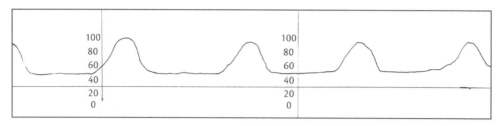

ask for the clock to be covered (the monitor, too) to reduce the attention on numbers and keep the focus where it belongs.

So forget everything you've learned about stages and patterns of labor. Think of labor as a series of contractions that ease open your cervix and push out your baby. When you become immersed in labor, the very nature of labor dissolves ordinary boundaries of time and space. You and labor become one.

Relax, breathe, feel the earth—and then do nothing extra

What does a hen have to do to ensure the birth of her chicks? Just four things: relax, breathe, feel the earth beneath her, and then do nothing extra. For example, during the hatching process, the hen often gets up and turns the eggs over. Doing nothing extra means she does nothing unnecessary. She does not jump up and down on the eggs, poke holes to see if they are ready to hatch, or take ten-minute breaks. She simply instinctively turns them over.

Chickens, like most creatures in nature, learn how to live without any coaching. They know how to relax, breathe, feel the ground, and do nothing extra.

[At first you may find] doing nothing extra the most difficult of these four elements. It simply means carry out each task as naturally and instinctively as you can, allowing nature to meet you halfway. The less you do, the more nature will do for you.

—Emily Lee, Melinda Lee, Joyce Lee, Martin Lee

Laborland's Native Language

With few exceptions, the further along in labor a woman is the more difficult it becomes for her to ask or answer questions, make decisions, or even respond with a simple yes or no. Only after the rational, verbal part of her brain comes to a screaming halt does the intuitive, unconscious part of her fully take over

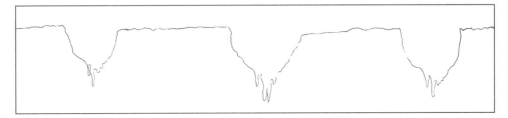

Figure 27.5

As an artist, I began to draw and paint an "inverted hill" pattern to mirror a different aspect of women's experience of contractions. When women (and perhaps birth attendants) see the inverted pattern, it serves as a reminder to direct their attention inward and downward to follow baby, who is moving downward with each contraction. In addition, as labor progresses a woman who is prepared and supported to cope with the intensity of labor finds her thinking mind melting and opening to a deeper knowing, tapping into her vast unconscious resources and even universal knowing. It seems to me the hill pattern then reflects movement toward conscious knowing.

Does the direction of labor contraction waves send messages?

to carry her through a journey that can't be navigated intellectually. This shift from thinking to feeling, from conscious to unconscious (and unselfconscious), helps women surrender to active labor. Without this shift, where mind and ego melt into the background, most women could not endure the intensity of labor. For modern women, the shift is facilitated when everyone is fluent in the language of Laborland: speaking softly and slowly, and using simple phrases to avoid disrupting the woman's labor trance or concentration.

MASSAGE AND REFLEXOLOGY

Nurturing touch during labor releases endorphins that reduce stress, fatigue, and anxiety.[29] New research shows that massage and reflexology in labor can lower blood pressure and significantly decrease anxiety, fear, and pain.[30, 31] Most women in labor appreciate slow, firm touch—especially on the lower back, sacrum, or legs—that is synchronized to the rhythm of breathing and body movements.

WARMTH

New research shows that a tiny part of the brain that processes physical temperature also perceives "warmth" from, and trust in, another person. In one study, participants who briefly held a cup of warm (versus cold) coffee had increased feelings of trust in another and also felt more caring and generous.[32]

Stress hormones are lower and more oxytocin is released when the laboring mother is warm. Shaking and shivering do not always indicate being cold (hormone surges or medications can also make a mother shake in labor), but often a woman in labor will appreciate a cozy blanket, hot packs, and warm hands touching her.

Hospital rooms are often chilly, so bring along:

- Extra layers: short- and long-sleeve shirts, sweatshirts, and wool socks

- A cozy comforter, blanket, or robe for the mother and her partner

- Packets of organic broth, miso, and tea for warm drinks in labor or postpartum

WATER

Many women in labor enjoy being in warm water—either resting in a hot tub or hanging out in the shower—which lowers stress hormones and increases oxytocin levels; the sound and sensation of running water can feel soothing, as well. Warm water also provides counterpressure, which helps many women relax and cope with pain. Additionally, research shows that laboring in water reduces epidural and Pitocin use.[33] It's usually recommended not to soak in a tub until labor is active and progressing (getting in too early may slow contractions) and that caution be used if the bag of waters has broken. Lots of fluids are important in order to avoid dehydration.

Many plans made before labor, including wanting to be in water, may not actually work out as hoped. Some women end up not liking being in water, or the tub doesn't get filled in time, or the circumstances of labor necessitate remaining on dry land. In such instances, the power of water can be brought into the birth room through music with water sounds, visualizations using water imagery, or moist hot packs for an aching back.

MUSIC

Listening to music reduces both the perception of and the distress from labor pain[34] and cues rhythmic breathing and movement. Music is also effective in reducing stress and analgesia use during and after cesarean surgery.[35, 36] The use of headphones or earbuds helps decrease stimulation from the unfamiliar sounds in the operating room. Music calls you to return to yourself, to your center, to what you know; it leads you to where you want to go. Find music that transports you from linear thinking and feeling stressed to positive imagery and feeling calm. Allow the music to enter you; listen from a quiet place within you. Music can also help you move your body in rhythm with labor. If you are exhausted, upbeat drumming might help you keep going. If you are anxious and stressed, soothing music might help you rest between contractions.

ART

Hang your own birth art in your birthing space. Or if you made or have a labyrinth, bring it with you. For example, your drawing of "opening" can be a visual meditation (see pages 177 and 213) or your drawing of a labyrinth placed at eye level can help strengthen your concentration and ability to cope with pain.

AROMATHERAPY

Aromatherapy can increase your feelings of well-being during labor. Dip a towel into cool rosewater with a few drops of lavender, and wipe your forehead, face, and neck with it. A little aromatherapy oil goes a long way: put one drop of aromatherapy oil in a dispenser or on a cotton ball; breathing in the fragrant scent will send you away from the pain.

Relieve tension
with peppermint, rosemary, lavender, or clary sage.

Enhance labor and open your cervix
with lavender, myrrh, jasmine, or geranium rose.

DOING THE NEXT BEST THING

Doing the next best thing without comparing it to what you wanted or expected, and without second-guessing yourself is a quality of a Birth Warrior and a hallmark of Birthing From Within. In the midst of the intense experience of birthing, you can only make decisions based on what you know and feel in the moment. So commit yourself to laboring passionately in the direction of your intentions while not being attached to a specific plan or outcome.

"When you go into a tight place and everything goes against you until it seems that you cannot hold on for a minute longer, never give up then, for that is just the place and time that the tide will turn."

—HARRIET BEECHER STOWE[37]

This practice is very difficult for many people to fully grasp. The idea of not knowing what to do until the moment arrives can seem passive and risky. And yet, in truth it is spontaneous, mindful, and energizing; it is the ultimate manifestation of trusting yourself. Even if you had a general plan before starting out, being willing and flexible enough to change course when necessary takes courage and self-love.

Don't let a detour stop you

If you find yourself in a cascade of decision-making (for instance, during an induction or long labor), it will be impossible to avoid thinking and analyzing. As a Birth Warrior, gather the necessary information, make the decisions, then recommit to doing whatever coping practices have been working for you. A supportive birth environment featuring privacy, warmth, darkness, and a partner's loving touch and words of encouragement can help you return to the trance of Laborland.

Fathers and birth partners: You'll want to read the e-book *Field Guide to Laborland.*

KEY TO THE ANCIENT MAP OF LABOR: KEEP GOING

Giving birth is a mystery; some aspects are unknowable. After filling your Gathering Basket with tips on how to navigate your way through Laborland, be sure to leave some space for self-discovery, intuitive flashes, and surprises. When you come to that inevitable threshold where you think you don't know what to do, do something and see what happens.

THROUGH
THE SEVEN GATES

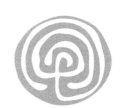

In the story "Inanna's Descent," the warrior queen encountered seven gates. In old legends and myths, wherever there is a gate there is the promise of something valuable behind it. As a Birth Warrior, think of each gate as an invitation to know and value yourself more deeply.

Because birth is a rite of passage, you will pass through many gates as you move through the twisting pathways of your Laborinth. Imagine that each turn reveals a gate where you meet something unexpected. It might be a moment you could not have anticipated, like a sudden encounter with the Birth Fairy, or a new sensation, perspective, or insight.

Before birth, you cannot know or choose the gates you will encounter, the order in which you will pass through them, or how you will respond to each one. An essential task of a Birth Warrior is to accept this. Once you do, you begin to let go of attachment to specific outcomes or "getting it right." Instead of trying to strategize to avoid gates of doubt, fear, or difficulty, cultivate

The Significance of Seven

The number seven symbolizes:

Initiation

Learning

Hardship

Determination

Wisdom

a mindset of flexibility, taking action, coping, and self-love. A rite of passage, by nature, brings you to your knees—that is, to the edge. By passing through the gates, you develop a wisdom that cannot be gained in any other way.

No one can predict how any woman will respond, emotionally or physically, to unexpected events while giving birth. What is surprising, upsetting, or difficult for one woman may not be for another because her preparation, expectations, knowledge, support, and belief system will have created within her a different way of perceiving and reacting to the gates she encounters.

Let's explore some of the different kinds of gates in Laborland. A woman who is overconfident may eventually find herself at the Gate of Doubt. A woman who anticipates conflict with hospital staff but then has a kind, helpful nurse may find herself at the Gate of Mercy or the Gate of Gratitude. A woman who meets the very thing she's been hoping to avoid may find herself at the Gate of the Tiger. In transition, almost every woman finds herself at the Gates of Holy F#%ki*g Terror and Great Determination.

Initiation begins when you decline the temptation to remain comfortable, safe, or nice. It begins the moment you decide that, whatever the price—personal loss, time, money, relationship, blood, sweat, or tears—you will do the "One Forbidden Thing."[1]

The threshold is either outward beyond the horizon or inward under the surface. You cross a threshold when you do the One Forbidden Thing.

—JOSEPH CAMPBELL

In hero myths and stories, the protagonist faces a moment when he or she must break the rules to go on. Perhaps she is warned not to eat or drink anything in the other world, but she does it anyway. Bluebeard warns his bride not to open a certain door, but she opens it anyway. If the heroine is cautious or follows the rules, she remains a Good Girl, unchanged—end of story. But if she is a Birth Warrior, she does the One Forbidden Thing, even if she is terrified or faces uncertain consequences. Her journey continues, her soul grows, and rebirth is assured. That is what makes a Great Story.

As you cross each threshold, the gate fades away and the path opens in front of you. Nearing the center of the Laborinth, there is a mounting sense that something deep within you is forever changing—there is no turning back.

> Upon passing through the
> Seventh Gate,
> Inanna was humbled and
> bowed low.

TASKS OF PREPARATION

Carolina Quintana, one of our dedicated mentors in Guadalajara, Mexico, understands the importance of preparing women for their inner journey through labor. She recounted this story of transformation:

> Sofia, a pregnant woman began leaving childbirth class before she had finished her mariposa (butterfly) mandala. I spoke to her by the door, "You can leave. But you need to understand that making a mariposa mandala is like labor. It takes time. You finish when you are finished." Sofia thought this over, went back to her seat, and continued working until her mandala was complete. After giving birth, she told me that finishing the mandala taught her something about herself: like the butterfly who cannot rush her transformation in the cocoon, she, too, had to be patient and keep working—however long it took—until it was finished.

Like Sofia, when building stamina, endurance, and patience for labor, find ways to do what you have been avoiding or to finish projects that are hard for you.

GATES OF BIRTH

Imagine the gates you may be facing or passing through in Laborland, or ones you have already crossed in your childbearing year. Paint, draw, or sculpt one or more gates, or sketch seven gates within your Laborinth. What or who is behind, around, or in front of each gate? If you wish, add a guardian, a gatekeeper, a symbol for the price of passage, or a treasure that lies beyond each one.

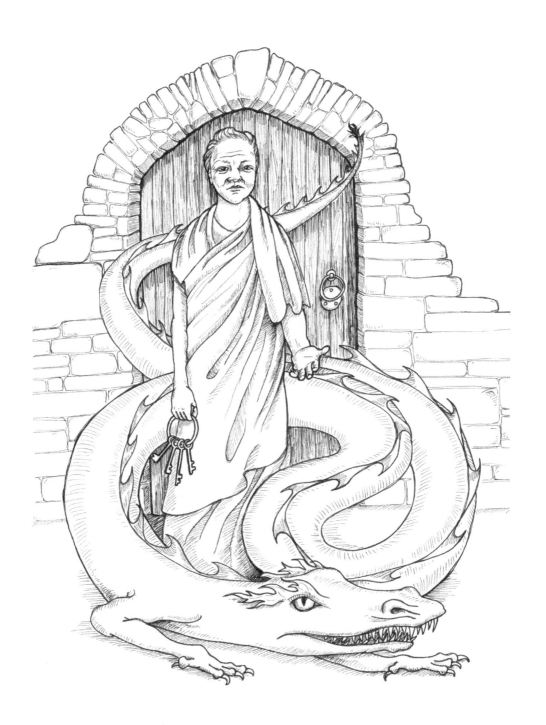

29

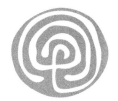

The Gatekeeper

In old stories and fairy tales, a gatekeeper guards the entrance to important realms, often containing hidden treasure. He appears in such forms as a three-headed dog, a dragon, a magical being, or a human. Whatever forms the gatekeeper and the gate take, they mirror part of your psyche and story.

In the story "Inanna's Descent," Inanna was a woman of power. In the upper world, she was a warrior queen who had seven temples and was successful in the arts of assertion, persuasion, and achieving her goals. Her skills, power, and knowledge, however, were tested as she descended to the underworld, for in a rite of passage everything that is known and valued is called into question. During her journey, Inanna encountered Bidu the Gatekeeper. Let's look at their relationship and how it is relevant to your journey as a Birth Warrior.

Bolting the Gates

When Inanna arrived in the underworld, Bidu bolted the seven gates. Locked gates represent obstacles in mind or circumstance that the Warrior must overcome to reach the goal and complete the rite of passage. Bolting the gates is a symbolic gesture of compassion to slow down an eager initiate, to pace her descent.

When circumstances force you to pause before a "bolted gate," rather than thinking you are stuck and not making progress know that beneath the surface you are growing the strength, resolve, and understanding needed to descend further into the unknown and complete your rite of passage to grow into your emerging role as Mother.

> To turn her attention inward, Bidu asked Inanna two soul-searching questions:
>
> "Who are you?" and "Why has your heart led you to this place from which you will not return unchanged?"

Your inner Gatekeeper is on duty when:

- You face a threshold and meet the unknown

- Your habit mind, rigid beliefs, or emotional patterns block access to the treasure you seek

- Your readiness and resolve are tested to ensure that you are ready for the riches that lie beyond

- You decide it is time to bust through the Gate and go for it

The Gatekeeper abides within you. Your birth attendant is not a Gatekeeper. Do not equate a nurse with Bidu just because she takes your clothes and puts them in a bag or denies you something that is on your birth plan. Yet these unwanted moments become threshold moments when the Gatekeeper within inquires, "Who am I without my robe? Who am I when my birth plan is not followed? Who am I when birth doesn't follow my plan?"

WHO OR WHAT UNBOLTS THE GATE?

It is never someone else who has the "key" or authority to unbolt a gate of birth. The gate is within you, and so is the key. When your inner eye opens, when your heart expands, when your fist opens to release fear or attachment to a long-held belief—a locked gate begins to open.

In the Greek myth of Psyche and Eros, Aphrodite commands the pregnant and abandoned Psyche to gain the strength she needs by accomplishing four tasks, the last of which is to single-handedly retrieve beauty ointment hidden in the underworld. Fearful of dying in the underworld, Psyche is told to bring two cakes with her to help ensure her return. Guarding the ointment is Cerberus, a three-headed dog. Psyche throws him one cake, allowing her to enter the cave to retrieve the ointment; to escape, she throws Cerberus the other cake. Emerging from the underworld more conscious of her abilities, Psyche enters a new phase in her life.

Unbolting the gate of birth is a task also associated with the Hindu deity Ganesha, a Gatekeeper who dwells in thresholds. He is invoked at the beginning of new endeavors because he destroys vanity and pride. In his left hand is a prod he uses to push away obstacles; in his right hand, a rope for lassoing difficulties. With his huge ears, he hears prayers. In his trunk, he holds a sweet delicacy symbolizing the joy of self-discovery.[1]

THE PRICE OF PASSAGE

To receive the treasure (such as, wisdom, compassion, a child), the Gatekeeper exacts a price: The

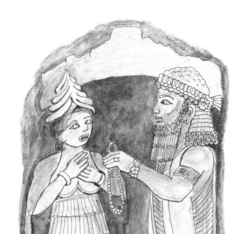

*At the Second Gate,
Bidu took from Inanna her
necklace.*

*Inanna protested,
"What is this?"*

*Bidu answered,
"Quiet, Inanna. The ways of
the underworld are perfect
and may not be ques-
tioned."*

Warrior must part with something of value. It is this exchange and willingness to sacrifice that creates the energy and momentum required to open and pass through the gate. This is how the Maiden evolves into the Warrior Mother.

Like most of us, Inanna wanted to receive all the benefits of her journey without having to give anything in return. She assumed she could keep her *mehda** (her crown, lapis bead necklace, breastplate, robe, beliefs, plans, and lapis measuring rod)—all the valuable things she carried to announce her royal status and protect her from difficulties in the underworld—without having to sacrifice anything.

Nonetheless, at each gate Bidu took one thing from Inanna, lifting from her the trappings of innocence and beliefs she no longer needed to complete her journey. Each time, the proud queen protested, "It isn't fair! Give it back!" Gate by gate, Bidu reminded Inanna that the ways of the underworld, of Laborland, are ancient and may not be questioned.

*In exchange for giving up (or losing) something as you pass through
the gates of Laborland, in this rite of passage your Birth Warrior
is awakened and you give birth to a child.*

A TASK OF PREPARATION

*Seven Mehda from the Cradle of Civilization
to Your Baby's Cradle*

Make a list of seven birth *mehda* you are gathering—
things you hope will protect and sustain you in labor. Some
will be tangible, like special clothing, jewelry, or objects you
plan to bring or wear (such as a birth plan, music playlist, or
aromatherapy oils). *Mehda* can also be intangible (such as attitudes and deeply held convictions and beliefs like pride, suffering in silence, or ladylike self-control).

For each of your seven *mehda* write a sentence describing
the power or value it provides in helping you achieve your
goals in birth. The meaning could be positive, negative, or a little of both.

Next, imagine that at one of the gates in Laborland Bidu (or circumstance) seizes one of your prized
birth *mehda*. Imagine how you might respond. Like
Inanna, you might first resist, demanding, "What
is this? Give it back!"

Now ask yourself, "In the absence of this birth
mehda, who am I?"

> "Janie stood where he left her for
> unmeasured time and thought.
> She stood there until something
> fell off the shelf inside her. Then she
> went to see what it was."
>
> —ZORA NEALE THURSTON[2]

*After Inanna lost all her worldly possessions,
her mehda of power and protection,
what remained that could not be taken?*

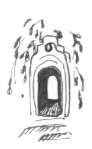

OPTIMAL POSITIONS IN LABOR

As you navigate through Laborland, progress can more readily be made when you are moving and in optimal positions. So "don't just lie there like a latke," as a woman at a workshop admonished. Take one small step at a time, both psychologically and physically.

For generations our dominant image of labor was of a woman being confined to a hospital bed. Even if you don't agree with it, or hope to escape it, the first thing you will be asked to do upon admission to a hospital is get in bed and lie still so the baby can be monitored. But there are other, more optimal positions for labor, as expressed in the following story about alternative birth positions.

Meria gave birth to her three children at home with a midwife. The first time, she gave birth on her back, which was more painful than she had expected. So when she became pregnant with her second child she sought advice from her grandmother Meta, a German immigrant who still lived in the house in which she had birthed and raised her children.

Meria's grandmother told her that in 1919 she, too, had given birth lying on her back and also found it very painful. During her second pregnancy, Meta asked her midwife for advice, and her midwife said, "Stand up." So during that labor Meta pushed while standing and holding on to her buffet—and she found it was much easier and less painful. Like her own midwife, Meta advised Meria to "stand up and hold on to your buffet."

As it happened, Meria had a buffet much like her grandmother's, about four feet high by six feet long, with drawers to hold silver and dishes. She recounted:

> A table could be a bit too low to lean on in labor, but the buffet was just right! I was up and about in labor. It was only two hours before the urge to push came. I held on to the buffet and pushed, then walked away and pushed in a squatting position, and finally pushed holding on to my husband… and my baby was born! It was the easiest and least painful of my three births. During my next birth, the midwife made me lie down to deliver the baby, and it hurt much more.

Baby Not Engaged?
Try Walcher's Position

Baby has to get into the pelvis to get through the pelvis.

To be born, a baby first has to drop down into the pelvis. For a first-time mother, often this happens days or weeks before labor starts. If when labor begins the baby is "high" or "not engaged," this does not necessarily mean that he is in an abnormal position or too big. However, it does mean that his head will not be pressed against the cervix, which could cause dilation to take longer and increase the mother's chance of having a cesarean.

As early as the 1600s, midwives observed this problem and discovered a position that would help a baby move down into the birth canal.[1] This position was written about as early as 1795 in Venice,

Gail Tully, of Spinning Babies, uses the "Three Sisters" techniques to get babies to drop and engage: "sifting" (using a rebozo), a side-lying release, and an inversion. Refer to her website for instructions and illustrations.

but it did not become popular until the late 1800s when Dr. Walcher in Germany wrote about it, and consequently the position was named after him.

If you are in labor and you know your baby hasn't "dropped" yet, try Walcher's position to encourage your baby to move down past the pelvic rim: lying on your back on a bed, let your legs hang off the bed unsupported so that the weight of your legs increases the diameter of the pelvis at the inlet. Your buttocks should be aligned with the edge of the bed. Sustain this position for three consecutive contractions.[2]

UPRIGHT POSITIONS
Standing Up

Standing up during contractions allows your hips to release tension and move in a variety of ways, from micro-movements to a full range of motion. Circle your hips, do figure eights, or rock your pelvis forward and backward or from right to left while leaning over furniture or a birth ball. Turn on some music, and sway to the rhythm. With both hands, grasp a long cloth belt (like a yoga strap or martial arts belt) looped over a door (figure 30.1), then go up and down into half-squats; this lifts your rib cage and increases space between your ribs and pelvis, which gives your baby room to spin. You can also accomplish this while being suspended by the strong arms of a birth companion (figure 30.2).

Sitting Upright in Optimal Maternal Posture

Sitting upright provides rest for your legs and still gives you the benefits of gravity. When you sit upright in a chair, on a birth ball, or on the edge of a bed— with your hips higher than your knees—your diaphragm can move, allowing you to breathe freely. Rest your feet flat on the floor or on a stool so you don't have to tense your psoas and abdominal muscles to keep your balance.

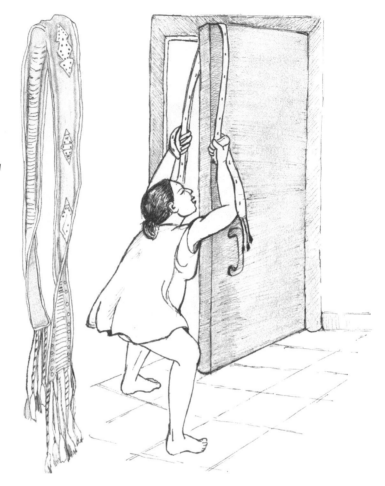

Figure 30.1

Sitting on a Toilet

Sitting on a toilet, facing in either direction, is good place to be in labor because you benefit from privacy and gravity, and it is a place where you already know how to release and let go. When you are laboring on a toilet, your caregiver can still check in on you—and there is almost always enough time to give birth elsewhere.

ON HANDS AND KNEES

On hands and knees in labor, you benefit from a full range of motion in your hips while releasing tension in your back, abdomen, and thighs. This position also facilitates use of touch, back massage, counterpressure on the sacrum, hip squeeze, and being gently rocked with a rebozo. Being on hands and knees can help rotate a baby in posterior position into a more favorable occiput anterior position (see pages 252–253). Between contractions, try draping your body over a birth ball or peanut ball to help you rest and relieve pressure on your wrists.

SQUATTING

Near the end of dilation and while pushing, women who are walking or standing will naturally go up and down between standing and half-squats. This releases the psoas and makes more room in the pelvis. Rather than stay in a squatting position after the contraction is over, rest your legs by standing up or sitting on the edge of a chair. Avoid a deep squat, where your knees are higher than your hips, because this may close your pelvis a bit and also tighten your perineum, increasing the chance of tearing during pushing.

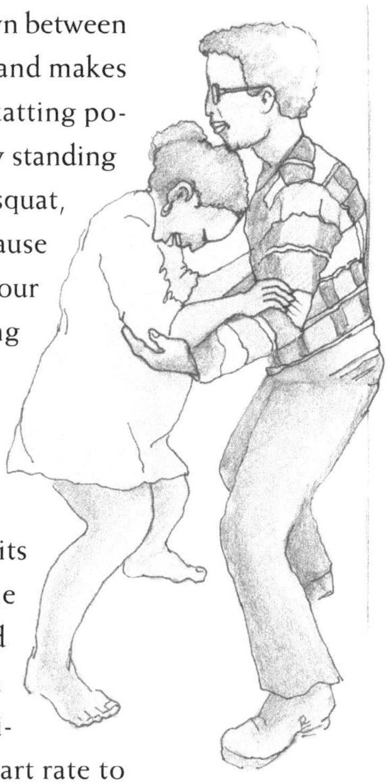

OPTIMAL POSITIONING IN BED

When a laboring mother lies on her back, the natural shape of the pelvis is compressed, decreasing its diameter by as much as an inch. In addition, the weight of the baby can put pressure on major blood vessels (aorta and vena cava), decreasing oxygen flow to mother and baby—which may lead to dizziness and shortness of breath, and cause baby's heart rate to drop. For this reason, when pregnant and laboring women must be in bed they are encouraged to lie on their sides or to recline.

Figure 30.2

SIDE LYING USING A PEANUT BALL

In one study, the labors of women who used a peanut ball were ninety minutes shorter than the control group; pushing stage was twenty-three minutes shorter, and cesarean section rates were reduced by 13 percent.[3] A side-lying position is ideal when you need to rest, when labor progress

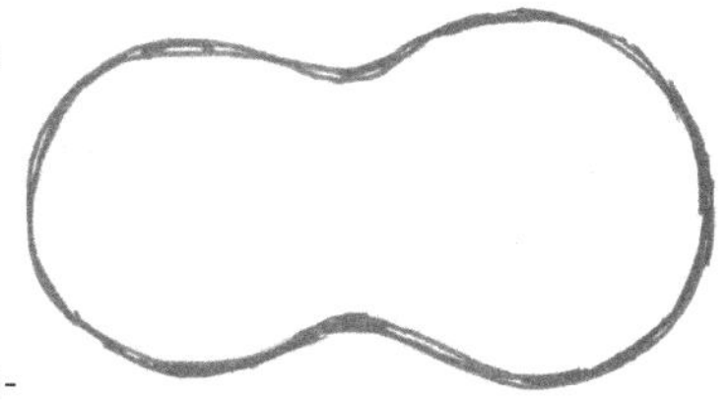

40–45 centimeters

has slowed down, or after an epidural when you can't get up. When positioned with a peanut ball between your legs, your psoas releases, thus opening your pelvic diameter and making more room for your baby to rotate and descend. (If your hospital or doula does not have a peanut ball, use a stack of pillows between your legs to release the psoas and help your baby out.) Position your top leg forward and over the dip in the ball, and extend your bottom leg back. Or reverse this so your bottom leg is positioned forward and your top leg is back (figure 30.3). Turn from side to side every thirty to sixty minutes. You can also use the ball to support your upper body while kneeling over it; in this position you can then rock back and forth on the ball, and even push.

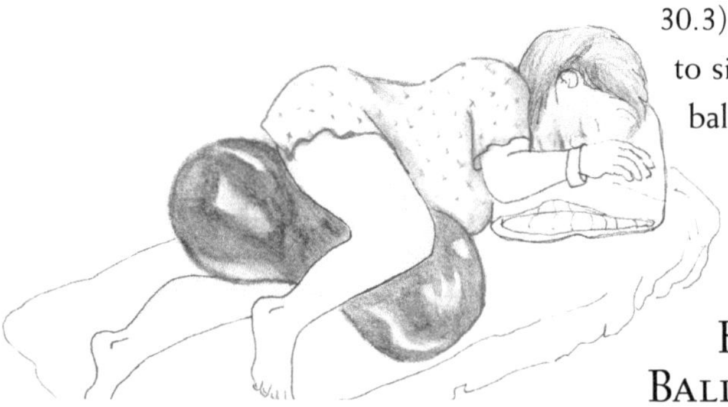

Figure 30.3

HOW TO USE A PEANUT BALL WHEN LYING ON YOUR BACK

Most women find lying on their backs more painful during contractions. However, if you are in this position because it feels right to you (and not because someone told you to lie on your back) try putting a peanut ball under your knees to help release your psoas and increase comfort.

Avoid Reclining

Half-sitting up, or reclining, does not provide the same benefits as being upright or lying on your side. Reclining increases the pressure on the sacrum and immobilizes the normally mobile coccyx, thus decreasing the mobility and diameter of the pelvis. It also prevents the pubic arch from widening (figure 30.4).

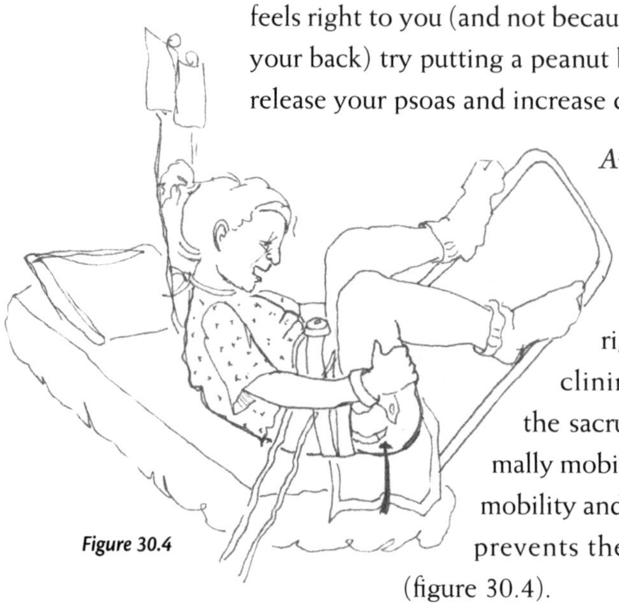

Figure 30.4

POSITIONING YOUR MIND FOR LABOR

Ultimately, the exact positions you are in during labor matter less than changing positions regularly. Changing positions (especially to upright or active postures) can increase the power and effectiveness of contractions. And yet, in spite of all your prenatal learning about the benefits of being active and in upright positions, when labor is actually underway part of you may want to maintain a comfortable position in bed or in the bath to avoid stimulating new or more intense sensations. Whether or not this occurs, let go of the notion that changing positions will make you comfortable, or that the goal is comfort. In fact, often it is an uncomfortable position that leads to labor progress. Your doula and birth companion may need to encourage you to "keep moving" in order to keep labor moving.

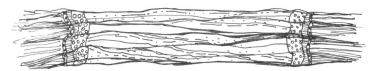

The Traditional, Versatile Rebozo

For three centuries, the rebozo, a long piece of cloth, has been used to bundle up newborns close to the heart; to carry older children, bundles of merchandise, or other goods on the back; and as an essential part of the traditional wardrobe of Mexican women. An excerpt from a poem by Ricardo López Méndez describes the many uses of a rebozo:

This section was written by Carolina Quintana de Oropeza and Leticia Loza, Certified Birthing From Within Mentors in Guadalajara, Mexico.

Cuando fuiste niña cubrió tu cabeza
Y entrabas al templo con el a rezar
Cuando fuiste novia cubrió tu belleza
Y enjugó tu llanto si te vio llorar

When you were a little girl, it covered your head
And you entered the church with it to pray
When you were a bride, it covered your beauty
And wiped away your tears if it saw you cry

Tu rebozo madre, me sirvió de cuna
Se inició en tus hombros, como en un trigal,
Con el me cubriste del sol a la luna,
El era mi cielo y era mi jacal . . .

Your rebozo, Mother, was a crib for me
It started on your shoulders, like in a wheatfield
With it you covered me from the sun and the moon
It was my heaven and my hut . . .[4]

For centuries the rebozo has also been used by *parteras* (midwives) during labor to relieve pain or to help the baby move into the best position. These movements are known as *sobadas* and *manteadas*, a combination of massaging and movements done with the rebozo. Several years ago Doña Queta, a *partera* from the ethnic group of the Zapotecs of Oaxaca, started transmitting her knowledge to midwives, childbirth educators, and doulas. Some time after, Guadalupe Trueba, a childbirth educator and midwife with years of experience and one of our mentors, made videos showing how to use the rebozo during labor.[5]

Guadalupe Trueba's video and others demonstrating use of the rebozo during labor are available on YouTube.

In our classes at Magenta Educacion Perinatal, we always have rebozos at hand. This allows future fathers to experiment and learn various ways to comfort their partner before and during labor.

Here are just a few of the ways to use a rebozo during labor:

- With the mother on hands and knees, leaning over a birth ball or a chair, wrap a rebozo around her belly. Stand behind her and hold each end of the rebozo, then rhythmically rock her belly from side to side. The woman can offer feedback on how slow or fast she likes it.

- With the mother sitting on a chair or ball, place a warm

rice pack or an ice pack on her lower back, then wrap the
rebozo around her body and tie it.

- To help induce a deeply relaxing state: fold the rebozo in
  half lengthwise, and spray or sprinkle a few drops of
  aromatherapy oil on the fringe. With the mother lying
  comfortably on her side, slide the rebozo slowly over her
  body—from head to toe—while shaking it; the light touch
  of the fabric helps release tension. Do this several times.
  Then cover her with the aromatherapy-scented rebozo
  while she continues to rest.

- To help the mother focus her attention inward or to release
  a headache, wrap a rebozo snugly around her head,
  covering her eyes and ears to shut out distractions. She can
  lean on her partner or doula, or be lying down.

- Enhance childbirth preparation by using a rebozo with
  Birthing From Within mindfulness practices during "ice
  contractions."

In recent years, a modern version of the rebozo called *fulares*
has emerged. It is longer than a regular rebozo and is used as
a sling to carry babies. So now we also have a monthly session
called Rebozarte, where parents-to-be and new parents bring
their babies to learn different ways of using the *fular* and share
with other parents the joys and difficulties of parenthood.

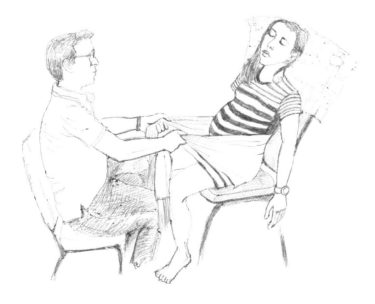

WHAT TO DO FOR STALLED LABOR AND BACK LABOR

A long labor, often with back pain, that eventually stalls and then involves medical management (Pitocin augmentation, epidural, or cesarean)— the "labor from hell"— is traumatizing, especially for parents who are unpreprepared for certain events, intense pain, or lots of technology. Fortunately there is usually something less interventive to try in the face of a challenging labor.

Midwives and birthing women have long explored practical ways to deal with the problems of stalled labor and back labor. Today, however, if labor is slow birth attendants are more inclined to suggest drugs and interventions. This is when you need to call on your inner Birth Warrior. She won't tell you that you failed somehow or that there is nothing more you can do; instead, she would ask, "If there is one small thing I could do to help my baby out, what would it be?" She would review the age-old wisdom and make one more effort. In so doing, even if the baby does not rotate, descend, and slip out, you will know you did your best, and that may give you some peace of mind.

Back labor occurs when the pain during contractions is felt in the lower back rather than in the lower abdomen. It was once thought that back labor was only caused by a baby lying in the face-up, or occiput posterior (OP), position, which presses the back of the baby's head, the occiput, into the mother's sacrum during labor (figure 31.1). However, women may also experience back labor with a baby in the more common face-down, or occiput anterior (OA), position (figure 31.2).

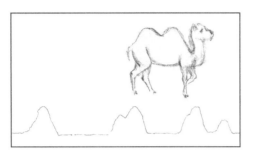

Some women experience "camelback" contractions. Before a contraction completely ends, another one, usually less strong, begins, making the double contraction about ninety seconds in duration.

Babies can rotate in unpredictable ways over the course of labor. The baby's head tilts and turns as she makes her way through the birth canal, navigating the angles and planes of the pelvis. At the time of birth, most babies are in the more favorable OA position. For babies who are in the OP position at birth, over two-thirds were not in the OP position at the onset of labor.[1] Of the 15 to 30 percent of babies who begin labor in the OP position, less than 5 percent are still OP at the time of birth,[2] suggesting that early efforts taken to help such babies rotate may be successful.

MORE TIDBITS FOR YOUR BACK LABOR BASKET

When a baby is in the OP position, her head may not be well applied to the cervix. This may cause contractions to be irregular and short, slowing progress to active labor. Women in this situation might experience "false" labor or a prolonged prodromal labor, both of which can lead to discouragement and exhaustion. If action is not taken early in labor to help the baby rotate, the slow pace of labor may result in interventions, such as epidural, Pitocin augmentation, or cesarean.

Try the following measures to get a jump-start on coping with back labor and increase the chances of your baby rotating into an optimal position (and speeding up a slow labor):

Leave the bag of water intact. Sometimes providers will artificially rupture the bag of water in an attempt to speed up labor. The bag of water provides a cushion between the baby's head and the cervix, which may allow the baby's head to spin more easily and thus be advantageous when a baby is in the OP position. If the water breaks before the baby rotates to the OA position, the sudden descent of the baby's head, which accompanies the release of amniotic fluid, might lock the baby into a persistent posterior position or possibly result in a deep transverse arrest.* This leads to prolonged, nonprogressing labor and may necessitate a cesarean. It is common, with a baby in the OP position, for the bag of water to release before labor starts, but if your bag of water is still intact it is best to leave it this way.

Try knee-chest position. In her book *The Labor Progress Handbook*, Penny Simkin describes this position as a good one to try if labor stalls, with or without back pain.[3] Get on your knees, lean forward, and lower your chest to the bed (figure 31.3). Your knees should be only hip-width apart. In this position, the distance between the pubic bone and sacrum widens. Use lots of pillows for support, including one under your knees. Maintain knee-chest position for approximately forty-five minutes or as long as you can tolerate it.[4]

In knee-chest position, the baby can slide back out of the pelvis up to a centimeter, an important occurrence if the baby's head has been "jammed" in the pelvis in a less than optimal position (asynclitic* or posterior). This position can also decrease an early urge to push. If there is an anterior lip* or swollen cervix, tipping forward can move the baby off the cervix during contractions, which helps reduce the swelling and facilitates completing dilation. Helping the baby "back up" while contractions become stronger and more regular and the pelvic outlet opens, gives the baby's head a "second chance" to rotate into a more optimal position. In addition, knee-chest position can reduce back pain while allowing your birth companion to massage your back or apply counterpressure to your sacrum. When you get out of this position, you can further assist rotation of your baby by lying on your side, or getting up and leaning over a table, or taking a warm, relaxing shower.

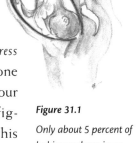

Figure 31.1

Only about 5 percent of babies are born in occiput posterior position.

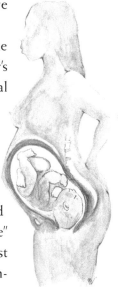

Figure 31.2

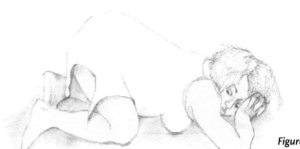

Figure 31.3

Try side-lying position. Lie on your left side, with two pillows or a peanut ball under your bent right knee with your left leg extended straight down.

Use a peanut ball (40–45 centimeters). When resting in bed or if you've had an epidural, use a peanut ball to lift your upper leg, which opens the pelvis and helps the baby rotate (see figure 30.3 on page 244). One study showed that among women who used a peanut ball, compared with those who did not, the first stage of labor was shorter by ninety minutes and the second stage was half as long.[5]

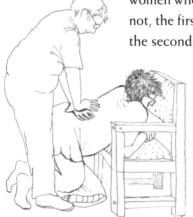

Figure 31.4

Try hands-and-knees position. This position uses gravity and the weight of your baby's body to help spin him to an OA position. You may experience some degree of relief when on hands and knees, because your baby's head will put less pressure directly onto your sacrum. It is also easier for your birth companion to massage or apply counterpressure to your sacrum or hips (figure 31.4).

Do labor lunges. Put one foot on a chair or stool, off to one side. Keep your other foot flat on the floor. During contractions, rock gently from center toward the bent leg (figures 31.5 and 31.6).

Avoid lying-flat or reclining-backward positions. When a mother lies on her back or reclines in bed, her baby's occiput rests on her sacrum, with the baby's weight pressing along her back (figure 31.7). If she remains like that for any period of time, gravity can hold the baby in the OP position, preventing him from rotating to an OA position. Furthermore, back labor is extremely painful when the mother is semi-reclined or lying

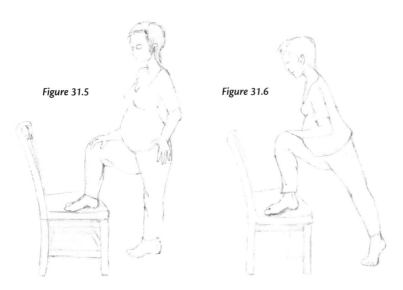

Figure 31.5   *Figure 31.6*

flat. This may increase her desire for an epidural, thereby starting her down a slippery slope of decreased mobility, less ability to use the positions that favor rotation, and consequently, less opportunity for the baby to rotate with gravity and movement.

TEN ABDOMINAL LIFTS

In her book *Back Labor No More*, Janie McCoy King explains why abdominal lifting can be crucial in relieving back pain and helping labor progress when the baby is in the OP position.[6] Lifting the abdomen changes the alignment of the baby's head and body so that the force of contractions is directed along the center line of the baby's head and body down toward the cervix, instead of back toward the mother's spine (figure 31.8).

Figure 31.7

Place your hands on either side of your belly, slightly above your hips. When a contraction begins, let your hands follow the tightening of your uterus until the heels of your hands are in front of your hip bones. To prevent slipping, lock your fingers together under your belly. Now your hands are in position to lift your abdomen and pull it toward your spine during contractions (figure 31.9). Let your forearms do the lifting. Your upper arms should remain fairly still while your elbows serve as hinges. Do not lift by raising your shoulders or upper arms.

A vector is a straight line, like an arrow, possessing both force and direction. A force (contraction behind the baby's head) directed at an obstacle (sacrum) meets and creates pressure, resistance, and pain. When the baby's head and body are in alignment with the opening cervix and pelvis, the head does not meet bony resistance with a contraction. Therefore, you experience less pain and more progress. Author Janie McCoy King uses the analogy of thrusting your fist through open space: your fist has direction but meets no resistance, generating no pain. However, when thrusting your fist into a wall you will experience pain. This is why doing the abdominal lift and other position changes may help. When you change the direction of the baby, he can get past an obstruction and find his way down through the pelvis and

When the contraction is over, you can either relax or maintain the baby's new vector by continuing to lift and support your abdomen with your hands. A rebozo can also help secure the belly in this position. In her book *The Belly Mapping Workbook*, Gail Tully suggests repeating the lift for ten contractions.[8]

COMPASSIONATE EPIDURAL AND/OR CESAREAN

If you have tried all these positions and techniques and labor is still slow, you may be too exhausted to continue or unable to relax enough for your baby to accomplish her rotation. While it may be the last thing you planned or desired, a compassionate epidural may allow you to rest, hydrate, and relax. This, in turn, may help the cervix to dilate and your labor to progress. After a long, hard struggle, an epidural may enable you to birth vaginally. However, even after doing everything humanly possible, the baby may still not rotate and slip out, in

Figures 31.8 and 31.9

• Apply an ice compress or heating pad to your sacrum.

• Apply steady counterpressure on your sacrum or hips (figure 31.5).

which case a cesarean may be the answer. Do what needs to be done next and know that your baby's position or having back labor is not your fault.

OP and Epidurals
What's the link?

A positive correlation exists between a baby being in an OP position and the mother having an epidural and/or cesarean. However, there is insufficient evidence to say for certain what is cause and what is effect. Does having an epidural make mothers more likely to have a posterior baby? Or does having a baby in OP position, which often entails a longer and possibly more painful labor, make it more likely for mothers to request an epidural?[10, 11] Most likely, both factors are at play. Many people believe that women given an early epidural may not feel the pain of back labor and therefore might not have the instinct or ability to change position.

Furthermore, epidurals cause a profound relaxation of the pelvic floor muscles, which otherwise provide a necessary resistance against which the baby's head can spin. Think of the pelvic floor as a funnel guiding the baby's head into position. Being immobilized in bed, combined with relaxation of the pelvic floor muscles, may lead to a posterior or transverse arrest.

Modern management has begun to eclipse the old knowledge of midwives and birthing women about how to solve the problems of stalled labor and back labor; yet we can still benefit from modern medical support when our own efforts are not enough. Here is another example of building a bridge between the ancient map and the terrain of modern birth.

When a baby is OP at the beginning of pushing, there is a significant increase in the odds for use of a vacuum extractor or birth by cesarean.[9] To avoid either outcome, do what you can to help your baby rotate early in labor.

Cephalo-pelvic disproportion (CPD) is a term is used when birth attendants believe that "failure to progress" in labor is due to the baby's head being too big to fit or turn in the mother's bony pelvis. It's a touchy subject in the birth world, as it cannot be an absolute diagnosis (often a mother who gives birth by cesarean for CPD later gives birth vaginally to an even bigger baby).

Labors that are slow or seem to stop progressing are frequently attributed to CPD. However, other factors, often ignored or downplayed, also impact the pace of labor, such as a stressful environment, fear, immobility due to electronic fetal monitoring or standard hospital protocol, dehydration, and "the clock." Since there is no billing code for complications due to these factors, care providers tend to blame the mother—either her bones, her baby (CPD), or her uterine contractions.

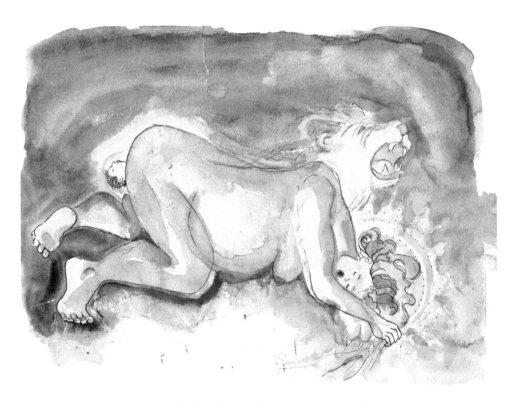

Pam England, Pushing Lucien Out © 1990, *watercolor*

32

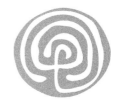

PUSHING BABY OUT

It seems like pushing should be absolutely natural and intuitive, and sometimes it is. Lots of variables will shape your experience of pushing. Get your Gathering Basket—it is time to harvest essential pointers for pushing your baby into the world.

Pushing begins after the cervix is completely dilated and has moved out of the way. Transitioning from the first stage of labor (dilation) to the second stage (pushing) frequently goes unnoticed. More often, however, it feels like a hairpin turn in the labyrinth of birth when sensations and mood change dramatically and you pass through the Gate of Change.

THE PUSHING EXPERIENCE

After yielding to contractions for hours, you may suddenly find yourself responding to a primitive, uncontrollable urge to push, energized by a rush of adrenaline, possibly making you feel out of control. Yet some women do not feel a strong urge to push and need guidance from their birth attendant. Although some babies "slide out" with very little effort by the mother, pushing usually requires hard work on her part.

Most birth attendants will want to confirm, via a vaginal exam, that the cervix is completely dilated before a woman begins actively pushing. When the cervix has moved out of the way, contractions normally slow down from every two minutes to every three to five minutes, giving the woman time to catch her breath and rest between pushes.

The urge to push does not always come immediately after reaching complete dilation. Some women experience a natural "lull" in their labor at this point, which can last an hour or longer. Renowned childbirth educator and author Sheila Kitzinger calls this lull "the rest and be thankful stage."[1] A mother may be told she can wait until she feels the urge to push, in which case she might not have to push as long. Alternatively, the mother can start pushing even though she doesn't feel a strong urge to do so. If you have an epidural, you might wish to ask that it be turned down at this point so that you can tune in to your body's sensations of the need to push.

Figure 32.1

During the lull, your baby is inching his way down and wiggling his head into position. Before labor begins, your baby's skull bones are "like big pieces of a puzzle: they fit together, but they are not firmly attached"[2] (figure 32.1). As your baby moves down through the birth canal, his skull bones move closer together and may overlap a little to reduce the circumference of his head, a development called "molding" (figure 32.2). Molding does not hurt your baby or his brain, because compression in one direction is naturally balanced by expansion in another. But after birth your baby may have a "cone head" until the skull bones slide back into their normal position (figure 32.3).

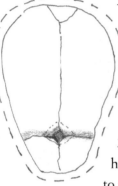

Figure 32.2

As a Birth Warrior, your willingness and intention will play a significant part in your pushing experience. Keep in mind, however, that other factors beyond your control will also influence turns in your labyrinth of birth, including length of labor, exhaustion, hydration, the strength of uterine contractions, your ability to try dif-

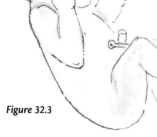

Figure 32.3

ferent positions, support from birth attendants, the structure of your pelvic bones, the position of your baby, and possibly his size.

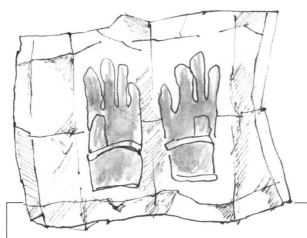

The second stage of labor consists of three seamless phases.

Phase one: The lull.

Phase two: The pelvic phase, identified by the strong urge to bear down.

Phase three: The perineal phase, or "crowning,"* associated with gentle pushing and the birth of the baby.

How gloves changed birth

The first pair of rubber gloves that could be sterilized repeatedly was produced in 1890 by Goodyear Tire and Rubber Company for Johns Hopkins University. In 1964, an Australian rubber company began mass-producing disposable latex gloves. This invention of disposable exam gloves changed birth in our culture, as they allowed for vaginal exams during labor with less risk of transferring germs between the mother and birth attendant.

Before such gloves were invented, no one knew exactly when a woman's cervix was completely dilated. Birth attendants and practitioners would wait for the mother to begin pushing, at which point they would assume her cervix was fully dilated since she was feeling the urge to bear down. After the invention of disposable exam gloves (along with the concurrent introduction of the electronic fetal monitor and a significant increase in obstetric spinal and epidural anesthesia), our experience of the second stage of labor changed profoundly—for both birth attendants and mothers.

> Of course, disposable sterile and nonsterile exam gloves have made a positive contribution to medicine, surgery, and labor by greatly reducing the risk of infection. However, consider how this one invention shifted mother-directed pushing to authority-directed pushing simply because it allowed the birth attendant to know before the mother that she was completely dilated.

Push less, push more effectively

When allowed to push spontaneously, women naturally bear down two to four times during each contraction. Each effort lasts between one and six seconds. This is far different from directed pushing, during which women are coached to hold their breath and push with force continuously for ten seconds, three times, during every contraction.

How Long to Push

In 1861, a doctor published his opinion that the pushing phase is dangerous for the baby. In declaring, without any evidence, that a mother should never push longer than two hours during labor, he established a mindset that has endured for over a century.[3] It has prompted generations of doctors to rush mothers with forceful pushing and to hurry the births of babies using forceps, episiotomy, vacuum extraction, and cesarean surgery. Fortunately this outdated, fear-based model, founded on the belief that pushing is risky, is now being questioned and reevaluated. Midwives have long been proponents of patience and watchful waiting; and now ACOG,* having looked carefully at the evidence, has recently updated its recommendations for how to manage pushing and how long it can safely take:

> Defining what constitutes an appropriate duration of the second stage is not straightforward because it involves a consideration of multiple short-term and long-term maternal and neonatal outcomes....Adverse neonatal outcomes generally have not been associated with the duration of the second stage of labor.[4]

Patience is becoming policy

Before arrest of labor* can be diagnosed in the second stage, multiparous* women should be allowed to push for at least two hours and first-time mothers for at least three hours. Many women push even longer, especially those with an epidural or with a baby who is not in an optimal position. This is not a problem as long as progress is being made.[5] To increase the number of vaginal births, doctors are also being encouraged to revive the lost arts of manually rotating baby's head and using forceps. Our hope is that eventually this new consensus statement will lead to real change in how pushing is seen and managed, decreasing cesareans for so-called second-stage arrest.[6]

PUSH WITH AN EMPTY BLADDER

When your baby is deep in the pelvis, his head may compress your bladder or urethra, making it difficult for you to fully empty your bladder. In labor, a woman can urinate every hour or two and still retain urine. To address this condition, try warm or cold "perineal showers" or putting your hand in running water. If over time your bladder becomes full like a water balloon, it can prevent your baby from descending and also increase pain during pushing. When the bladder is overdistended, the reflex to urinate becomes impaired, making it hard or even impossible for a mother to urinate. The next best thing to do at this point is utilize a single-use catheter to drain the urine and allow labor to progress normally.

USE GRAVITY TO HELP YOUR BABY OUT

Upright positions increase the diameter of the pelvic opening, harness the power of gravity, and strengthen uterine contractions so your baby can slide down and out more easily. In positions where

Distended Bladder

"I thought I was peeing, but I was just dribbling. I pushed and pushed for hours but made no progress. Finally, one of the midwives noticed a bulge above my pubic bone and realized my bladder was very full. She put in a catheter, and the pee just kept coming. There were 850 cc (just over three and a half cups) in there. Afterward, there was less pain with contractions, and every push made progress."

—GABRIELA

Get Up! Open Up!

When a laboring woman is in an optimal maternal position (a half-squat with her knees lower than her hips), her pelvic outlet is 28 percent greater than when she is lying on her back. Lying flat or reclining collapses the diameter of the pelvis one half inch to an inch![7]

Getting a little help from an experienced old bat!

Bats usually give birth hanging with their heads up and their feet down (which is upside down for them). On one occasion, Thomas Kunz, a biologist at Boston University, witnessed an inexperienced fruit bat struggling with labor while hanging in the wrong direction. A female bat (a bat midwife or doula) flew over to her and, for three hours, repeatedly "tutored" her by getting in the correct position for bat birth while imitating bearing down as if she were giving birth. The midwife bat also fanned the birthing bat with her wings and licked her, perhaps to cool and stimulate her. Finally the laboring bat got the message, turned around, and delivered her pup. Afterward, the assisting bat helped maneuver the pup into a nursing position.[8] Scientists have also observed midwifery—older females assisting younger mothers in birth—among Indian elephants, Afghan hunting dogs, and bottlenose dolphins.

your hips have full range of motion as you push, you may be able to find the exact position that is most effective for you and your baby. You can't know what your optimal pushing positions will be until you are in labor. Most women find that they try a variety of positions as pushing progresses and as the baby moves down through the birth canal.

Intuiting your pushing positions

Without an epidural, you may feel how even a slight shift in your position—leaning as little as an inch in one direction or the other—enhances the strength of each push. Of course, sometimes it all feels the same, and you just have to keep on pushing.

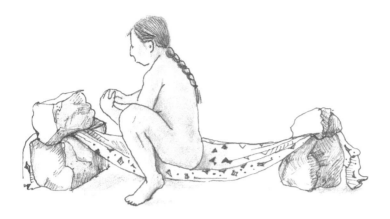

A woman in one of my childbirth classes who had lived in El Salvador described a birth hammock. The laboring mother squats over the hammock, and her child is born into its soft cloth.

Instinctively arching your back

During pushing, moving your hips backwards while arching your back may open your pelvis and help your baby move into a better position. Arching, rather than rounding, your back may be especially helpful with a baby in occiput posterior position. Women often instinctively do this while on hands and knees or squatting. If you are reclining in bed, placing a rolled towel under your sacrum will support your arched back through a few contractions. Be aware that birthing women are often told not to follow their instinct to arch their backs but instead to curl their backs inward, into a C curve. This is one way but not the only way.

> "I have noticed that when women are left to birth instinctively, they will often move from a squatting position, if they got into one, into a hands-and-knees position just before the head crowns. In forward-leaning positions, any tearing that occurs will usually be labial rather than vaginal. Labial tears sting like mad but heal well."
>
> —ROSANNA DAVIS
> LICENSED MIDWIFE, BFW MENTOR

Lying down

Although there is emphasis on upright positions due to their effectiveness, pushing while on your back can work. Lie down if you are tired or intuit that this is the right position for you. Women with epidurals always give birth lying on their backs or sides in bed. If you've watched the British TV show *Call the Midwife*, you might have been struck by the fact that most women in 1950s London (even at home with midwives) birthed while lying in bed. Side lying can be a good position—sometimes exactly what is needed—for slowing down pushing and for mothers who are confined to bed or are very tired.

On your hospital tour, the demonstration of how the fancy hospital bed breaks down may give the impression that the bed will allow you to get in a variety of positions; however, lying in any bed limits your freedom of movement and requires you to lie on your hip bones. When you are pushing while reclining in bed, you are sitting on your sacrum with your legs usually held up or resting in "leg rests." If you are pushing in bed, you can still get up on your hands and knees and have a full range of motion in your hips.

Early Urge to Push

I had this overwhelming urge to push and could not control it. I was excited that my time had come and I would soon see my baby. But my midwife kept telling me not to push because I wasn't completely dilated yet. I couldn't not push, and I didn't know what to do.

— Leslie

When a baby's head is deep in the pelvis (at +1 station or lower) before the cervix is completely dilated, the pressure can stimulate an early urge to bear down. At such times, sustained and rigorous pushing doesn't feel right, so a mother instinctively pushes gently at the peak of each contraction until she is fully dilated. There is little risk that short, grunty pushes will cause the cervix to swell. However, sometimes the reason a woman is told not to push is that her cervix has swollen or she has an anterior lip* around 9 centimeters dilation just before it's time to push. This is usually because the baby's head is in an occiput posterior position.

If it's important for you not to push, here are some things that can help you stop: changing position to decrease the pressure of the baby's head on your cervix (side lying, hands and knees, or knee-chest tilt), open-mouth panting or blowing, and having a support person at your side making eye contact to reassure you. Usually the need to resist the early urge to push is short-lived; with patience and change of position, swelling of the cervix is reduced or dilation becomes complete—and it's full steam ahead.

Birth Sounds

You may be surprised at the wonderfully primal sounds that come from the core of your being as you push and give birth. Hearing your unique birth sounds (moaning, grunting, growling) lets you know your baby is almost here. There's no right sound to make. Letting the sounds out lets your baby out. Don't allow social inhibitions—yours or anyone else's—to change the natural course of your birth.

What to Do When Your Baby Is Crowning

Women often intuitively alter their breathing and stop pushing (or push hard) as the baby's head crowns. The slow birth of your baby's head allows your perineum to gradually stretch as your baby moves down with each contraction. Pushing and birthing your baby's head between contractions slows the emergence of your baby.

Women who have an overwhelming urge to push vigorously as their baby is crowning may benefit from the guidance of a birth attendant who can remind them to pant or push gently. For others, however, being told when to push or stop pushing, to pant or "give little pushes" is distracting as they may prefer to tune in and push their babies out without guidance. If this approach works better for you, you (or your partner) may have to tell your birth attendant to be quiet so that you can find your own way.

When your baby's head is crowning, your birth attendant or companion can lubricate your perineum generously with oil. Be aware that not all hospitals provide oil, so consider bringing your own olive oil or any unscented oil to be sure that there is some available.

The best positions to decrease your chance of perineal tearing are being on hands and knees or lying on your side. These positions do not spread your thighs wide open and therefore do not stretch your perineum. Many people assume squatting is a great position for bringing the baby down during pushing, and indeed it can be; however, during crowning, the pelvic opening closes a bit while squatting with the knees higher than

Find out for yourself

Lie down on your back. Bend your knees and open your legs wide, pulling on your thighs to bring your knees back toward your chest; feel how your perineum tightens. Now close your legs a little and bring your feet to the floor; feel how much more "give" there is in your perineum when it is not stretched tight.

Note to Birth Partners

Sometimes a mother benefits from touching her baby's head while crowning and wants to do it, but she can't remember to do it or cannot get herself into a position to do it. So do your part to make this possible.

the hips, and there is more stress on the perineum, which can lead to prolapse of pelvic organs and more severe tearing.

Feel your baby emerge with each push

It may be helpful to reach down and feel how much each push is moving your baby so you will know how strongly or gently to push. Your partner or birth attendant can remind you to reach down and touch your baby's head. Some women are eager to do so, while others are so focused on the hard work of pushing that they choose not to.

Looking in a mirror

Some mothers enjoy watching the birth of their baby in a mirror. Others find it distracting. Most unmedicated women squeeze their eyes shut to help them concentrate while pushing.

PERINEAL SUPPORT

Part of birthing vaginally may include the perineum giving way a bit, ranging from superficial grazing (sometimes called a "skid mark") to tearing. Tearing can't always be prevented, even with optimal positions, oil, warm compresses, and pushing gently. Some factors that may make tearing more likely include a first baby, the unique architecture of the pelvic floor, the birth attendant's approach, and the size and position of the baby. One factor you may have some control over is your position when pushing. Lithotomy position (lying flat on the back with legs pulled back) and deep squatting tend to increase the likelihood and severity of tearing. A natural tear is usually less painful than an episiotomy, and it heals more quickly. But an episiotomy may be necessary when a baby needs to be born quickly or when forceps or a vacuum is used.

Steep decline in episiotomy

When *Birthing From Within* was published in the late 1990s, the episiotomy rate was about 70 percent in the United States. Since then, birth activists' efforts and increased cesareans have led to a dramatic decrease in episiotomies. In 2006, the national episiotomy rate was 12 percent.[9] Of course, episiotomy practices and rates vary widely from country to country, and even from practice to practice. Ask your care providers how often they perform episiotomies and what they do to protect the perineum during delivery.

Perineal massage

Gentle pushing and pouring oil over the perineum during crowning can help reduce tearing; massaging the perineum, on the other hand, probably will not make a difference. Perineal massage while the baby is descending can be very distracting, abrasive, and painful. If you don't like it, say so.

Directed Pushing ☺ Forceful Pushing ☺ "Purple Pushing"

When a woman is directed to hold her breath and push forcefully to the count of ten, capillaries in her eyes and face burst, causing a purple discoloration known colloquially as "purple pushing."

A woman who has seen directed or forceful pushing in the movies or on TV may assume this is how she must push to get her baby out: lying on her back with her knees pulled back, legs open, feet in the air, while a nurse takes on a cheerleading role, coaching her throughout each contraction by instructing her to take a deep breath and hold it, tuck her chin, and ""PUUUSH...1...2...3...4...5...6...7...8...9...10!" No mother would inflict purple pushing on herself; it is completely unnatural and can be disadvantageous for both baby and mother. Women who aren't coached during pushing, hold their breath for shorter periods of time and are just as effective.

When asked about their episiotomy philosophy and statistics, birth attendants' responses can be interesting. One OB, when asked about her approach to episiotomies, replied, "It depends."

"Depends on what?" the pregnant woman asked.

"It depends on if I've had a really bad tear with a patient. If so, I cut everybody until I get over it."

Waterbirth or warm, wet washcloths pressed firmly against your perineum can be soothing during crowning and can reduce the likelihood of tearing.

Researchers who completed a recent study on how to decrease tearing found, "The [hands-off] technique appeared to cause less perineal trauma and reduced rates of episiotomy. The hands-on technique resulted in increased perineal pain after birth and higher rates of postpartum haemorrhage."

—P. PETROCNIK AND J. E. MARSHALL[10]

Directed or Purple Pushing Defined

Directed pushing is also called "purple pushing" because the mother's face literally turns purple, her neck veins distend, and her eyes get bloodshot from bursting capillaries. The following day her face and chest are speckled with clusters of tiny purple or red spots (petechiae), indicative of oxygen deprivation.

Having a nurse in a cheerleading role coaching a mother through pushing may create feelings of anxiety and urgency, perhaps undermining her self-confidence. The tension that fills the room from the forceful counting to ten often makes a mother think that if she doesn't push as hard as she can her baby will not be born "in time" or be healthy or the doctor will resort to the use of vacuum extraction, forceps, or a cesarean. Also, forcefully holding her breath for ten to twelve seconds while bearing down causes the pressure around the mother's heart and lungs to increase above healthy levels and the amount of blood returned to her heart to decrease. In response, her heart pumps less blood to her uterus and placenta, causing her blood pressure to drop, which results in the baby receiving less oxygen.[11] Decreased oxygen may lead to a drop in fetal heart rate; once this happens, vacuum extraction, forceps, or cesarean may be used to save the baby. Babies born after purple pushing tend to have lower APGAR* scores.[12] Strenuous pushing can also interfere with the baby's descent and rotation.

In addition, purple pushing can cause mothers to experience sore muscles, fatigue, and psychological stress. Some mothers, exhausted from purple pushing, give up and say, "I just can't do this anymore!" Such a response may trigger more cheerleading ("Yes, you can! P-U-S-H!") or more interventions to finish the birth for her since prolonged forceful pushing increases pressure on the pelvic floor, which may cause the mother structural damage.[13] You can ignore prompts for directed pushing or tell your well-intentioned birth attendant to stop counting to ten. It is ultimately up to you.

PUSHING WITH AN EPIDURAL

Because an epidural numbs the legs and lower back, women given this form of pain relief cannot try upright or active positions for pushing and thus typically give birth lying in bed on their backs or sides. Although they usually do not feel much of an urge to push, sensing pressure during contractions may cue them to push. Women with epidurals are either directed to push strenuously or allowed to "labor down." Even when laboring down, when the baby is beginning to crown mothers are usually directed to pull their legs back and push forcefully. Read more about birthing with an epidural in chapter 35.

"BREATHING THE BABY OUT"

A prevailing idea in natural birth circles is "breathing the baby out." While there is value in having the mother tune in to her breath and allow the power of her uterine contractions to do their work, the phrase "breathing the baby out" often projects a narrow picture of what a mother should or should not do during pushing. Naïve first-time mothers may internalize a passive approach to their birth or think that all they need to do is "relax" for their baby to be born. There is also a risk that women will believe something is wrong with them if they feel a strong urge to push. We encourage mothers, educators, and birth attendants to avoid making rigid rules about what a mother's response should be.

NEARING THE CENTER OF THE LABYRINTH

You have cradled your baby in your womb and carried him under your heart for months; thus, only you can feel his head moving through your pelvis, and feel your pelvis opening with each contraction. Sometimes the transitions from dilation to pushing and from pushing to birth are straightforward and quick. At other times in second stage you may feel lost in your Laborinth. During pushing, the pathway rapidly winds back and forth as you near the center of the labyrinth—the place of birth, death, and rebirth. You are so close! The path seems to suddenly turn you away from the goal.

Midwifethinking blog says it best: "Pushing is physiological and instinctive, and a feature of all mammalian births. To tell a woman that if she pushes she has given in to external programming and her baby will not enjoy a gentle birth, is disempowering, especially for those who fail to override their 'conditioning.' A powerful, primal, loud and 'out of control' birth is just as amazing and valid as a gentle, quiet 'in control' birth."[14]

Time seems to stop. You may or may not "trust" that you will get there. It doesn't matter whether you trust or not; every effort you make will bring you toward the center of the labyrinth.

ANOTHER LITTLE LESSON IN OBSTETRIC HISTORY

Until the late 1700s, women the world over labored and gave birth in the position of their choice, typically upright or sitting on a birthing chair. Lying flat on the back on a table was first made popular in France in 1738 by François Mauriceau, physician to the queen, who proposed it as an updated alternative to the "old-fashioned" birthing chair. Mauriceau encouraged women to lie on their backs not because it would help them birth, but because it allowed him to use forceps during problematic deliveries. (Before cesarean surgery, forceps were the only alternative to vaginal delivery.)[15]

Others attribute the beginning of birthing on the back to King Louis XIV of France (1642–1715). During his time, women preserved their modesty by giving birth dressed and sitting on a birthing chair, their laps covered with a sheet. King Louis engaged the court physician to convince women of the court that giving birth would be easier if they lay on their backs on a high table. Little did they know that their king was secretly watching the births from behind a curtain, gaining some perverse sexual gratification from seeing the women exposed.

Further, women were discouraged from choosing their own positions in labor and birth by American physician William Dewees, who invented stirrups in 1826. Stirrups are metal frames with straps that fix a woman's legs in the wide-open lithotomy position.

The invention of the fetal stethoscope around 1850 further ensured that a women's place in birth would be on her back—even during normal labor and birth—because it is easier to hear fetal heart tones when a mother is lying still on her back.

Over time, more and more emphasis has been put on monitoring the fetal heart rate, leading to more bed-ridden laboring mothers.

To date, most doctors are trained to deliver a baby with the mother on her back, with or without stirrups. It has become so familiar and comfortable for them they cannot imagine how to arrange their hands or what to do for women in any other position—even when they agree that upright positions are better.

Voice of the Birth Warrior

It begins with a single bark or two…Then silence. Suddenly, there's an answering yip, a yap…and…a howl introduces a primordial coyote symphony: Screams, yips, yaps, barks, and wails blend into ever-changing music. No phrase is repeated. —LAURAY YULE

Arising as a Birth Warrior means doing what needs to be done without inhibition or overthinking. In the western United States, the coyote has inspired us to think about what it means to be wild and spontaneous, even within the confines of urbanization. She is an inspirational symbol for birthing mothers who are searching for ways to connect with their intuitive selves and find their authentic and powerful voices in labor.

A widely accepted notion, though disastrously incorrect, is that all women do, or should, respond to labor pain in the same way: quietly and calmly. Ironically, dealing with labor pain quickly and calmly usually means behaving in a most unnatural way: breathing in controlled patterns, refraining from moaning or wailing, and lying still rather than writhing or rocking. Sounds that suggest the sexual nature of birth may unfortunately be left out of such a woman's birthing repertoire.

A woman in a workshop told us that she labored at home, moaning and "howling" through the wee hours of the morning. At dawn her dad opened the front door to get the paper and saw three coyotes in the yard, howling in sympathy.

Yet many women have discovered that one of the unexpected gifts of birth was finding their "voice." Perhaps it was the first time in their lives they said, "No!" "Stop it!" "Don't touch me. Go away!" or simply screamed primitively, constituting the first, but probably not the last, time they screamed in motherhood. This does not mean that every woman needs to be vocal in labor. Working with thousands of women has taught us that those who are naturally quiet and introspective are more likely to be quiet in labor, while women who are verbally expressive daily may naturally be that way in labor.

Birth customs and attitudes about vocalization have their own idiosyncratic roots, both individual and cultural. Sometimes those expectations, whether internal or external, shape and suppress a woman's vocalization in labor. Be aware of the beliefs you and those around you hold, and approach your birth with an openness to do whatever your body and voice need you to do.

Chanting

Some women in active labor who are not naturally quiet become like coyotes in their varied vocal expressions during contractions. This is an aspect of birthing that you can't plan, practice, or control. Chanting in labor is primordial, beautiful, and effective. Chants are effective because they unify body and mind, leaving no room for doubt, fear, or self-pity. In labor, you may feel as though your cervix has something to say about its incredible stretching and opening, perhaps: "Ouch, o u c h, o o w w w w ..." Or perhaps the sound is a deep, long moaning, such as "A a a a h h h O h h h h OOHHH ..." Or you might talk to your cervix, saying, "Cervix, open, O-O-O-O-O-P-E-N," as you simultaneously envision your cervix opening with every contraction. Or you might speak directly to your baby, saying, for example, "Baby, come o-u-t! Baby, move d-o-w-w-w-n!" Whatever sounds or words you utter, their uninhibited expression will momentarily dissipate pain.

Oh F@K!*
Swearing Reduces Pain

For some women, profanity may connect them to their forceful core and help labor. Their vocalizations may be along the lines of "!*$h!T…%F*@K!*"

Swearing is a common response to pain; when you hit your thumb with a hammer, you probably say, "Ouch!" or shout some profanity. Fathers-to-be who work in construction often playfully ridicule the notion of stoically breathing through intense pain, knowing that vocalization when in pain can be a release. In fact, strong labor may require power and aggression, which increases oxytocin.

> "When faced with the forces of labor, we can't hide the fear, the anxiety, the responses to pain.... All the inhibitions and trappings of our social selves are peeled away as our bodies thrust and heave, vomit and grunt, cry and leak. The animal is there for everyone to see."
>
> —SUSAN DIAMOND[16]

Research has shed light on how swearing can reduce the perception of pain and increase endurance and pain tolerance. One study shows that swearing as pain reduction is more effective in women who, before labor, swear fewer than sixty times a day.[17]

Interestingly, the first words that ancient people spoke may have been expletives in response to pain. New research shows that the part of the brain responsible for swearing is separate from, and much older than, the part of the brain that composes grammatically correct sentences. The normal speech center in the brain is located on the outer layer of the left hemisphere, whereas swearing arises from an ancient structure buried deep in the right half of the brain.[18] The hormones of labor (in addition to pain and exhaustion) inhibit cognitive and verbal functioning, but they allow free access to the primitive parts of the brain, including the part connected with swearing.

In some Birthing From Within classes, women immerse their hands in bowls of ice to experience how vocalizing releases pain.

Labor is full of surprises, and how you vocalize when consumed by the power of giving birth may be one of them. Your authentic expression, whatever it may be, can help you move through pain rather than feel trapped by it.

Listening

It's as natural and powerful to quietly listen in labor as it is to vocalize. When sung to, laboring women are often calmed. Turning their attention to the lyrics, they allow the sounds of the words to penetrate their bodies, helping them transition from pushing to birth.

While pushing out their babies, mothers at the Bumi Sehat (Healthy Mother Earth Foundation) birth center in Bali listen to midwives softly sing a song of greeting that is said to be sung in all the village temples. The lyrics mean: "May we bow to the excellent glory of God the divine rising Sun, as manifest in your Soul. May our prayers protect us from harming one another on our journey home to the illuminated light."[19]

Midwife Birth Songs

We all came to welcome you
We all came to your birth
We all came to welcome you
To welcome you to earth.

And I was there to love you
I was there to love you
I was there to love you
And give my body forth.

Your quick and easy entrance in
Through heaven's open door
Your quick and easy entrance in
Through Heaven's open door.

I am opening up in sweet surrender
To the luminous love light of this child.
I am opening up in sweet surrender
To the luminous love light of this child.

I am opening.
I am opening.

These lyrics are generally credited to midwives in Colorado.

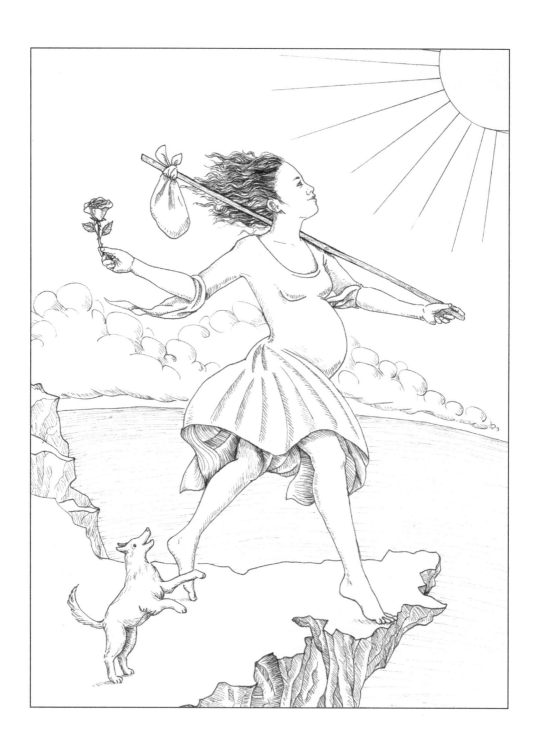

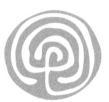

THE FOOL

Coyote, a revered mythological figure among some Native American tribes, creates, teaches, and helps humans, often using his cleverness and wit to "turn the tables" on the powerful or knowing. In the royal courts of Europe, jesters were allowed to express what needed to be said to the king when no one else could without fear of punishment. The archetypal Fool, or Trickster, wise in an innocent way, has performed an important ritual function in cultures through the ages. Examples of contemporary Fools are Jon Stewart and Stephen Colbert.

In their book *Riding the Horse Backwards*, Arnold and Amy Mindell describe how one of the Native American tribes had a funny clown member called "the reversed one." His horse walked forward, yet he rode it facing backwards and, even without holding the reins, moved forward optimistically. This powerful image can inspire us to examine our habitual patterns and perhaps loosen our grip on the "reins" of our plans.[1] During the intensity of birth and postpartum the rules change, and familiar landmarks may be difficult to see or out of reach.

In your journey through pregnancy, birth, and motherhood, you can ride forward in the same direction as all the voices. Or part of you may ride your horse backwards and do something different or next to impossible. The wise Fool inside is comfortable living beyond ordinary boundaries and rules, loves challenges, colors outside the lines, is playful, and likes to experiment.

> *Disorder can be a source of order…and growth is found in disequilibrium, not in balance. The things we fear most in organizations—fluctuations, disturbances, imbalances—need not be signs of an impending disorder that will destroy us….Fluctuations are the primary source of creativity. The most chaotic system never goes beyond certain boundaries; it stays contained within a shape that we can recognize. Throughout the universe, then, order exists within disorder, and disorder within order.*
>
> —MARGARET WHEATELY

The Fool is willing to start the journey with nothing and without having to know how long it will take or where it will lead.

START ACTING THE FOOL

Start acting the Fool by considering what the Fool within wants to do today. Here are a few ideas:

- If you typically plan your day, do not plan it.

- If you tend to "go with the flow" through your day, make a plan and rigidly stick to it.

- If you normally ask twenty questions of your caregiver, ask none at the next visit.

- If you usually hold your tongue and wish you didn't, speak your truth on the spot without apology.

- If you are a calorie or nutrient counter, count the flavors you enjoy instead.

- If you always go to work by turning left, turn right and find a new route, without using GPS.

- If you think making birth art is a waste of time, put on your art smock and paint without planning the picture, draw without an eraser, or sculpt with feeling.

Breakthroughs in learning frequently occur when we are at the edge of chaos.

—JOHN L. BROWN AND CERYLLE A. MOFFITT

Birth Fairy is the name we give to the Trickster who appears on the path of the Birth Warrior. She keeps you on your toes, sprinkling her fairy dust (surprises) when and where you least expect it. Sometimes she emerges for just a few moments, or she may choose to stick around a while. The Birth Fairy's gift may be delightful or very challenging. It's nothing personal; she is not karma, punishment, or reward. Her visit—the unexpected surprise—is part of your rite of passage.

For pregnant and birthing women, there can be a huge emphasis on being in control, being informed, making plans, and doing it right. This intention has its place, but there is also a point of diminishing returns. If you believe there is only one way you can birth, you limit yourself and your preparation. No matter how much you know, study, and plan, you are going to be surprised by at least one occurrence in birth or postpartum. The more rigid a woman is in her birth plan, the more of a magnet she may be to Birth Fairy dust.

WHEN THE UNEXPECTED HAPPENS— GET BACK ON YOUR HORSE!

Birth was a time of honor for most tribal mothers. A woman in childbirth was treated with the same respect as a man in battle. In fact, in the tribal mind, there was a metaphysical equation between the two acts.

—JUDITH GOLDSMITH

*L*ong ago, warriors trained daily to strengthen their mental focus and hone their physical skills in preparation for meeting any situation in battle. Never knowing exactly what to expect, a warrior has to be spontaneous, creative, and ready to respond to what is happening in each moment.

Picture a woman riding into battle on her decorated warhorse. She is engaged in a fierce battle, then suddenly loses her balance or is knocked off her horse. She hits the ground hard, but the battle continues. What can she do? She can feel defeated or ashamed for falling off her horse and risk getting trampled while waiting to be rescued. Or she can get back on her horse and continue doing her best, moment by moment, without attachment to success or even survival. When she returns to the village, she will be received as a Warrior who did her best; everyone will accept that falling off her horse is just part of what happens on the battlefield and does not diminish her honor.

Metaphorically, being in labor or on the postpartum Return can feel like a spiritual and psychological battle. Imagine you are riding a spirited labor horse that is taking you to the edge of your physical, mental, and emotional limits, a place where you question everything you thought you knew about labor and yourself, and experience doubt and fear of losing control. Your battleground is between your mind and your heart— between what you imagined you would do in labor and what you are actually being called to do. Falling off your labor horse represents the moment you think you can't do it, or aren't doing it "right," or find that you're doing something you thought you would—or should—never do. In this moment, your ego hits the ground hard. Labor will not stop for you to process, strategize, or be comforted. Another contraction is riding toward you. There is only enough time to take a breath, focus, and mentally get back on your labor horse and ride to meet the next contraction.

Labor Math

Don't Believe Your Labor Math

The modern map of labor presents dilation as a steady progression from one to ten, which can lead many parents to reduce labor to a linear numbers game. I coined the term "labor math" to express this impulse to quantify labor and "figure out" how long and how hard it will be, which can create a lot of suffering and confusion.

For the majority of women, labor is most intense toward the end of dilation, often referred to as "transition." Since early labor usually has a slower pace than later labor, when the rational mind is flooded with endorphins many women don't realize how far they've come, or how close they are to meeting their baby. Believing they still have a long way to go, or that "it will never end," they lose hope and start looking for a way out. They also scare themselves when they do time calculations in their heads that go something like this: "It took twelve hours to get this far, so it will take another twelve hours to get the baby out. I can't keep doing this for twelve more hours." When immersed in the timelessness of Laborland, the woman may not realize that it might just be a few more hours before she holds her baby, especially if no one checks and corrects her miscalculations. When labor is progressing and almost over, a woman may need reassurance that she is opening and that's why it is so intense.

By contrast, when a mother does these calculations in a second labor, the math might be based on the length of her first labor. For example, if her first labor was twenty hours, she might think she is still in early labor with many hours to go when, in fact, pushing might be right around the corner. These women may need reassurance that they are progressing more quickly than before, as is common in a second labor.

When birth partners suspect that labor math is negatively impacting a laboring mother's state of mind, they can suggest goals to cope with it that involve brief periods of time before making any decisions about pain medication. For instance, they can have an objective to "Keep going for just six more contractions" or "one more hour" rather than the ten, twenty, or more hours the mother might be imagining. Women who are committed to birthing without drugs and who are in normal labor will often commit to coping with labor for short periods. Birth partners can also focus on new methods of coping, such as getting in a shower or tub, turning up music, or dismissing some people from the birthplace.

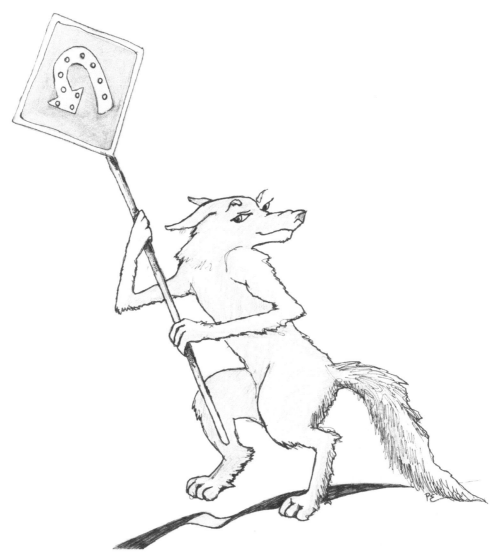

Labor Trickster might show up at the last minute and put up a U-turn sign in Laborland. Suddenly, a mother can find herself going in the opposite direction of what she envisioned; she may feel disoriented and bewildered if circumstances require her to cope in a way for which she is wholly unprepared.

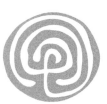

35

EPIDURAL

If you are pregnant, one of the questions you are probably asked is whether you plan to have an epidural in labor. To answer this question, you have to envision yourself either having an epidural, avoiding an epidural, or taking a "wait and see" approach. Making this decision during pregnancy influences other decisions, such as where you will birth, who will support you, and how much effort to put into preparing to cope with pain. Knowing in advance what is involved in having an epidural during labor, as well as the pros and cons of having one, can help you make a more informed decision when the time comes.

Women often feel pressured to make a decision about pain relief while pregnant and stick to that decision in labor. It's as if you have to pick sides—Team Epidural or Team Natural—and then condemn the other side. This creates a division among women that is polarizing both before and after birth.

Epidural analgesia does not necessarily guarantee satisfaction with childbirth. Some women say they

"A friend of mine said, 'You didn't choose what I would have chosen, but that didn't matter.'

I answered, 'But you can't know what you would have chosen. I didn't choose what I thought I would have chosen either.'"

—TREYA KILLAM WILBER[1]

felt powerless due to their lack of mobility and personal control. Others say that having an epidural gave them a sense of control. Expectations and beliefs play a role in how a woman experiences an epidural. The author of a systematic review of women's subjective experiences in birth states, "The influences of pain, pain relief, and intrapartum medical interventions on a woman's satisfaction with labor are neither as obvious, as direct, nor as powerful as the . . . attitudes and behaviors of the caregivers."[2]

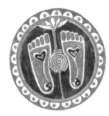

Your Birth Warrior is not afraid of being ostracized based on the decision you make about an epidural and how you deal with labor pain. Instead, your Birth Warrior will gather information about epidurals and other pain-coping practices so that you are prepared for anything during labor.

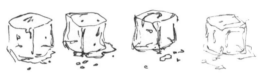

Be sure to learn the mindful pain-coping practices appearing throughout this book. Regular and dedicated practice (with "ice contractions") will help you build confidence and a mindset for coping, resilience, and focus. In the end, whether pain medication is a part of your birth or not, mindfulness will be an asset.

WISE AND COMPASSIONATE USE OF EPIDURALS

Rather than assume that epidurals are "good" or "bad," think about them in a more nuanced way and, as a result, begin to understand the potentially compassionate use of epidurals for yourself and others. Epidurals are given not only as pain relief but as merciful medicine for many other situations that influence the course of labor, such as the following:

- *Prolonged labor and accompanying exhaustion.* An epidural can decrease the release of stress hormones, thereby helping labor progress and increasing chances of a vaginal birth. An exhausted mother also needs to sleep.

- *Failure to progress.* Prolonged stress not only exhausts mothers physically but can invoke fear, elevating adrenaline levels, which neutralizes oxytocin, weakening contractions and slowing or arresting cervical dilation. In cases where dilation has stopped, even though strong, regular contractions have been continuing for more than four hours and every effort has been made to augment labor naturally, an epidural may normalize labor and prevent unnecessary psychological birth trauma.

- *Induction with Pitocin.* Artificially stimulated contractions tend to be more intense. In addition, a cervix that is unripe (long, thick, firm, closed, or dilated just a little) is likely to dilate slowly when labor is induced, resulting in a long, painful process. Coping also becomes more difficult and stressful due to the mother's reduced mobility, especially over a long period of time. An epidural can bring relief from pain and allow the mother to rest.

- *Baby in undesirable position.* A baby in asynclitic or posterior position can cause back pain and slow progress. Relief and relaxation from an epidural can help the baby rotate and descend.

- *Cervical scarring from a previous surgery.* Cervical scarring can inhibit dilation, and if natural strong labor is not enough to dilate the cervix, Pitocin administered to augment exhausted labor may not be effective. An epidural, on the other hand, can increase dilation by helping the mother relax and lowering her stress hormones.

- *Trauma during previous birth.* A woman who was traumatized by the pain, length, or intensity of a previous birth may decide that she "can't go through that again" and choose an epidural to avoid being traumatized again.

- *Previous medical or traumatic experiences unrelated to birth.* Previous medical or traumatic experiences unrelated to childbirth may interfere with a woman's ability to trust her body, trust others, or trust the natural process of birth. An epidural can interfere with triggers from sensations and traumatic memories, potentially allowing the mother a more satisfying experience.

- *Preexisting emotional and physical exhaustion.* When a birthing woman does not have the mental, spiritual, or physical strength or emotional support to cope with more uncertainty and suffering, an epidural becomes a solution to more than just labor pain.

- *Part of a cesarean birth.*

TIDBITS FOR YOUR FACT-GATHERING BASKET

There are two types of epidurals: "continuous" and "patient-controlled." With a continuous epidural, medication is delivered continuously by a pump into the epidural space to provide steady pain relief. When it is time to push, the pump can be turned down or off to allow the mother to begin to feel sensation. With a patient-controlled epidural, after the epidural is inserted the mother is given a button to push whenever she feels the medication wearing off and wants more medication. With upper limits set, she is unable to overmedicate. In fact, with a patient-controlled epidural, mothers tend to use 30 percent less medication,[3, 4] which allows them to feel pressure and a mild sensation of pushing.

A Typical Epidural "Map"

- First, the mother has an IV started; she receives several pints of IV fluids to counteract the anticipated drop in blood pressure after the epidural anesthetic is injected and will continue receiving IV fluids throughout the rest of labor.

- When an epidural catheter is being inserted, the mother has to sit very still (through several contractions) on the edge of the bed with her back rounded or lie on her side. Partners and doulas are usually told to leave the room while the epidural is being placed.

- A thin flexible tube is inserted into the epidural space in the mother's back. The tube remains in for the rest of labor, taped to the mother's back so it won't fall out when she moves about.

- The mother is positioned on her side, propped up with pillows.

- The mixture of medications flows into the mother, and the effects of the anesthetic are felt within a few minutes. If her relief is incomplete or she experiences side effects, the anesthesiologist or nurse may make adjustments to her position, or to the amount or mixture of medications, or, if necessary, take the tube out and start the whole process again. Laboring women receive more effective relief with less medication when the anesthetic bupivacaine is combined with an opiate such as morphine or fentanyl.

- Because epidural anesthesia numbs the bladder, a catheter is inserted to drain the mother's bladder.

- The epidural greatly restricts the mother's freedom of movement. She stays in bed while attached not only to a catheter but to an IV, a blood pressure cuff, and a fetal monitor. She needs assistance to be moved from side to side about every thirty minutes to ensure even distribution of the medication.

- After the epidural takes effect, the mother's energy and mood, as well as the atmosphere of the birthing room, generally shifts, becoming quieter. Data is collected and monitored by nurses. If the mother has labored long and hard, and she and her partner are exhausted, the lights are dimmed and they take much needed naps. The doula may feel there is nothing more she can do and no place for her to rest, so she may leave, at least temporarily.

Side Effects, Concerns, and Drawbacks

Epidural analgesia is used by more than half of laboring women, yet there is no consensus about what unintended effects it causes. In addition, few studies control for the confounding factors that result because women who request epidural are different from women who do not.

—ELLISE LIEBERMAN AND CAROL O'DONOGHUE

Many mothers picture being comfortable in labor with an epidural, without understanding the possible side effects, concerns, or drawbacks. Although the sensation of pain is localized in labor, analgesic or anesthetic drugs cannot target,

---

Another Little Lesson in Obstetric History

Several generations ago, many women grew up not hearing stories of their birth because their mothers had been drugged with "Twilight Sleep," a combination of morphine and scopolamine that erases all memory of labor. Not remembering labor did not mean women did not feel it: they went wild in labor, screaming, fighting the nurses, or trying to run away. So doctors and nurses gagged them and restrained them to their beds with leather arm straps, knowing the women wouldn't remember this either.

In the 1960s and 1970s, Western women rebelled against being routinely medicated, restrained to the bed (even when they weren't medicated), and discouraged from breast-feeding. Their demand for information and autonomy in labor fueled the movement for natural childbirth and participation in birth. As a result, many daughters heard stories from their mothers who coped with pain by either "just getting through it" or using Lamaze breathing. When the daughters grew up and began families, many just expected to be able to cope and birth naturally.

Then obstetrics changed again, and with it the birth stories that women passed on to their daughters. With the rise of inductions and cesareans in the 1990s, more women needed analgesia or epidurals. Consequently, most contemporary women and birth attendants grew up hearing birth stories that included analgesia, epidurals, induction, and operative deliveries. Currently in the United States, six out of ten first-time mothers who birth vaginally have an epidural in labor.[5] If cesareans are included, the rate is close to 90 percent.

isolate, and eliminate pain without also affecting other systems in the body, including the baby. Some physiological considerations are the following:

- There is a misconception that the drugs used in an epidural do not reach or negatively affect the baby. To varying degrees, every drug or medication you take into your body during pregnancy and labor passes through the placenta to your baby. Within minutes of being injected into the mother's body via epidural, opiates cross the placenta and enter the baby's bloodstream. However, one group of researchers has reported that "continuous infusion of epidural analgesia for up to fifteen hours does not result in significant drug accumulation in either mother or neonate."[7] Currently, there is limited information on drug accumulation in the baby during labor.

- There is a risk of a sudden drop in maternal blood pressure, which decreases oxygen flow to the baby and lowers the baby's heart rate. If the baby's heart rate slows down, the mother must breathe oxygen through a mask. In addition, an internal scalp electrode may be inserted into the baby's scalp to obtain a reliable reading of the baby's heart rate. If fetal distress is persistent or severe, the baby's birth will be accelerated through the use of forceps, vacuum extraction, or cesarean section.

- Epidurals cause vasodilation (relaxation of arteries), which leads to a sudden drop in the mother's blood pressure. The mother's body compensates by constricting arteries to bring her blood pressure back up. However, that vasoconstriction includes the uterine artery, so even when the mother's blood pressure seems normal, perfusion of the placenta and the supply of oxygen to the fetus is still diminished, causing a decrease in the fetal heart rate.

- Several hours after an epidural is started, maternal fever over 100.4°F (38°C) is five to eight times more likely.[8, 9] In one study, after eighteen hours of epidural 36 percent of women had fevers.[10] When a mother's temperature is elevated, so is

Just like any other medical technology, the safety and effectiveness of epidurals is not 100 percent guaranteed. Although the majority of epidural catheters placed in labor work well, at least 10 percent of epidurals do not provide complete relief, and about 13 percent need to be redone one or more times[6]—another good reason to cultivate a mindset of resilience and flexibility.

her baby's, but a fetus has no way of cooling down and becomes stressed by any elevation of temperature, whether by infection or epidural. An overheated fetus shows a dramatic increase in heart rate. Before birth, it is impossible to be certain whether the temperature elevation and fetal distress are due to epidural fever or to an infection. Since an infection can be life threatening to a fetus, even though the majority of fevers in labor are due to epidurals, proactive measures are taken when a mother runs a fever in labor. In case the fever is the result of an infection, mothers and babies are treated with intravenous antibiotics, and birth may be hurried along with Pitocin, forceps, vacuum extraction, or cesarean.

- An epidural interferes with natural oxytocin production, so it is common for contractions to slow down after an epidural; the next step is usually to administer Pitocin through an IV. Pitocin can cause unnaturally strong and prolonged contractions, which sometimes decreases the oxygen supply to the baby. If this happens, the Pitocin drip will be slowed down or stopped, the mother may need to breathe oxygen through a mask, and/or she may have an emergency cesarean.

- A mother with an effective epidural usually has little or no sensation of her contractions or the urge to push. Instead of coaching a mother to push when she has no sensation, many hospitals recommend "laboring down," a term used to describe the passive movement of the baby through the birth canal without the mother actively pushing.

- Some studies have shown an increase in the incidence of cesareans in mothers with epidurals.[11] Other studies found insufficient evidence that an epidural increases the risk of cesarean birth.[12]

TWO EPIDURAL-RELATED ISSUES FOR THE NEWBORN

1. Epidural "fever"

Fevers in newborns caused solely by epidurals are common and not harmful, typically lasting less than five hours. A baby may be born "warm" due to the mother having an epidural fever in labor or as a direct effect of the epidural medication in the baby's body. Sometimes after an epidural the baby has a temperature even when the mother does not,suggesting that the anesthetic may affect a baby's autonomic nervous system and ability to regulate its temperature.[13] Whatever the cause, warm babies are taken to the newborn intensive care nursery for observation or a septic workup to rule out infection.

A septic workup may cause days of emotionally painful separation, stress and pain for the baby, worry for the parents, and interference with breastfeeding. It involves drawing blood every few hours and a spinal tap. A spinal tap entails inserting a needle into the outer covering of the baby's spinal cord to remove and culture a sample of the spinal fluid that bathes the spinal cord. Even before the lab can confirm whether an infection is present, most babies with an elevated temperature receive antibiotics.

2. *Breastfeeding and epidurals*

There is now clear evidence that mothers who receive pain medications in labor, whether they go on to have a vaginal or cesarean birth, experience a higher risk of breastfeeding problems, including a delay in their milk coming in and babies losing weight.[16, 17] It is essential that a mother who has a complicated birth (use of pain medications, Pitocin, lots of IV fluids, cesarean, and so forth) receive prompt help and good support with breastfeeding in the first few hours and days. Lots of skin-to-skin contact, frequent breast stimulation (via nursing or pumping), and reassurance can mitigate side effects from birth interventions and help her milk come in sooner, build up her confidence, and reduce infant weight loss.

Gut microbes are established after birth and remain fairly stable throughout life. Babies given antibiotics within forty-eight hours of birth show a decreased number of beneficial bacteria in their gut a month and two later.[14] Antibiotic treatment early in life may affect long-term health, increasing the risk for asthma, allergies, and obesity.[15] Exclusive breastfeeding from birth helps the newborn's microbiome be as normal and healthy as possible, even if he received antibiotics.

EPIDURAL CULTURE IN THE HOSPITAL

Near the end of labor most women birthing in a hospital think, say, or even wail, "I can't do this anymore," "Make it stop," "Cut it out of me," or "I need an epidural." Women say these things in home births, too, but there are two major differences with support at home. The birth attendants and the laboring woman are in agreement to (1) support the intention to birth naturally and (2) discern whether a woman at the Gate of Doubt is truly asking to be transported to the hospital for an epidural or simply needs more encouragement.

In the hospital, a woman can ask for many things: "I want to labor without an IV," "I don't want continuous monitoring," "Let me get up and push," or "Just cut it out of me"—and nobody jumps to fulfill her requests. But when a woman is at the Gate of Doubt and cries out for drugs her wish is their command. The core of her desperate plea is usually a need for more or a different kind of support, yet that is rarely offered. Instead, her support people get scared or feel powerless, and an epidural is ordered up, even if the mother is within an hour or a few hours of birthing naturally.

Note to Birth Companions

For more suggestions on how to help a mother through the Gate of Great Doubt, see page 230.

Even before labor, during pregnancy and hospital childbirth classes epidurals may be "pushed" by hospital staff. A woman with an epidural is an easy and quiet patient to manage; while she is comfortably sleeping or watching TV, every element of her physiology and labor are regulated and monitored by machines that can be observed from a central location. As most births take place with an epidural these days, this is the norm that nurses and OBs are trained to manage. They are uncomfortable or even anxious when a mother does not have an epidural, because they may not possess the skills or experience to effectively care for an unmedicated laboring woman. Natural birth has gradually become a new terra incognita within our culture.

When weighing the benefits of pain relief near the end of labor, consider whether the added stress of being confined to a bed and enduring further interventions is worth a few hours of rest and lessened pain.

INVOKE YOUR HUNTRESS

Discover more about your motivations concerning an epidural by asking yourself the following questions:

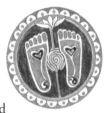

- What is motivating me to plan to have, or to avoid having, an epidural?

- How do I view other women who have epidurals in normal labor?

- What am I (already) telling myself it would mean about me if I had an epidural in labor?

After an epidural takes effect, the hard work and rhythm of labor suddenly ceases. Understandably, after the pain stops, most women and their birth companions disengage from the birth process and begin to watch TV, read emails, engage in social media, and have visitors. Even though she no longer appears to be in labor, a woman with an epidural still needs emotional support, physical touch, and company. Foot massage is enjoyed by many women

"My mom was not prepared for her role as my labor support person. She felt anxious and helpless seeing me in pain; she didn't know how to make me comfortable. Suddenly she said, "If you don't have an epidural, I'm going to leave."

—FRIDA, FIRST-TIME MOTHER

Frida did not want an epidural, but even more, she did not want her mother to leave or to be upset with her so she had an epidural to alleviate her mother's discomfort.

True Surrender

"The last thing I wanted was an epidural. I knew I could get through labor. Everyone who knew me knew I could. I am the strong one in the family and among my friends. I hike, kayak, swim, and ride my bike without tiring. I always do what I say. But I didn't plan on a four-day prodromal labor, a painful Pitocin augmentation, and not dilating. It was when I said, "'I need an epidural," that I experienced the deepest surrender I have ever known. Before labor, I envisioned surrender very differently. To know that an epidural was what I needed, and to ask for it—that was surrender."

—*Alita, first-time mother*

confined to bed by an epidural, and it may speed up labor too.
Effort also needs to be made to influence the rotation and
position the baby's head, so every half hour or so two people
need to turn the woman from one side to the other and position
her legs with pillows or a peanut ball. Although an epidural
involves extensive medical management, it is still possible to subsequently have a positive, even joyous birth.

Huntress Tracks
Her Postpartum Return

While the side effects and management of a labor epidural
are fairly predictable, every mother's experience of an epidural
is unique. If during labor you felt that having an epidural was
right but during your postpartum Return feel doubt, ambiva-
lence, or regret, view the epidural in the context of your whole
labor and not as an isolated decision. While exploring your
decision and experience, try not to defend, explain, or apologize
for your epidural. Rather, look inward to discover what you are
telling yourself about yourself because you had an epidural in
labor.

It takes a certain kind of courage to labor without drugs,
and it takes a certain kind of strength to ask for and accept
a drug you hoped you would not have.

36

INDUCTION

Induction is sometimes necessary and life saving. Other times it is just a routine part of a crazy trend. Whether you are considering an induction or planning to birth naturally, it is wise to learn what you can do to decrease your chances of being induced, as well as how to be mentally prepared should induction be recommended.

The majority of women do not really know what is involved in an induction, or how risky and traumatic it can be. Many assume that because induction is so common it must be safe, or safer than waiting for labor to start on its own. With this misconception, it is easy to give consent to the scheduling of an induction without being fully informed.

Since over 23 percent of labors in the United States have been started artificially with drugs over the past decade, many birth stories begin with "I was induced . . ." The great number of labor induction stories has subtly but powerfully influenced cultural beliefs and behavior. Induction is common and considered either benign or traumatic, depending on the perception of the storyteller, whether it is your sister, childbirth teacher, doctor, or subjects

Labor Induction Rate

1990: 9.6 percent

2010: 34 percent

2011: 24 percent

2013: 23 percent[1]

in a film documentary. Pregnant women internalize these polarized messages and may become confused, fearful, or dogmatic in their approach to induction.

Consider the impact on pregnant women when induction policy is routinely mentioned during early prenatal appointments, for example, with such comments as, "We'll induce you if you go to 39 weeks and haven't gone into labor." A mother might replay such a comment in her mind or recount it to friends and family, possibly reinforcing the idea until such a circumstance becomes a reality. Although the extent of the connection between mind, body, and health is still unclear, it is wise to be aware of what you are hearing, telling yourself, and repeating to others. Also, don't slip into magical thinking, believing that you can avoid an induction if you make the "right" choices or don't learn or think about inductions.

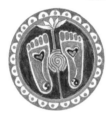

If you are worried, prepare as a Birth Warrior: Go on a Birth Tiger Safari (chapter 21), read about epidural and cesarean birth (chapters 35 and 37), and practice the modified Simonton Process (chapter 27).

Why Women Have Inductions
Medical indications for labor induction

> "The decision to induce is 'socially contagious.'"
>
> —Dr. Michael Kramer[2]

Regardless of potential risks, there are circumstances when induction is medically indicated, including: hypertension, preeclampsia, eclampsia, insulin-dependent diabetes, premature or prolonged rupture of membranes (particularly if GBS+), severe fetal growth restriction, postdates (defined by ACOG as a pregnancy past 41 completed weeks), decreased amniotic fluid, and poor placental function (see page 309). Whenever the idea of induction is suggested, it is imperative to distinguish between having an informed consent dialogue with a care provider and listening to a care provider use fear tactics to persuade you to consent, such as giving only worst-case scenario possibilities.

Elective Induction
(also called **social-pressure or convenience induction**)

An elective induction is chosen by the mother and/or care provider when there is no medical indication for labor to be started. A woman's personal reasons may include eagerness to meet her baby; feeling uncomfortable or tired of being pregnant; wanting to schedule her baby's birthday for astrological, financial, or other reasons; or social pressure. Many women who otherwise consider themselves informed and autonomous may elect to be induced for social reasons, such as to have a birth coincide with when their doctor, doula, or mother will be available, or to avoid birthing on a holiday.

Whether a woman should schedule an induction for the sake of convenience is controversial; what everyone agrees on is that she be completely informed about the potential risks to herself, her baby, and the course of the birth. Concern about having a "big baby" is not a valid medical reason for induction (see chapter 9). Timing a birth to circumvent the doctor's weekend, holiday, or vacation schedule or to coincide with an out-of-town family member's visit are also not good reasons. Keep in mind that if an induced birth, especially an elective one, turns out to be long, difficult, or complicated the mother may feel guilty or blame others.

WHEN IS BABY REALLY READY?

The technical term for a woman's due date is "estimated due date" (EDD), but often the "estimated" part is forgotten and the EDD date gets written in a woman's chart and in her mind. And because it is used to determine when and what kinds of tests are done it can gain a significance that is out of proportion to its actual importance. Expectant parents, and their family and friends, can fixate on the date, leading to anxiety

"My first baby, my daughter, was born at 37 weeks. I was carrying twins during my second pregnancy, and I was concerned about them coming early. So every morning while still lying in bed, I'd talk to my boys. I'd say, 'Boys, stay in there till 37 weeks. Stay nice and comfy in there. You don't want to come out too early or you'll have to go to a nursery, and you won't get to nurse right away, and we won't get to spend time together.'

"I renewed that intention every day before I got up.

"On the morning of the 37th week, I stopped holding my breath. I told the boys, 'Okay, you can be born today.'

"Two hours later, my water broke, and the boys were born healthy."

—VIRGINIA BOBRO

Have the foresight to schedule your visitors for several weeks after your due date rather than right around it. Imagine how hard it is to feel like you are "keeping everyone waiting" when special guests are hoping to attend the birth and see the newborn and you are still pregnant for a week or more.

and pressure if the baby doesn't arrive when expected and possibly a decision to induce that can yield unfortunate results.

Until recently, the belief that babies were ready to be born by 36 to 37 weeks permitted inductions done for convenience or because the woman was "tired of being pregnant" to flourish. However, due to new research and concerns about the high number of babies induced prior to 39 weeks, ACOG revised its definitions of "term birth" in 2013.

There is now growing evidence that babies who are "early term" (born prior to the 39-week mark) are at considerably higher risk than previously thought of having complications such as fever, life-threatening infection, temperature regulation issues, problems with feeding and gaining weight, need for a ventilator, and jaundice.[3] Any of these complications increases stress for the parents, lengthens hospital stays, and therefore increases costs.

In addition to this risk of complications, there are numerous other reasons to keep your baby inside until at least 39 weeks. During the last weeks of pregnancy, antibodies from your body are passed to your baby, strengthening the baby's immune system and helping her fight infections in the first weeks of life. Each day your baby is snuggled inside you, she is gaining weight, storing iron, developing more coordinated sucking and swallowing abilities, and storing brown fat that will help her maintain body temperature after birth.

Another important reason to keep your baby inside until at least 39 weeks is to allow her lungs and brain—the last of the vital organs to completely develop—to mature. Your baby's lungs undergo a tremendous growth spurt in the final weeks of pregnancy. Before birth, the placenta "breathes" for your baby. Nature intends for labor to begin only after your baby's lungs are sufficiently mature to breathe outside the womb, at which point a signal is sent to

A Word about Due Dates

Babies born on their due date: 4 to 5 percent

Babies born between 40 and 41 weeks: 34 percent

Pregnancies that progress past 41 weeks: 7 percent

Pregnancies that progress beyond 42 completed weeks: 1.4% percent[4, 5]

Definition of Terms

In November 2013, the American Congress of Obstetricians and Gynecologists and the Society for Maternal Fetal Medicine recommended replacing the word *term*, which previously indicated gestation between 37 weeks and 42 weeks, with the following gestational age designations:

Early term: 37 weeks through 38 weeks plus 6 days

Full term: 39 weeks through 40 weeks plus 6 days

Late term: 41 weeks through 41 weeks plus 6 days

Post-term: 42 weeks and beyond[6]

your uterus that your baby is ready to be born.[7] Similarly, at 37 weeks your baby's brain weighs only 80 percent of what it will weigh at 40 weeks.[8] The cerebral cortex, the part of the brain that controls cognition, perception, reason, and motor control, is the last brain region to develop.

You may be uncomfortable during the last few weeks of pregnancy. If so, this is the time to invoke your Huntress, who is capable of waiting patiently for labor to begin on its own. Find ways to fill your time with activities you love and people you enjoy, knowing that these last few weeks of gestation are important to your baby's well-being.

Social Inductions May Soon Be Medical History

There is a growing movement to eliminate social inductions. A survey of 2,600 hospitals found that 67 percent have a formal policy against labor inductions that are not medically indicated. Doctors at hospitals that enforced this policy noticed that not only did babies not grow excessively big after a week of waiting, but there was a decrease in:

- Labor time (of about six hours)

- Cesarean section rates

- Admissions to the Neonatal Intensive Care Unit (NICU) for difficulties with breathing, sucking, or gaining weight

- Stillbirths[9]

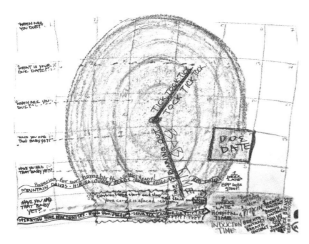

"TIME" AS A CENTRAL THEME IN LABOR INDUCTION

Kay was planning a home birth until she transferred to the hospital for a postdate induction. In her drawing of induction, "time" is the central theme. Her drawing began as a calendar and a clock. Neighbors and co-workers asked, "When are you due?" or "Haven't you had the baby yet?" During the last month, social pressure to be induced intensified. "The pressure," Kay recalled, "didn't only come from others; it began to come from within, too."

What You Can Do Now
Visualize Your Cervix Ripening and Opening

I've adapted the Simonton Process[10] (described on page 213) to help you visualize your cervix ripening and opening spontaneously or during an induction. You might like to listen to the guided visualization.

Methods of Induction

There are many ways to induce labor, from things that parents can do on their own at home to a medical induction in the healthcare center or hospital.

Home Induction

Always a hot topic in birth circles, there are many approaches to getting labor started at home. Encouraging baby to get into a good position and drop into the pelvis are good first steps (see chapter 16). Castor oil, herbs, and other natural remedies are popular, but keep in mind that just because something is labeled a "natural induction" doesn't mean it is without risks. Do your research and consult with your birth attendant in advance.

A popular way to induce labor is by making love. Intimate touch, kissing, orgasm, and nipple stimulation release oxytocin and stimulate the uterus to contract. For an infusion of natural, side effect–free prostaglandins on the cervix, go to the source: semen.

Medical Induction
How Ripe Is Your Cervix?

How "ripe" (ready) your cervix is indicates how responsive it is likely to be to a medical induction—information that can be gathered through an assessment called the Bishop Score. Determined from a vaginal exam, it reflects the position, dilation, thinning, and softness of

Operation Home Induction

"After 41 weeks, we began 'Operation Home Induction,' which included hiking, driving down a bumpy mountain road, sex, and nipple stimulation. Our midwife stripped membranes; we ate green chile and even considered old wives' tales."

—Kay and Matt

the cervix, and how far the baby has descended into the pelvis (station*). A score of eight or greater (out of thirteen), especially for a first-time mother, indicates an increased chance that vaginal delivery is likely. A score of six or less indicates the cervix is unripe, spontaneous labor is not imminent, and an induction may lead to a cesarean even if medicines or dilators are used to ripen the cervix.[11, 12] When a cervix is unripe, which means long, closed or barely dilated, and/or posterior, the induction process often begins by artificially ripening the cervix before starting the "active" induction with Pitocin. This can be done by sweeping, or stripping, the membranes or inserting a balloon catheter or drugs into the vagina.

- Sweeping or stripping membranes

Sweeping, or stripping, the membranes may be performed once or periodically after 38 completed weeks. It is a relatively noninvasive way to encourage cervical ripening and the natural onset of labor by releasing prostaglandins in the cervix and can be performed by a doctor, nurse, or home birth midwife. A birth attendant inserts a finger through the opening in the cervix and "sweeps" all the way around to separate (or "strip") the amniotic membranes from the lower uterus. This causes mild cramping or discomfort and occasionally may inadvertently rupture the bag of water.

Many women find this procedure uncomfortable, and sometimes it is done without prior consent as part of routine prenatal care. Talk with your care provider prior to 37 weeks to find out how often they do vaginal exams at the end of pregnancy and what they are hoping to find out by doing an exam. If you do not want a routine vaginal exam, or you do not want your membranes stripped, be sure to tell your care provider in advance.

A Cochrane review of the effectiveness of sweeping the membranes showed that when performed weekly on women at term the duration of pregnancy was reduced and the onset of spontaneous labor increased.[13] If the cervix is ripe, sweeping the membranes might be all it takes to kick-start labor.[14]

- Balloon catheter

Use of a balloon catheter is a low-risk, mechanical way to ease open a cervix (one that has already dilated to about 2 centimeters) before beginning a Pitocin induction. The procedure involves passing a catheter with a deflated balloon near the tip through the opening in the cervix and into the lower part of the uterus, and then inflating the balloon with sterile water. The catheter is taped to the leg, allowing the mother freedom to walk while the weight of the water balloon exerts steady, gentle pressure on the cervix and stimulates the release of prostaglandins. Mothers report mild to severe discomfort and cramping from a balloon catheter.

Because the balloon catheter poses almost no risk to the baby, only intermittent fetal monitoring is required. Hospital policies vary on whether a mother may go home with the catheter in place or must be confined to the hospital or even confined to bed with continuous fetal monitoring. Once the cervix softens and dilates a few more centimeters, the balloon catheter falls out spontaneously. Afterward, labor may start on its own or be induced with Pitocin. Compared to cervical prostaglandin drugs, there is almost no fetal distress reported with balloon catheter inductions, and there is a high rate of vaginal delivery.[15]

- Cervical ripening drugs

If your baby needs to be born before natural ripening has occurred, or if your cervix does not ripen naturally by 41 to 42 weeks, your birth attendant might recommend that a prostaglandin gel or slow-release tablet be applied to the cervix to help it ripen. Compared to labors induced only with Pitocin, inductions that begin with prostaglandin medicine show a lower cesarean rate and increased likelihood of vaginal delivery within twenty-four hours.[16]

There is one major risk to be aware of: certain cervical ripening drugs (Cytotec/ Misoprostol) can overstimulate the uterus, causing excruciating, prolonged contractions that come in quick succession and last more than a minute and a half, without sufficient time to rest in between. A hyper-stimulated uterus can decrease the amount of oxygen available for the baby, resulting in fetal distress, meconium,* amniotic fluid embolism,* uterine rupture, or even death. These side effects require interventions ranging from the mother breathing oxygen through a mask to an emergency cesarean. For this reason, mothers and babies being induced with prostaglandin medicines need close monitoring in the hospital.[17]

- **Pitocin**

Sometimes one or more of the above methods of cervical ripening will kick labor into gear without further interventions. Usually, however, Pitocin will be started once the cervix is considered favorable. At this point, the mother and baby will be continuously monitored (if they haven't been already) and the mother will receive an IV with fluids.

Oxytocin: Greek for "swift birth."

Oxytocin is the natural hormone that stimulates uterine contractions. Pitocin (also called oxytocin, Syntocinon, and "Pit") is a synthetic form of oxytocin used to start or augment labor. Pitocin is also used immediately postpartum to prevent or stop hemorrhage, making it one of the most life-saving inventions in modern obstetrics.

Of course, in certain situations the benefits of Pitocin induction outweigh the risks, such as when the water has broken but contractions are absent or too weak to advance cervical dilation, thus increasing the danger of uterine infection; when it is important that the baby be born soon; or when labor is stalled.

Although Pitocin induces uterine contractions, it is not the same as the body's natural oxytocin and can cause serious complications for mother and baby, even when they are closely monitored.

Keep in mind that it can take up to three (twelve-hour) doses of cervical ripening drugs for labor to start or the cervix to be ripe enough for Pitocin to be administered. This is the primary reason medical inductions can take up to three days.

Things to Bring for Labor

In addition to everything you are already planning to bring, be sure to include:

- Comfortable pillows (with your name written on them)
- A warm blanket
- Battery candles or fairy lights
- Your Warrior Bundle
- Headphones
- Music or a book on tape
- Sunglasses
- Healthy juices and snacks

Natural vs. Synthetic Oxytocin

NATURAL OXYTOCIN	SYNTHETIC OXYTOCIN—PITOCIN (ALSO SYNTOCINON)
Oxytocin, a hormone produced by the pituitary gland in the brain, contracts the uterus during orgasm and labor, stimulates the "let-down" response during breast-feeding, and increases maternal feelings.	Synthetic oxytocin works by stimulating the smooth muscles of the uterus and blood vessels, bringing on or strengthening uterine contractions. Changes that normally occur over days or weeks are condensed into hours.
The mother's body naturally releases oxytocin in spurts, which allows her and her uterus to rest completely between contractions. When the uterine muscle relaxes, it also allows the baby and placenta to receive ample oxygen before the next contraction. A feedback loop is created: the contraction increases the pressure of the baby's head on the cervix; cervical stretching stimulates more oxytocin release; more oxytocin triggers more contractions; and so on.	Pitocin, the synthetic oxytocin most widely administered, is given continuously by IV, with the dosage regulated by a pump. Even with careful monitoring this continuous infusion can cause uterine contractions to be too strong or closely spaced, preventing the uterus from completely relaxing between contractions. When this happens, a baby can suffer from oxygen deprivation. Pitocin can be decreased or turned off at any time, and some mothers have found that once a good contraction pattern kicks in, they can ask to have the Pitocin turned off.
The biofeedback loop in the mother's body responds to the pain from contractions stimulated by her own natural oxytocin with the release of beta-endorphin, an opiate-like substance that helps counteract pain and contributes to the hazy feeling many women experience in labor.	Once Pitocin is given, the mother's natural biofeedback cycle is interrupted, and her own production of natural oxytocin and beta-endorphin (a natural pain-reliever) decreases, despite the fact that she is in pain.
In keeping with another built-in biofeedback mechanism, oxytocin gradually increases throughout labor. During active labor, when pushing can become too intense or painful, high levels of beta-endorphin, which reduce oxytocin levels, are produced. This slows down labor, making it possible for the mother to cope just before and during pushing. When it is time to push, a surge of oxytocin, beta-endorphin, and catecholamine produce within her a feeling of euphoria and a much needed "second wind" to help her push the baby out.	Pitocin does not enter the brain, so no matter how high the dose it cannot signal the brain to produce beta-endorphin. A mother receiving Pitocin will require continuous fetal monitoring and is usually confined to bed. Without the natural endorphin high, the intensity of induced contractions, coupled with restrictions on movement, make it difficult for even the most determined and prepared mother to cope. An epidural becomes a compassionate partner in a long induction.
After the placenta is expelled, oxytocin continues to flow, contracting the uterus and minimizing bleeding. Oxytocin, along with prolactin, are key hormones in breastfeeding and contribute to mother-baby bonding.	A long induction with Pitocin increases the likelihood of postpartum hemorrhage because over time the uterine muscle becomes less responsive to both natural and synthetic oxytocin.

Blessing of the Pitocin

A mother's labor was stalled; she was given the choice of strengthening her labor contractions with Pitocin or giving birth by cesarean. She had hoped to do neither; she chose Pitocin.

When a Pitocin order arrives from the pharmacy two nurses check the label together to make sure the dosage and patient's name are correct. Knowing the mother was disappointed, I spontaneously said, "I bless this Pitocin." As soon as I said it, something shifted. Who knows what or why. I asked other nurses at the desk, "Who else wants to bless the Pitocin?" As I carried the bag of Pitocin through the nurses' station and down the hall, it was "blessed" by the receptionist, several nurses, and a housekeeper. One by one, each laid a hand on the IV bag—and gave a blessing. One nurse prayed, "Dear God, please let this Pitocin be powerful and safe for this mom, and may her labor go quickly." I told the mother her Pitocin had been blessed by all these people. Hours later, the mother gave birth, vaginally.

—DONNA MOORE

⑥

Induction is a major medical intervention and poses a risk for all women and babies. The safety and effectiveness of labor induction depends on so many factors that it is impossible to predict with certainty the benefits or risks for any individual woman.

> *Inductions, whether medically indicated or elective,*
> *employ the same methods and carry the same risks.*

Once started, regardless of whether an induction is medically or socially motivated, a continuous chain of medical interventions and monitoring is required to keep mother and baby safe from potential side effects and complications. Inductions are often referred to as a "cascade of interventions" because each step can lead to unintended side effects, which then need to be managed with still more interventions or drugs, each of which can have its own side effects. Therefore, inductions create a cascade of decisions. "I never knew there could be so many decisions in a day, one after another. It was more exhausting than the contractions," observed Lana, a first-time mother induced for social purposes.

Taking an Induction Break

Kay, being induced for postdates, was disappointed at having to let go of her plan to birth naturally, and her mounting stress at having to make decisions while "running out of time," in addition to her pain, immobilization, and exhaustion, was overwhelming. "At one point," Kay recalled, "I learned I was not even dilating. I broke down. My nurse said I needed a little break, so she stopped the Pitocin and prepared a warm bath for me." After the bath, the induction resumed.

Here's how induction breaks work: At the end of pregnancy, increased estrogen enhances the sensitivity of the uterine muscle cells. The surface of each uterine muscle cell is covered with receptors for oxytocin. When the receptors are saturated with oxytocin or Pitocin, the uterine muscles should begin to contract. When contractions do not start or are not strong enough to dilate the cervix, more Pitocin won't necessarily make a difference. So turning off the Pitocin IV for an hour or more allows the uterine receptors to unload and the mother to rest, eat, shower, and walk around. When the Pitocin drip is started again, the uterine muscle receptors will reload; this time the uterus may get the message, and labor will begin.

Releasing Residual Body Stress

The uncertainty, pain, exhaustion, procedures, and worry during labor all release stress hormones that produce the fight, flight, or freeze response, leaving new parents tightly wound, both physically and mentally, sometimes for weeks, following a birth induction. A mother, along with her partner, will need rest. But they won't get it in the hospital because there will be an endless stream of staff coming into her room day and night, as well as visitors. So for at least a week after the parents return home, the best medicine is nourishing food, massages, baths, naps, and restricting visitors to help integrate the experience and release residual body stress. If the mother received lots of IV fluids or birthed by cesarean, she may require more support with breastfeeding and may need to reach out for help sooner rather than later. If either parent feels dissatisfied or traumatized by the birth experience, consider scheduling a birth story session with a Birthing From Within Mentor.

WHAT YOU NEED TO KNOW
ABOUT THE PLACENTA'S EXPIRATION DATE

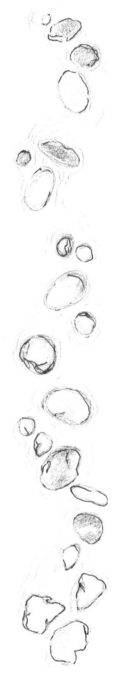

Your baby's placenta is a temporary organ that has an expiration date. Although it is not an exact date, most caregivers agree that after 41 to 42 completed weeks, a biophysical profile (BPP*) should be done to carefully assess placental health and determine whether watchful waiting or induction is the next best step. Your baby's placenta, like all living tissue, ages over time. After 40 to 41 completed weeks, placental function gradually diminishes. In most healthy, well-nourished women, placental function is adequate until 42 completed weeks. Depending on maternal health, nutrition, and accuracy of dates, placental function may diminish a bit earlier or remain good even at 43 weeks.

There is no way to assess placental function unless you have a BPP, which evaluates placental function by measuring amniotic fluid and fetal well-being. Ample amniotic fluid is one sign of a happy, healthy baby and placenta. Typically, amniotic fluid volume peaks at 37 weeks with about 1,100 cc, then gradually decreases to about 300 cc by 42 completed weeks. When amniotic fluid is less than 300 cc, placental insufficiency becomes a concern.

What happens in a postdate pregnancy
when the placenta is not working optimally?

Your baby depends on a healthy placenta for oxygen and nutrients. So if placental function is decreasing day by day while you wait for a natural or home birth your baby may suffer neurological damage or even death. In such a situation you should have a BPP to assess the health of your baby and placenta.

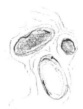
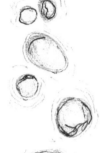
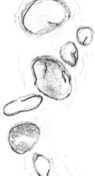
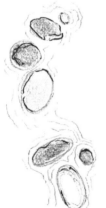

1. Get the most accurate reading

Low amniotic fluid can be caused by moderate dehydration, which does not put your baby at risk. To avoid confusion and an unnecessary induction, drink plenty of water the day before and the day of your ultrasound or BPP. It may also help to take a warm bath before your ultrasound.

2. Don't ignore the results and hope for the best

As with any test, there can be false positive results with a BPP. However, if amniotic fluid is low or absent, or there are early signs of fetal distress your baby needs to be born in the hospital—sooner rather than later.

Even if a BPP is assuring, if labor is slow and there is fetal distress—meaning decreased heart rate and/or meconium—you should go to the hospital immediately. During labor, at the peak of uterine contractions, blood flow in the uterus and placenta is reduced. As each contraction releases and the uterine muscles relax, blood begins to flow freely through the uterus and placenta again. Fortunately, like our lungs, a healthy placenta has an oxygen reserve. So even though the supply of oxygen to the baby is diminished for ten to fifteen seconds, babies with healthy placentas show no sign of distress. Your midwife can determine that your baby is doing well by listening to your baby's heart rate; a healthy baby's heart rate is normal at the end of and between contractions.

Babies tell us when the placenta is not at peak performance and there is diminished oxygen reserve through a change in their heart rate pattern called "late decelerations." Even with a stethoscope at home, a midwife who is listening at the end of a contraction and between contractions can detect a drop in the baby's heart rate that recovers slowly. If this happens, the mother should receive oxygen by mask and be transferred to the hospital. There is a possibility that decelerations will continue to be minor and a normal birth will follow. But there is also a risk that the baby heart rate will continue to decelerate, causing neurological damage or even death. These warning signs cannot be ignored.

If there is dark or thick meconium in the amniotic water, you should go to the hospital immediately as it indicates low oxygen in the baby, a sign of fetal distress. This is an even greater concern if you are postdates. If a newborn breathes in meconium in labor or at birth, it can cause difficulty breathing and pneumonia.

At the hospital your baby can be monitored, and there are specially trained baby doctors and nurses in case you need them. You may be able to deliver vaginally; however, a cesarean birth might be the safest way for the baby to be born.

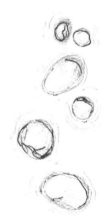

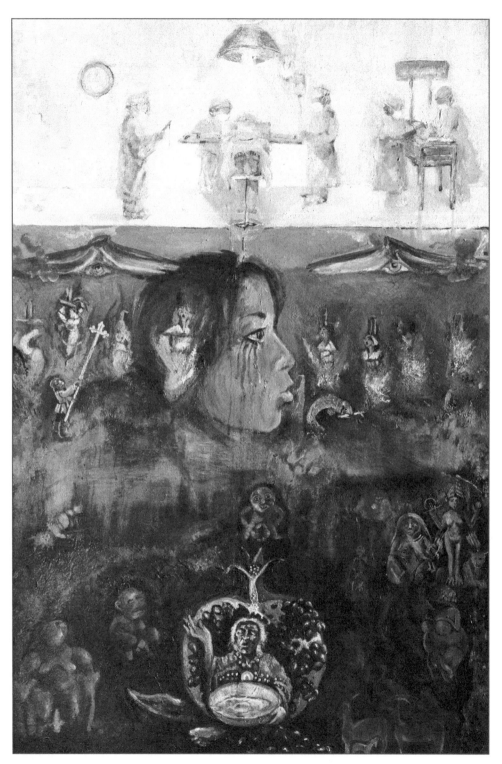

Pam England, Faith Based Birth, *2004 © acrylic on canvas.*

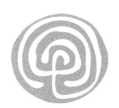

37

CESAREAN BIRTH

In many communities, about one out of three women give birth by cesarean. Therefore, an essential part of your holistic preparation is learning what to expect, how to decrease your chance of cesarean surgery, and how to cope if you experience a cesarean birth.

Thirty years ago, as a home birth midwife, I refused to teach about cesareans in my childbirth classes, thinking it might lead to more cesareans or scare mothers. Even as a nurse-midwife, when I unexpectedly had a cesarean my partner and I were freaked out and unprepared. It was only then that realized I was doing a grave disservice to expectant parents. Almost immediately after my recovery I began teaching what I then called 'spiritual cesarean.' I explained step-by-step what happens, from the parents' perspective, and how to get through the experience both practically and psychologically. Mom and dads were riveted, not afraid. Some cried out of relief and release. They thanked me for finally explaining what to expect and how to cope. For those who later had a cesarean, there was less anxiety and trauma; their process of emotional healing and postpartum integration was easier.

So for the past approximately seventeen years, Birthing From Within has been teaching educators, midwives, and doulas how they can change the conversation about cesareans in their community by teaching honestly and compassionately about cesareans from the perspective of uninitiated mothers and fathers. This chapter presents our holistic approach.

EVERY BIRTH IS A RITE OF PASSAGE

There is a common misunderstanding that birth as a rite of passage is limited only to those who birth "normally"—vaginally and without interventions. As a result, many people believe that women who birth by cesarean miss out on this rite of passage. Yet a rite of passage is any event, whether ceremony or crisis, that marks a significant personal transition, including that from Maiden to Mother, no matter how it happens.

Every birth is a rite of passage. A cesarean birth is in no way less valid or meaningful than any other birth, even though it may take the mother longer to integrate her birth experience. A mother who births naturally may feel her power immediately after birth, partly due to the surge of adrenaline and oxytocin, while a mother who gives birth by cesarean may be exhausted and feel a range of emotions at first, such as relief, gratitude, disappointment, and confusion, especially if she also endured a long labor or an induction. However, in whatever way her labor and postpartum Return unfolds, a woman comes to know something about herself she did not know before her ordeal—the mark of a true rite of passage. In fact, we might say that a woman who desperately wanted a vaginal birth, who did everything she could to achieve one, but had a cesarean is a true Birth Warrior—one who made a great sacrifice to bring her baby into the world.

WORDS MATTER
C-section versus cesarean birth

The words used to refer to a cesarean can profoundly influence what you picture in your mind, how you approach the topic, and how you feel about cesarean surgery. Birthing From Within Mentors have seen this over the past two decades of conducting simple experiments in our childbirth classes. We ask first-time parents to make two quick drawings about cesareans, then compare them and talk about what comes up. The instructions are first to sketch, for 1 minute, whatever image comes to mind when they hear "C-section," "A woman was sectioned," or "I had a C." Then they are asked to sketch for 1 minute what comes to mind when they hear "cesarean birth," "I gave birth by cesarean," or "My baby was born by cesarean." Next, parents are encouraged to have a lively discussion about the differences in their perceptions, attitudes, and imagery for "cesarean section" versus "cesarean birth."

Drawings of cesarean section are dominated by surgical images, such as bright overhead lights, incisions, blood, surgical instruments, clocks, and doctors and nurses. The mothers almost always have incomplete bodies and unhappy, fearful, or tearful expressions (figure 37.1). While drawing a "C-section," parents typically feel powerlessness, fearful, loss of control, failure, loneliness, or disappointment.

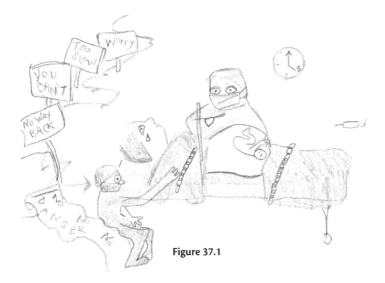

Figure 37.1

By contrast, the parents' second drawings (figures 37.2 and 37.3) contain fewer medical and surgical symbols, and medical staff is less prominent. The mothers are drawn with complete bodies, facial expressions, and hair; their families are represented; and fathers and babies (often absent in the "C-section" drawings) appear close to the mothers. Parents share that linking the word *birth* to the word *cesarean* helps them envision a more complete image of the experience and makes them feel more connected to themselves, their births, and their babies. In particular, the pregnant women had a powerful sense of being "mothers," not just surgical patients.

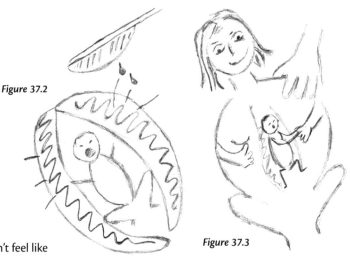

Figure 37.2

Figure 37.3

"After my cesarean, I didn't feel like I had given birth. Since I work in the birth field and teach natural birth classes, I felt like an imposter, so I never told my birth story. At my first Birthing From Within workshop, I heard the term "cesarean birth" and everything changed. Until that moment it had never occurred to me that I had given birth to my daughter. For the first time in ten years, I acknowledged myself for having been strong in labor and doing what needed to be done. The shame and guilt melted away just by adding that one word: *birth*."

—MATI

"She ended up with a cesarean."

The commonly spoken phrase "she ended up with a cesarean" shapes and conveys our collective attitudes about cesarean birth. When telling a cesarean birth story, a narrator who focuses on details of the labor leading to the culminating moment and then uses this phrase implies that the mother's efforts were all for nothing and suggests regret, failure, even judgment. By contrast, when a woman births easily we say, "She had a fast birth," not "She ended up with a fast birth." Often the reality is that the cesarean was "the next best thing" and that the mother made every effort to avoid one. Consequently, it seems preferable to say, "She gave it her all and gave birth by cesarean."

AVOID AVOIDING

Many pregnant women know and accept that a cesarean may become necessary and do not resist learning more about it or considering the possibility, even if they don't want to have one. Other women actively avoid thinking about cesareans out of a misguided attempt to prevent a cesarean from happening. Their birth support team may even reinforce this risky approach. Unfortunately, neither wishful thinking nor a strategy of avoidance prevents cesarean surgery—or any other unwished-for outcome. They do, however, increase the chances that the woman will be unprepared if a cesarean actually happens.

If you have been avoiding the topic of cesarean birth, begin exploring what is motivating you to avoid learning about or talking about cesareans and how you can prepare for this scenario should it occur. Consider the following: What have you already done to decrease the likelihood that a cesarean might happen? What do you want to know about cesarean birth? What do you want your birth companions and attendants to know if you have a cesarean? How do you envision getting through a cesarean—what would you want or need?

Cesarean section rates in US hospitals range from 7 percent to 70 percent.[1] Internationally, rates range from less than 1 percent in many African countries (with associated high maternal and infant mortality rates) to 45 percent in Brazil.[2]

The WHO report in 2010 concluded: "Worldwide, CS [cesarean sections] that are possibly medically unnecessary appear to command a disproportionate share of global economic resources. CS arguably function as a barrier to universal coverage with necessary health services. 'Excess' CS can therefore have important negative implications for health equity both within and across countries . . . its use follows the healthcare inequity pattern of the world: underuse in low income settings, and adequate or even unnecessary use in middle and high income settings."[3]

THE CESAREAN RATE

The World Health Organization (WHO) recommends that the cesarean rate should be between 5 and 15 percent.[4] However, cesarean birth has become the most common surgery performed in the West. About 1.4 million women in the United States give birth by cesarean each year, a rate of 33 percent.[5]

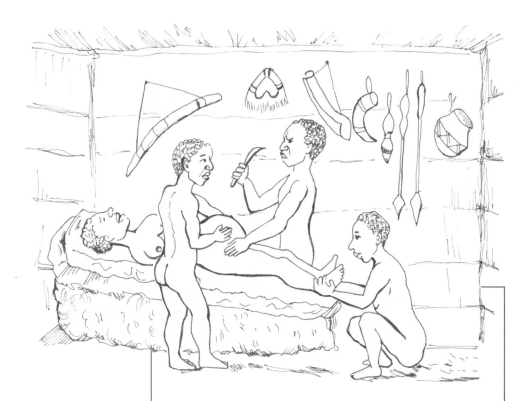

**Successful cesarean performed by
indigenous healers in Kahura, Uganda**

In 1879, Robert William Felkin, a British medical
missionary and explorer, witnessed a cesarean section
performed by Ugandans. The healer used banana wine
to semi-intoxicate the woman and to cleanse his hands
and her abdomen prior to surgery. He made a midline
incision and applied cautery to minimize hemorrhaging.
He massaged the uterus to make it contract but did not
suture it; the abdominal wound was pinned with iron
needles and dressed with a paste prepared from roots.
The patient recovered well. Felkin concluded that this
technique had clearly been employed for a long time.
Similar reports come from Rwanda, where botanical
preparations were also used to anesthetize the patient
and promote wound healing.[6, 7]

Another Little Lesson in Obstetric History

The term "cesarean section," coined in the 1500s, per-haps originates from Lex Caesarea, an imperial law in ancient Rome.[8] This law forbade burial of a pregnant woman, so if a woman died while pregnant the child was to be cut out of her abdomen. It is a common belief that Julius Caesar was born by cesarean, but he probably wasn't. Pliny the Elder wrote that the name "Caesar" came from the Latin word for cut, which is *caedere*.

The first cesarean . . . and VBAC

"The first record of a successful cesarean comes in the year 1500, when the wife of Jacob Nufer, a Swiss swine-gelder, went into labor and could not seem to deliver. Thirteen midwives (so the story goes) had tried and failed, at which point Jacob collected his tools of the trade and did what needed to be done: he made an in-cision. Is it possible he had the intuition to wash his hands and clean his tools first? We will simply never know how it was done. All we know is that both mother and child did very well. In time Mrs. Nufer gave birth to six more children, including twins, all of whom she delivered normally. She lived to the fine age of seventy-seven."

—*Nancy Caldwell Sorel*[9]

DECREASING THE LIKELIHOOD OF CESAREAN

Before delving into the details of cesarean birth, take some time to notice what you are already doing to decrease your chances of having a cesarean. Many women who birth by ce-sarean have, indeed, done "everything right," but the cesarean Birth Fairy—the unexpected—paid a visit anyway.

Some steps you can take to decrease the risk of having a cesarean

- Stay healthy, eat well, and exercise frequently during pregnancy.

- Find out the cesarean rates of potential birthplaces and birth attendants in your community (see sidebar).

- Choose your birth attendants mindfully.

- Learn pain-coping practices to help you persevere during tough moments and a long labor.

- Rest your body and unwind your nervous system by walking in nature, dancing, doing yoga, meditating, creating art, working through fears, and more.

- Be in optimal maternal position as often as you can during your third trimester and in labor.

- Have excellent continuous labor support, ideally from a skilled doula.

- Know when and how to ask questions to determine when an intervention or induction is necessary.

- Labor at home as long as you can.

- Labor and push in a variety of positions.

- Get a second opinion when in doubt about a recommendation for a cesarean.

"At an obstetricians' conference, some 125 members of the audience were asked to raise their hand to indicate their C-section rate.

'Less than 15 percent?' Two hands went up.

'15 to 30 percent?' Half the hands went up.

'More than 30 percent?' The rest.

Then the speaker asked, 'How many of you care?'

No one raised a hand, and the room broke out in laughter."

—DR. ADAM WOLFBERG[10]

Being patient may prevent a cesarean

Although one in every three first births "stalls" in active labor, this does not mean a cesarean is inevitable. About one out of every three of these women goes on to achieve a normal vaginal birth. Nonetheless, in our birth culture a lack of progress for two or more hours increases the risk of cesarean by up to sixfold.[11]

Research and new ACOG statements strongly support the idea that patience is the number one way to decrease the cesarean rate.[12] It is estimated that "watchful waiting" alone could eliminate 130,000 cesareans a year in United States. Parents, nurses, and doctors all need to become more comfortable with waiting when labor hasn't started "on time" or isn't progressing as quickly as hoped. If your labor stalls, rather than consenting immediately to a cesarean consider various alternatives such as waiting and doing something different, such as hydration by IV; changing positions; or having an epidural to rest. (See chapter 31 for more information about stalled labor.)

Preparing for Cesarean Birth

Giving birth by cesarean means having major abdominal surgery, a reality that cannot be downplayed. While we may be able to use intuition as a guide through natural labor, we don't have an internal map for cesarean surgery. Even when a cesarean is medically necessary and a mother gives her consent to surgery, it is not necessarily something she "chooses." For this reason, as soon as the decision is made many women, feeling they have lost control, give up participating emotionally and just wait for the birth to be over, hoping their baby is okay.

Due to the high cesarean rate, hospital staff have become accustomed to performing cesarean surgery, which may explain why they often do not clearly and calmly explain to parents what is happening. Many parents have told us that their stress and anxiety were increased by not knowing what was happening or why. Although each cesarean birth is unique, certain procedures typically take place.

Overview of Cesarean Surgery

Once the shift toward cesarean begins, the intimate "cocoon" parents made in labor dissolves. Even when there is no emergency and no need to rush, there is often a sudden flurry of activity among the staff in preparation for surgery. Many parents have told us that when medical professionals seemed anxious and were rushing, they assumed that something must

Potential risks of cesarean surgery[13]

For mothers:

- Longer hospital stays
- Higher rates of infection and other complications needing treatment or hospitalization
- Pain, often lasting more than six months
- Adhesions
- Breastfeeding problems (delayed and/or lower milk supply)
- More likely to have complications in future pregnancies and births, including infertility, uterine rupture, or problems with the placenta
- Perception of delayed maternal-infant attachment
- Higher rates of postpartum mental health issues, including emotional trauma, PTSD, or depression
- Visible scar on the lower abdomen

For babies:

- Accidental surgical cuts
- Respiratory complications
- Higher rates of NICU* admissions
- Longer hospital stays and more frequent readmissions
- More weight loss in the first week; more trouble with breastfeeding
- Compromised immune systems
- Higher rates of asthma, allergies, type 1 diabetes

be terribly wrong or that their baby was in danger. If you are ever concerned about your well-being or that of your baby, ask for more information or reassurance.

When it is time to go to the operating room (OR), the mother and her partner are separated for a brief time. While waiting twenty to thirty minutes, her partner is asked to put on scrubs, booties, and a mask. This is a good opportunity for her partner to update family members on the situation or make sure there is a camera handy. It can also be calming to do Breath Awareness or another mindfulness practice.

In the OR, nurses drape the mother in sterile sheets and prepare her and the room for surgery. Operating rooms are sterile, cold, brightly lit, and sometimes full of medical personnel. Depending on the hospital and circumstances, there could be between six and twelve medical personnel in the room. Many women who enjoyed friendly prenatal visits are surprised when their doctors aren't as "warm and fuzzy" in the operating room since they are focusing primarily on surgery rather than their bedside manner.

The mother lies on a firm, narrow operating table. A wedge is placed under one of her hips, or the table is tilted to one side, to relieve compression of the inferior vena cava and maintain good circulation to her baby. Her arms are supported on narrow armrests extended out to her sides; this keeps her arms relaxed and out of the surgical area, while allowing access to her IV and monitoring equipment. A sterile cloth is hung between two poles at the level of the mother's breasts; everything on the other side of the screen is the "sterile field" where the baby will be born. The anesthesiologist (the only staff member on the mother's side of the sterile drape) sits by her head, which is where her partner will also sit when brought into the room.

Usually the woman's partner is brought into the OR just a few minutes before the birth of the baby; there's no time and no need to peek over the drape. Her partner sits close to her head so they can both witness the arrival of their baby. Her partner's presence and touch can be immensely reassuring for her.

The incision is made as small as possible. The baby is snug in the womb or, depending on the position of the baby and how far labor progressed, even deep in the mother's pelvis, so she may feel pressure, a tugging sensation, or being rocked back and forth for a minute as the doctor helps the baby out through the incision; this might feel weird or uncomfortable,

Partners and doulas:

Read more about your role in cesareans in the e-book *Field Guide for Fathers and Partners.*

Are Your Birth Partner and Companions Prepared for Cesarean Birth?

If a cesarean is recommended or becomes necessary, it is important that your birth partner and companions understand what it is, what they can do to help you cope, and what questions to ask the practitioners so you will be supported. Birth partners and companions should read about informed consent (pages 179–188) and support for a difficult labor (pages 249–254).

but it shouldn't be painful. Just minutes after the surgery begins, the baby is born. A special nurse takes the baby to the warmer to dry and assess him, making sure he is adapting well to his sudden arrival.

Having a Cesarean in Awareness

There is no "right way" for a woman to experience a cesarean; indeed, a mother's range of emotions can be wide and varied. She may feel spaced out, nauseous, or very present. She may simultaneously feel relief, grief, and confusion; she may fear for her own or her baby's well-being; or she may want to close her eyes and connect with her baby or have someone narrate to her what is happening. Many mothers have told us that the mindfulness practices they learned prenatally were a source of comfort and help in coping during their cesarean birth, making them feel close to their baby, handle the physical discomfort, and feel more grounded and safe.

Beginning of Baby's Immune System

As a baby moves through the birth canal, he swallows and breathes in millions of bacteria (microflora) from his mother's vaginal fluids. A mother's vaginal flora and her newborn's intestinal flora are "compatible."[14] Passing into the birth canal and being born vaginally supports healthy bacterial colonization of his intestines for life. Colonization with normal flora at birth has a significant impact on the development of the baby's immune response. Whatever the mode of delivery, a core gut microbiota is well established within a few weeks of life and persists largely intact into adulthood.[15]

During a (sterile) cesarean birth, a baby does not benefit

from immediate exposure to his mother's vaginal and intestinal flora on the way out. Furthermore, the baby may be initially "seeded" with the foreign microbiota from the hospital environment, which then populates his skin and intestinal tract. This seems to cause a mild inflammation in the baby's gut that appears to increase the risk of asthma and eczema—as well as diabetes, obesity, and other chronic health conditions—later in life.[16]

In addition, cesarean-born babies' colonization with beneficial bacteria is delayed for weeks to months. One study found that at six months of age cesarean-born babies had a colonization rate of one strain of beneficial bacteria that was only half that of six-month-olds in the vaginally-born group.[17]

"If you're going through an identity crisis, you might not want to consider the fact that, at the cellular level, you're really more microbe than human. A hundred trillion single-celled organisms, representing some four hundred bacterial species, inhabit the adult human gut, out-populating the cells in your body by a factor of ten. Nonetheless, it might comfort you to know that in exchange for room and board, your microbial cohorts offer several essential services, from pathogen protection to nutrient metabolism, and likely others yet to be discovered."

—LIZA GROSS[18]

Helping the baby's gut colonization

New research on "seeding" cesarean-born babies with vaginal swabs of mother's healthy bacteria shows that their microbiome is more similar to vaginally-born babies. (A small population was studied; more research is needed.) If a cesarean is being recommended, ask your birth attendant to help you follow this procedure:

1. Saturate a piece of gauze with sterile saline solution.

2. Roll it up like a tampon and insert it into your vagina for an hour before surgery, time permitting.

3. Remove the swab before surgery and place it in a sterile container.

4. Immediately after birth, let your baby suck on the microbiome-rich swab to "seed" his gut.

5. To also help colonize his skin with beneficial bacteria, do not wash off your baby's vernix; instead, rub the swab on his face, hands, and body.[19]

CHANGING TRENDS IN CESAREAN SURGERY

In an attempt to increase patient satisfaction, and perhaps preserve the spirit of birthing, there is a new trend to humanize cesarean surgery. Ask your doctor about the possibility of implementing some or all of these changes:

- Warming the cesarean operating room

- Dropping the drape at birth to permit mothers and their partners to watch the baby emerge

- Playing music in the operating room; if permitted, bring a CD or MP3 player and earphones

- Allowing skin-to-skin contact and breastfeeding in the operating room

- Decreasing separation from the baby, who stays with parents in the OR and in the recovery room

Amy Haderer, First Kiss © 2011, mixed media.

CESAREAN BONDING

One of the biggest concerns that women have about cesareans is bonding with their baby. In reaction to routine, unnecessary, or prolonged separation of the infant from his mother, there has been a growing emphasis on the importance of immediate mother-baby attachment, especially through skin-to-skin contact. Of course, for many reasons this should be encouraged and facilitated whenever possible (see chapter 42). However, the downside of this heightened awareness among parents and birth activists is a subtle pressure on mothers to "do it right" and a resulting feeling of failure and fear when this immediate contact doesn't occur in the way they hoped. After cesareans (or any time there is unwanted early separation), mothers can carry the unhelpful story that they didn't bond for a long time, negatively impacting their maternal behavior and self-image. It is important to keep in mind that infants, as well as mothers, are highly adaptable and that attachment in humans is not instantaneous but rather a process of "falling in love" that takes place over weeks and months through ongoing care, touch, and feeding. No matter how the birth or early postpartum period unfolds, the window of bonding does not close—not for mothers and not for babies.

After Zeus married Metis, she became pregnant. An oracle predicted Metis would bear a son who would overthrow Zeus. So Zeus sweet-talked Metis to gain her trust. Metis, now tricked, was hypnotized into being small, which allowed Zeus to swallow her and the child whole. Nine months later, Zeus was in terrible pain, moaning and groaning with a splitting headache. Much as a mother births from her womb, Zeus (representing the male medical model) tried to birth from his head, but he could not do it. So Hephaestus, son of Zeus and blacksmith of the gods, was called. With his ax, he split open Zeus's head, and out popped Athena already wearing armor and shouting like a warrior—the first human mental cesarean.

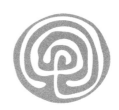

BIRTHIN' AGAIN
AFTER CESAREAN

After a difficult labor or cesarean birth, especially if the baby is not born healthy, the mother's psychological journey "home" can be a long one; it often takes several years or longer to fully integrate the experience and heal. To further complicate matters, if you are still wending your way out of the labyrinth of cesarean birth when you become pregnant again, you will be entering a new labyrinth of birth. In this case, in addition to completing the Tasks of Return from your cesarean birth, you must also perform the Tasks of Preparation for birthing again after cesarean. You may feel you are coming and going in two labyrinths at once. Whether you plan to have a vaginal birth after cesarean (VBAC) or another cesarean birth, be receptive to cultivating a fresh perspective.

*E*ven if it is accepted that cesarean surgery is necessary or life saving, the sudden interruption of the momentum of emotional anticipation, physical changes, and exertion that begins before labor and naturally builds as labor progresses is a shock to the psyche of mothers, especially those who planned a nat-

Cesarean Acronyms

VBAC: Vaginal birth after cesarean
TOLAC: Trial of labor after cesarean
CBAC: Cesarean birth after cesarean

ural birth. At some point afterward, many mothers feel incomplete, confused, broken, or that something is missing.

The Cesarean Chasm

How cesarean mothers express their stories in line drawings

After my cesarean, I tried to draw what I was feeling, including what was missing.

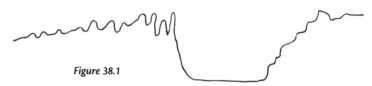

Figure 38.1

Over and over, I doodled a line tracing my journey. The line always began with optimistic anticipation, moving up and down through the hard work of labor and pushing, followed by a sudden drop into a chasm, representing the cesarean section, and finally a gradual return to the baseline, symbolizing my time in the recovery room (figure 38.1). I wondered if all mothers would draw "the line of birth" in a similar way depending on how they gave birth. To find out, I asked lots of mothers to draw their labor and birth experience as a line. To my surprise, cesarean mothers drew lines similar to the one I had drawn (figure 38.2). Mothers who birthed vaginally (regardless of other variations in labor, such as length of labor, difficulty, induction, use of vacuum extraction, home birth, or hospital birth) drew continuous lines that tended to go uphill as labor progressed, peaking at the moment of birth, then descending to the baseline (figure 38.3). The mother who drew figure 38.4 gave birth by cesarean under general anesthesia; her line of birth suddenly and completely breaks off, representing the time she was unconscious.

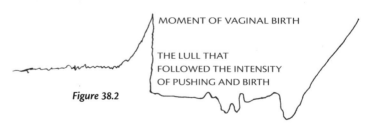

MOMENT OF VAGINAL BIRTH

THE LULL THAT FOLLOWED THE INTENSITY OF PUSHING AND BIRTH

Figure 38.2

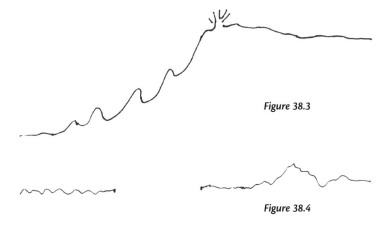

Figure 38.3

Figure 38.4

As seen in these cesarean "line of birth" drawings, to some degree and at some point during their return, many mothers feel incomplete, confused, and broken, or that something is "missing." Not all women who birth by cesarean feel this way, but if it is true for you, then whatever is missing is what you need to find and reclaim to feel whole again.

RECLAIM YOUR PELT

What is it that some cesarean mothers grieve and seek to resolve or recover? Many feel a loss of trust in their body's ability to do something it is meant to do. Others feel betrayed by promises about birth being natural and empowering, which turned out not to be true for them. Women who were discouraged from preparing for the possibility of cesarean may feel like they were caught off guard and ill-equipped to cope. On a more subtle level, still others may be grieving an incomplete initiation. What such mothers need to recover are their "pelts," a reference to a mythological story from northern Scotland and the Orkney and Shetland Islands. There, according to legend, seal people called "selkies," a name derived from the early Scottish word *selich*, live among humans, shedding their pelts when they reside on land. Variations of this folktale are commonly heard in other northern lands near the sea, including Japan, Iceland, Siberia, and the Northwest United States. They all offer a story that is useful for understanding the experience of cesarean mothers who grieve a loss.

The Story of Seal Woman

A lonely Scottish fisherman was walking along the beach one evening when his attention was drawn to strange voices and laughter in the distance. Looking up, he could barely make out what appeared to be a group of luminous, lithe beings dancing in the moonlight on a cliff. He wondered if they could they be selkies. He wanted a closer look, so he climbed very quietly up the backside of the cliff. There, tucked between the boulders, he discovered their seal pelts in all colors: black, gray, gold, and even pink. He decided to take just one pelt to prove he had indeed seen the legendary selkies. He quickly tucked it into his jacket and spied a little longer until the "beings made of moon milk with long hands and feet" put on their seal skins and slipped into the sea, yelping with joy.[1]

When he arrived home, he examined his prize. Then he stashed the pelt above the door jam and went about his evening routine of making dinner and mending nets. By and by, a strange barking and wailing outside his cabin broke the silence. He opened the door and was startled to see a selkie, beautiful and vulnerable.

A woman who trusts too much does not yet know to guard her "pelt" or identify a thief who looks safe and harmless. Some worrying and vigilance are important tasks of mindful pregnancy.

She introduced herself, saying, "I am a seal woman. I live in the sea, but today I was playing on the rocks with my brothers and sisters. I don't know what happened." She wept. "I can't find my skin. It's not where I left it. When I wasn't paying attention, somebody must have taken it. Without it, I cannot return to my home in the sea. Could you help me find it?"

Her fate was in his hands. He invited her in and weighed his options. If he returned her pelt, he knew she would immediately go back to the sea; without her skin, she would have to stay ashore. She was beautiful, and he was lonely. Out of her element, she would need him to survive. He wasn't malevolent; he just knew an opportunity when he saw it. He seized his opportunity and replied caringly, "Someone must have come upon it and taken it when you were distracted and amusing yourself. I don't know what happened to your pelt, but if you become my wife I'll take care of you. I'll provide for you and keep you safe."

She contemplated her dilemma. "I don't want to live on land; I want to live and love and birth in the sea. I'm at home there. But without my pelt, I will die in the sea, and without this man I cannot feed myself or survive on land." She consoled herself, saying, "He isn't so bad. He seems decent and caring. He will take care of me, feed me, and keep me safe." She looked around the alien surroundings and told herself, "Well, this is very strange, but I can learn to live here and make this work. I have to make it work, or I could die." And so, although she did not seek out or choose this arrangement, here it was. She did what she had to do: she consented to his offer.

When she wasn't tending to her wifely duties, Seal Woman often searched the rocks and shore for her skin. She looked out on the water and re-membered her former self, then wondered who she was now. Years passed. Out of her natural habitat of the deep sea, Seal Woman saw her skin begin to dry out and flake; her eyes became dull and red. No longer lithe and supple, she limped about. She made the best of it; she went about her daily chores as she slowly withered away.

One day, dark clouds gathered on the hori-zon—and within Seal Woman's soul. Her husband was away at sea. Inside and out, a storm raged. Rain lashed against the windows and washed away her apathy. In her solitude, she began to grieve all that she had lost. She wept and wailed, "This life is not what I wanted. I didn't really have a choice. It just isn't fair. I want my pelt back!" Powerful gusts of wind shook the cabin, rattled dishes, sent papers flying, and loosened the door. The door swayed back and forth, making an awful racket. She went to lock it when suddenly a gale slammed the door shut and knocked the sealskin from its hid-ing place above the door jam. It landed at her feet!

Seal Woman looked down and cocked her head. "What is

When a woman loses her "pelt," she is easily confined and made captive; she is vulnerable, has fewer choices, and also loses her voice.

Finding a hidden "pelt" is not easy. Even when the selkie's pelt was within reach, it was out of con-scious awareness—until the storm. Sometimes it takes an emotional storm to shake your "pelt" loose from its hiding place.

this?" she whispered to herself. She slowly picked it up and pressed it to her check. Upon smelling and feeling her pelt, Seal Woman began to remember who she was. Memories of the sea filled her mind and heart. She ran, yelping and barking, all the way to the beach, ripped off her human clothes, and slipped into her own skin. It felt familiar and unfamiliar at the same time. And it still fit, almost perfectly. Without a moment's hesitation, compelled by instinct she dove into the sea, leaping again and again until she was out of sight. Then downward she swam...Down, down, down into the deep sea she knew was home. At home, her healing began.[2]

When a seal woman has lived a full life, her pelt will have telltale signs of fights and struggles, scars and bald patches. Her pelt is a body map of where she's been.

Story Meaning, Story Medicine

Tuning in to the selkie's heroic journey may allow you to experience the deeper, poetic meanings of your own Birth Warrior's journey, and may be a means of healing. One way to find personal meaning is to discover its potential symbolic significance for you in the same way you might when interpreting a dream. For example, the sea might represent your psychic "home," access to deep and vast resources in your unconscious, or swimming in the Great Mother. The pelt could represent several things, such as power or a container for beliefs and assumptions. When her pelt is within reach, Seal Woman is autonomous on land and sea. To lose her pelt is to lose everything she knows and trusts to protect her.

The pelt being taken and hidden is another symbol potentially rich in meaning for a woman who has given birth. For example, a mother who has experienced a cesarean birth might describe how something was "taken," saying, "I missed out on pushing," "I missed being the first one my baby saw," or "I missed being able to say, 'I did it! I gave birth to my child.'" She often has conflicting feelings; one part of her is grateful to have a healthy child, while another part grieves a moment lost to her forever.

Another aspect of the story is that whoever has Seal Woman's pelt has the power, so the story is about a power struggle. The man will not give Seal Woman her pelt just for the asking, no matter how desperate or reasonable the plea. As long as he has the pelt, he enjoys and benefits from the power he holds over her and her dependence on him.

Like Seal Woman, as a wiser initiated woman you now know to watch your pelt. With your pelt of power, you can move easily between two worlds, your inner life and the external world. You know a new way to be in relationship with others or the system without being possessed by or in service to it.

Take some time to journal or make art about Seal Woman and her pelt, considering what parts of the story speak to you and what connections or questions arise.

⑥

SEVEN TASKS FOR CESAREAN MOTHERS PREPARING TO BIRTH AGAIN

Getting your "pelt" back is an internal process of recovery and healing and cannot be achieved by merely birthing "normally" following the next pregnancy. Being "in your skin" takes preparation. You will need to do the following.

1. **Heal emotional trauma from your previous birth.** Make it a priority to heal emotional trauma from your previous birth. There is no single way to do this. In different Seal Woman stories, how the pelt is recovered varies widely, although a consistent theme is that if Seal Woman keeps looking for her missing pelt, the odds are in her favor that she will find it, as will you if you try different ways of healing emotional trauma from a previous birth. One way is to consider having a healing birth story session with a special listener trained by Birthing From Within. Also read chapter 44.

2. **Renew trust.** Renew trust in yourself and your body by discerning whom, when, and how much to trust.

3. **Build confidence in your pain-coping ability.** To build confidence in your pain-coping ability, you need to prepare

again for the physical intensity and hard work of labor. If you took childbirth preparation classes during your first pregnancy, make it a priority to review the information as well as learn new pain-coping practices. If you plan to have an epidural, you still must be prepared to cope with pain before the epidural is placed, or in case there isn't time for an epidural, or in the event that it doesn't work well.

A Cesarean Mother's Map

A cesarean mother's Tasks of Preparation depend on her path. She may be:

• Scheduling a repeat cesarean (CBAC) for personal or medical reasons

• Lacking a "choice" because no local providers or hospitals offer VBACs

• Planning to labor and give birth vaginally but preparing for all possibilities

• Ambivalent about whether to schedule a repeat cesarean or commit to laboring and giving birth vaginally

4. Align your team and make decisions. Research the care providers and birthplaces in your community. In addition to speaking with your birth attendant about your unique circumstances and concerns, find out the benefits and risks of VBAC and CBAC. Additionally, talk with your birth partner about what's important to you and what you need from them; invite your birth partner to read the e-book *Field Guide for Fathers and Partners*.

5. Read chapters 10, 17, 21, and 30. The information and activities presented will support your physical and mental well-being.

6. Envision pushing. Read chapter 32. Imagine seeing and feeling yourself pushing your baby out.

7. Learn how to have a cesarean in awareness. Whether you are planning to have a VBAC or to birth by cesarean, read chapter 37.

CESAREAN BIRTH ART
Clay sculpting

Sculpting may reveal things that no other form of preparation can. Work the clay as you think about your upcoming birth, and feel what it will take. Try not to have anything particular in mind when you begin; rather, watch your intentions take shape. Preserve this heirloom for your child, if you like.

Many years ago, when I was preparing for giving birth after a cesarean, I took up this birth art assignment. I worked a large block of clay until it spontaneously formed a hollowed-out uterine cave, representing an enclosed retreat from the world. My fingers deftly made an opening with a labial door. Above this, I etched my cesarean scar and decorated it with leaves to represent my budding personal growth. I then sculpted a "newly born" mother holding her baby and emerging victoriously through the vaginal opening.

The birth cave and birth mother needed a protective guardian; a fiercely protective, primitive, furry-feather-winged and long-fanged creature surfaced. Realizing that this feral figure represented the part of me that would have to be fierce and primitive in my upcoming labor, I felt an energy stirring within me. Balance was needed. Someone had to hold the space of wisdom and calm during my upcoming ordeal within the womb cave. I shaped an unnerving wise woman elder. She needed a place to sit, so I smoothed out a spot for her to the left of the door.

My holistic approach included preparing for another cesarean. Finally, I sculpted a boxy figure that simultaneously represented a hospital building, the electronic monitor, and a surgeon wrapped in a tangle of fetal monitor wires. I liked that I could move him near or far as needed.

TIDBITS FOR YOUR GATHERER'S BASKET

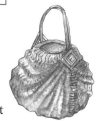

After having a cesarean, 45 percent of American women are interested in the option of VBAC.[3] Why? ACOG estimates that 60 to 80 percent of healthy mothers who attempt a VBAC would succeed; yet only one out of ten actually has a subsequent vaginal birth. Sometimes another cesarean is medically necessary. Some women choose a CBAC for personal reasons, including unresolved emotional trauma from the first labor or a lack of support from their partner, family, or friends. However, the majority of healthy women who have a repeat cesarean are never given the option of having a vaginal birth due to a hospital ban on VBAC, politics, policies of insurance companies, the fear of litigation, or a misrepresentation of VBAC risks.[4, 5]

If the hospital you are planning to birth in has a "no VBAC" policy, you still have choices. ACOG's 2010 Practice Guidelines for Vaginal Birth after Cesarean states:

> VBAC is a safe and reasonable option for most women, including some women with multiple previous cesareans, twins, and uterine scars.... Even if an institution does not offer trial of labor after cesarean, a cesarean cannot be forced nor can care be denied if a woman declines a repeat cesarean.[6]

Here's more good news: Numerous studies have determined that a VBAC is not associated with substantially more risk than any other birth. In many ways, the processes of labor, labor support, and assessment for a VBAC mother are similar to those for a woman who has never had a cesarean. The chance that a VBAC mother, whose labor begins spontaneously, will require emergency cesarean surgery is no higher than for any other laboring mother.

If the hospital has a no VBAC policy, don't sign the surgery consent form.

A Southern California county hospital has a no VBAC policy that applies to everyone—that is, everyone who goes along with it. Many of the immigrant women from Oaxaca, Mexico, simply refuse to sign the consent form for surgery; they therefore labor and have a VBAC.

Induction or augmentation with prostaglandins or Pitocin should be administered with extra caution, as these procedures are associated with a doubling of the uterine rupture rate.[7]

FACTORS THAT INCREASE YOUR CHANCES FOR A VBAC

- You've done work to heal emotional birth trauma from your previous birth(s).

- Your partner has resolved his or her emotional birth trauma.

- You eat well, exercise, and are healthy.

- Your care provider and birthplace are actively supportive of and knowledgeable about VBAC.

- Labor is not induced.

- The indication for your prior cesarean was breech.

- Your due date is at least eighteen months after your last birth (so your body and uterus have fully healed).[8]

- You've had a previous vaginal birth or no more than one cesarean birth.

MY PREPARATION FOR BIRTH AFTER CESAREAN

Counterintuitively, my preparation for my second birth began with the thing I least wanted: another cesarean. I reasoned that if my baby were to be born vaginally there was little more for which I needed to prepare as I already knew how to cope with a long, painful labor. But if the second birth were to be a cesarean I wanted to change my mindset so that I could embrace the experience, participate fully, and know I had done my best. No matter how my baby was born, it was my deepest intention to emerge emotionally and spiritually intact.

ICAN (International Cesarean Awareness Network) has been a leader in cesarean education and support for decades. Visit ICAN's website for information and current research on cesareans, VBACs, and support groups: www.ican-online.org.

I learned to sit quietly with my heartfelt questions and deepest fears as well as actively making birth art, contemplating birth stories and customs, talking over my "plan" with doctors, and keeping a journal. I also prepared my husband for what to expect and what to do during a cesarean. Finally, I arrived at a place where I embraced the unknowable and unplannable nature of birth.

I will never really know how all the work I did influenced my second birth. Lucien was born quickly and peacefully at home. In the end, I knew that birthing vaginally was not what healed me; rather, I credit my healing to the inner work I had done before labor. In a sense, finding my way back from cesarean birth trauma and through my second birth became a map that eventually grew into *Birthing From Within*.

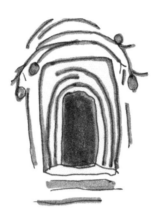

This book only contains part of the map;
the other part is in you.

39

DEATH OF THE MAIDEN, BIRTH OF THE MOTHER

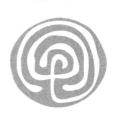

Every time one of my babies was about to be born, I'd think to myself, "You're going to die! This time you're going to die!" Then it'd come out. Somehow—I don't know how to explain it—but somehow it was like I had been born again.

—AN ITALIAN PEASANT

Preparation for your inner journey through Laborland as a Birth Warrior would not be complete without learning about the nearly inevitable "little death" that often precedes the death of the Maiden* and birth of the Mother. Although we seldom hear of a mother dying in labor, some women experience fleeting thoughts of dying near the end of labor, even when they are in no danger of dying physically. This is because by the end of (unmedicated) labor the mounting intensity—pain, hormones, and exhaustion—forces a profound surrender of the body and will, dissolving the ego until there is no self left to resist, to fear, or to try to control the labor.

"The moment a child is born, the mother is also born. She never existed before. The woman existed, but the mother, never. A mother is something absolutely new."

—RAJNEESH[1]

"During a pivotal moment in labor I cried out, "This is so hard! Why does it have to be so hard? I feel as though I'm going to die." My doula, who had told me the story of Inanna's descent a few weeks before, answered softly, "To be born as a Mother, the Maiden must die." In an instant, I understood completely. Those words gave me strength and renewed my determination."

—Sonja

"After giving birth, I felt as though the rug had been pulled out from under me. Suddenly a lot of things I took for granted didn't make sense anymore. I found myself questioning old beliefs and relationships. The void was unsettling, but during this time I began to construct a new me, a new belief system that came out of what I now knew about myself."

—Jada

Not every woman experiences a "little death," and most women who do don't talk about it, or may even forget about it. In fact, in many modern circles it is almost taboo for a woman to talk about feeling close to dying in labor or to explore the confusion, grief, or void that follows this "little death." However, when a culture denies this part of the inner journey of birth, women are unprepared, unsupported, and left feeling confused, terrified, and even ashamed. This part of the Birth Warrior's journey parallels Inanna's descent and initiation:

Inanna passed through the Seventh Gate and bowed low before the queen of the underworld, who represented the long denied and buried parts of her life. Inanna then "died" and was hung on a hook for three days and nights, where she underwent a life-changing transfiguration.

Several women have told me how thinking that they were dying actually increased their efforts to push harder to bring their child into the world. At that transcendent, selfless moment, a woman is no longer just in labor; rather, she becomes the activity of birth itself.

Part 6
THE WARRIOR
RETURNS

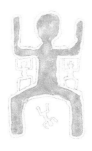

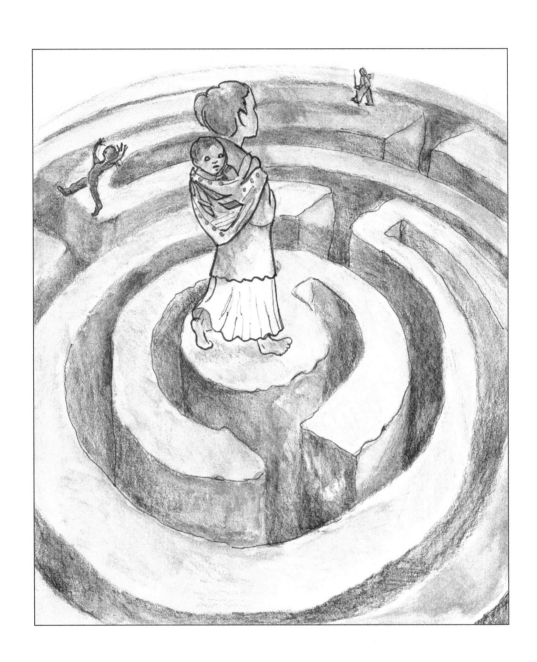

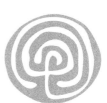

YOUR JOURNEY HOME

When you reach the center of your Laborinth, your journey is not yet over. Now you begin the final part of your journey—the Return. This is a vitally important part of your childbearing year as a Warrior; it should not and cannot be rushed. Fortunately there is a wealth of information to guide you holistically through your postpartum Return.

Just as you heard a Call to begin this journey, you will feel a Call to leave your birth cocoon and begin your Return. The Birth Warrior's Return is much more than just getting back to old routines and fitting into pre-pregnancy clothes. It takes time and involves integrating change at every level: physical, mental, spiritual, and relational.

One of the defining qualities of the archetypal Warrior is that she is steady and persistent, continually putting one foot in front of the other as she makes her way through the twists and turns of motherhood. At times, the impatient inner child will show up and say, "Are we there yet? I'm tired. This is hard! I just want to get back to where I was." But after being transformed by such life-changing events, she will never be exactly who she was.

When you reach this point, call on the compassion and patience of your Birth Warrior to acknowledge your inner child's impatience and lack of perspective. And summon the determination of your Birth Warrior to continue to do the next best thing.

Gathering Tips for Your Physical Recovery

Attention to physical recovery is an essential task of your postpartum Return. Following are tips to guide you.

Eat two dates immediately after your placenta is born

With the birth of the placenta, there will be uterine bleeding. A study shows that women who eat two dates immediately after the placenta is born lose less blood than women given a routine shot of Pitocin to control blood loss. In addition, loss of blood during birth leads to a drop in blood sugar. Dates are high in calories (glucose) and give an immediate boost to women exhausted from the hard work of labor.[1]

Drink date "coffee"

Dates are known as the "bread of the Sahara." People who live in the Sahara Desert roast and grind date fruit and seeds to make "coffee." Because date fruit is quickly converted into sugar in the human body, they add milk to slow down and sustain the rise in blood sugar.[2]

Avoid strenuous activity during normal involution and bleeding

In the first hours after giving birth, you can feel your firm uterus (about the size of a grapefruit) just above your pubic bone. The next day you can feel the fundus at the level of your belly button. Each day thereafter the fundus shrinks by one finger-breadth; by two weeks, your uterus will be deep in your pelvis.

During the first day or two after birth, blood flow is like a heavy period. It is normal to have gush of blood or pass a few small clots the first day or so, especially when you get up after lying in bed for a few hours or overnight.

For a couple of days after birth, you will experience after pains, menstrual-like uterine cramps that occur as the uterus begins its process of involution; they are strongest during nursing, stimulated by oxytocin, which is released when the milk lets down. A heating pad, warm baths, pain-coping practices, and ibuprofen can help ease their intensity.

For four to six weeks postpartum, while the placental site is healing, you will have vaginal bleeding and discharge (lochia), the color changing from red to brownish red, then pink and watery until it disappears.

In the first two weeks postpartum, when your uterus is still above the pubic bone and in contact with the abdominal muscles, excess activity—lifting anything heavier than your baby (such as laundry, groceries, a toddler), driving, or vigorous exercise—can slow down uterine involution and increase bleeding. To avoid a late postpartum hemorrhage or infection, take it easy during the first two to three weeks. Abstain from lovemaking until the bleeding stops completely; instead, enjoy other ways of being intimate and close. If, after doing too much, bleeding increases and becomes bright red but there are no other symptoms (see below), get a good book, go to bed with your baby, and stay put for a day. With rest, the bleeding should slow down and stop within a day.

Attend to abnormal bleeding

Uterine infection or a retained placental fragment can cause abnormally heavy bleeding. Both conditions require immediate medical attention, but with timely and appropriate treatment they are quickly resolved. See a doctor if: (1) your flow is heavy, bright red, saturating a pad in two hours or less, and isn't slowing down with rest or (2) you have a temperature of 100.4°, pain in your uterus or abdomen, general malaise, clots, or foul-smelling lochia.

HEALING MEASURES

Much can be done to accelerate perineal healing and ease the pain of hemorrhoids and breast engorgement in the first several weeks postpartum. Many of these healing measures can be applied at home.

Perineal Relief

Take herbal sitz baths

Herbal sitz baths will soothe your bottom and speed healing even if your perineum is intact after birth. You can buy premixed sitz bath herbs at an herb store. Alternatively, you can buy loose herbs and make your own mixture. To create an herbal infusion of your own, bring two quarts of water to a boil. Take the pot off the heat and throw in a large handful of soothing bath herbs. Let steep fifteen to thirty minutes. Strain the herbs out so the infusion is clear, and add to your bathwater.

For a week to ten days, take a daily twenty-minute warm herbal sitz bath. Sitz baths can be taken either in a shallow bath, so the herbs stay concentrated, or in a disposable plastic sitz bath that fits in your toilet.

Gather Herbs in Your Sitz Bath Basket

When preparing a sitz bath, use ½ to 1 oz. of the following herbs:

Comfrey leaves—softens, soothes, and builds new cells to speed healing

Yarrow flowers and leaves—has antibacterial properties and decreases swelling

Marshmallow root—soothes inflamed, swollen tissues

Uva ursi—has antibacterial properties and decreases swelling

Rosemary leaves—a mild antiseptic

Rose petals or lavender—a nice touch

Use homemade frozen herbal maxi pads

An ice pack on your bottom brings immediate relief right after birth, reducing swelling and tenderness. Get additional benefits by making six to twelve frozen herbal maxi pads before labor begins so they are ready to use right after birth. Prepare an herbal infusion (see page 348). Pour the herbal infusion over six to twelve maxi pads; arrange them on a cookie tray; and freeze. When frozen, pack the pads into sealable zipper freezer bags, three to a bag, with plastic wrap or waxed paper between the pads to keep them from freezing together, and store in freezer.

Before applying a frozen herbal maxi pad to your bottom, saturate a washcloth with warm water and wrap it around the frozen pad. The warmth will give way to the cold in a few minutes, and the ice and herbs will accelerate your healing.

Spray stitches

Fill a peri bottle from the hospital with your herbal infusion—or buy a disposable sitz bath that comes with a bag and tubing, and fill the bag with your herbal infusion. Then gently spray your stitches clean.

Apply raw honey

Raw honey has been used for millennia to heal wounds. Recent studies found it can sterilize a wound, decrease inflammation, stimulate tissue growth, and minimize scar formation.[3] Put raw honey on a pad (or a frozen pad) and apply it directly to your episiotomy. (A small amount of raw honey can also be applied to a cesarean incision.)

Hemorrhoid Relief

Apply witch hazel compresses, potato slices, corticosteroid creams, or local anesthetics to your bottom.

Breast Engorgement Relief

Between the third and fifth day postpartum, some women experience swollen, hard, and painful breasts due to water retention and lymphatic engorgement (not an abundance of milk). To relieve engorgement, try warm baths, showers, or a heating pad. If your breasts are so engorged the nipples are stretched flat, the baby won't be able to latch on; expressing or pumping milk can make the nipples erect before nursing.

Between feedings, apply a cold cabbage leaf to each breast to reduce interstitial fluid/swelling (not your milk supply). Roll or crush the spines of the cabbage leaf in your hands or under a rolling pin, and tuck it under your bra, changing the cabbage leaves every two hours. Or place frozen washcloths or ice packs against your breasts.

Cesarean Surgery Recovery

A cesarean birth is also major abdominal surgery. To prevent an early dehiscence, or separation of the scar after cesarean surgery, avoid straining abdominal muscles until the incision is well healed. Relieve incision pain with analgesics, a belly binder, and a soft ice pack over the incision. Many mothers find that acupuncture and other bodywork helps them heal more quickly.

Toning Abdominal Muscles

Begin abdominal exercises a week postpartum. It only takes a few minutes a day to begin toning your abdominal muscles. More tone will be restored if you exercise the first six weeks postpartum than if you begin these exercises later. Midwife and educator Robin Lim describes a full series of postpartum exercises in her book *A Complete Guide for Postpartum Women*.

Fertility and Birth Control

The day after you give birth you won't be thinking about having sex, so it may not seem relevant when your birth attendant asks you about your birth control plan. Yet it's a good idea to be aware of how fertility returns after giving birth. Here's what you need to know. Women who are not breastfeeding may ovulate as early as twenty-seven days after birth and should expect to have a period by twelve weeks postpartum. Women who are breastfeeding, especially when nursing exclusively and around the clock, have altered hormone levels, which delays ovulation and fertility. If you are interested in using breastfeeding as birth control, read up on the lactational amenorrhea method.

If you are not planning another pregnancy, use birth control. Some hormonal birth control methods should be avoided for the first six weeks or longer as they can interfere with milk supply. Discuss best options with your midwife or doctor.

Lovemaking

Lovemaking should not be resumed before bleeding has completely stopped and any stitches are absorbed, about four weeks postpartum. Even then many mothers, exhausted and preoccupied with the full-time care of their new baby, are not interested in sexual intimacy. When the baby is finally asleep, they are desperate to get things done or sleep themselves. Low libido, due to fatigue and low estrogen, is normal and common during the first year of motherhood. Maintaining intimacy as a couple, through massage and loving touch, date nights, and good communication is essential. The partner may need to take the lead in finding ways to stay connected as lovers and not just co-parents. Because breastfeeding lowers estrogen levels, nursing mothers often experience vaginal dryness. Try water-soluble lubrication. If you are extremely dry and tender, talk to your nurse-midwife or doctor about a prescription hormonal cream.

The Six-Week Checkup

It takes the uterus six weeks to return to its pre-pregnancy size. According to the standardized map of the childbearing year, the six-week checkup marks the end of postpartum. But every experienced mother knows that postpartum adjustment and healing takes much longer than six weeks; the journey out of the Laborinth can take several years. Patience and perspective allow you and your partner to fully integrate the social, emotional, and physical changes, as well as your new identity as parents.

For a Gentler Transition to Parenthood

Birth changes everything and everyone. The person you were when you began this journey cannot be the same "you" who returns. Neither your old wardrobe nor your shoes will fit the same. You and your partner are returning forever changed as a mother and father, not to your relationship as it used to be.

Acknowledge what you and your partner have "lost"

After the arrival of your baby, there is less sleep, spontaneity, money, and time to be together or to pursue individual interests. Try not to compete with your spouse regarding who has sacrificed more or who has the greater claim to total exhaustion. Recognize that your partner, too, is under stress, and make an effort to communicate well and practice lovingkindness with each other.

Allow yourself to rest

In early postpartum, napping is a necessity not a luxury. Allow yourself to rest during the day when your baby naps. It may help you to let go and get restful sleep if you ask someone you trust to care for your baby while you take a nap.

Turn your phone off. Hang a "Do Not Disturb" sign on your door. Give the dog a bone. Darken the windows. Fluff up your pillows. Kick off your shoes. Remove or loosen clothing that is constricting. Use earplugs and an eye mask. Dab some lavender oil on your pillow. Slip under the covers. Then "close your eyes and imagine that you are in a small boat, about to embark on a short journey. Pull up the anchor, and let the boat drift. The water may feel choppy at first, but soon the waves will diminish and you'll be sailing on a smooth sea."[4] When you get up, splash water on your face, stretch, and step outside to get a breath of fresh air.

Keep a healthy perspective

Laugh at your own frazzled floundering and incompetence. Don't worry about being, or even strive to be, a "perfect" parent—your baby doesn't have anything to compare you with. Don't judge yourself or be impatient if your Return is slow. Many parents say it took about three years before they felt they had completed their transition to parenthood and were "back" in body, mind, and soul.

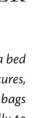

WARMING THE MOTHER

In Indonesia, the new mother is "roasted" on a bed over a smoking fire. In many traditional cultures, the birth room is warmed; heating stones or bags of warm sand are laid on the mother's belly to shrink the uterus and to bring in the milk. She also eats warm food.

—CAROL DUNHAM

*I*mmediately following childbirth, a new mother, shaken by the hard work of labor, rapid hormonal changes, and the power of giving birth, often shakes involuntarily. After a crescendo of intensity, the abrupt cessation of labor with the birth of the baby is a shock to a woman's body and mind. Birth shock is normal and is experienced by mothers during both home and hospital births. However, it is rarely talked about, so new mothers may be surprised and confused by how physically and emotionally vulnerable they may feel.

My labor was normal. Even though it wasn't that long, maybe seven hours, it was more intense than I ever imagined. As soon as my baby was born, he cried and was laid on my chest. I was so relieved it was over. I was not really "in my body" or fully aware of what was happening around me. The routines went on around me, to me, and to my baby. Fragments of conversations came and went. I was exhausted and in a dreamlike state. Giving birth to my child was kind of anticlimactic. After they cleaned me up, everyone left. My baby was taken away for hours. Everyone was gone so I could rest. But I couldn't rest. I was exhausted yet hyperalert. I was alone, thirsty, sweaty—and still not in my body.

—ALEXA

WATER OF LIFE, FOOD OF LIFE

After Inanna's descent, she was depleted and dehydrated. In his wisdom, one of the elders instructed two Allies to bring her the Water of Life and the Food of Life. The Allies fed and nourished Inanna until she was fully restored and strong enough to make her ascent back home.

"Until one is committed, there is hesitancy, the chance to draw back. Concerning all acts of initiative and creation, there is one elementary truth . . . that the moment one definitely commits oneself, then Providence moves too. All sorts of things occur to help one that would never otherwise have occurred. A whole stream of events issues from the decision... unforeseen incidents and meetings and material assistance, which no man could have dreamed would have come his way. Whatever you can do, or dream you can do, begin it. Boldness has genius, power, and magic in it. Begin it now."

—WILLIAM HUTCHINSON MURRAY[1]

After passing through many gates, having done everything in her power to birth, the Birth Warrior is spent. And yet if the Warrior collapses now her journey will be incomplete. This is when allies appear, offering physical and emotional assistance to ensure that the Warrior completes her journey.

The "Water of Life" perhaps represents the emotional and spiritual gifts that can be given to the new mother in the form of music, meditations, restorative yoga, bodywork, or energy work. Part of healing may include quiet introspection, a good cry, or perhaps a private birth story session. The "Food of Life" may stand for practical support to aid the new mother in her recovery. Apart from wholesome food, she will need light housekeeping, linen changing, laundry folding, errands, or the caring for older children while she naps. These are all things she could do for herself (and many women have to), but when they are done for her she is better able to complete her inner journey.

What is needed after a woman gives birth is loving attention from calm birth companions (allies) who can help restore balance in her nervous system by bringing the "Water of Life" and the "Food of Life." In many cultures, blood is considered "hot," so losing blood in childbirth makes a woman "cold." Care is taken to "warm" new mothers with warm savory food and hot tea. (In contrast, hospitals in the United States provide pitchers of ice water, soft drinks, and cold juice.) After a home birth, birth companions could wrap the mother in a blanket warmed in a dryer. In a hospital room, where blankets are often thin, warm the mother with items brought from home, such as thick socks, a comforter or blanket, and a robe. A partner who spends the night at the hospital will rest better under a warm blanket from home, too. Also be prepared to substitute warm drinks for cold ones; in addition to herbal teas, bring packets of miso, nutritious salty broth, or frozen homemade soup you can warm up. For the first few weeks after birth, the new mother should eat warm, easy-to-digest comfort foods such as mushy cooked whole-grain cereals, casseroles, soups, and rice and tapioca puddings. For extra warmth, the food and teas can be spiced with pepper, ginger, clove, and cardamom.

""Experiencing birth shock is like being a passenger in a racecar. Your body goes along for the ride, leaning with the curves to maintain balance at manic speed. When the ride is suddenly over, the car stops moving but your body and mind are still racing. Your heart is still racing; you are breathing fast; the muscles in your arms, hands, and thighs are tense and shaking. You are still stunned and cannot just get out and walk away."

—RACHAEL

SPINNING A COCOON FOR THE MOTHER AND BABY COUPLET

Following birth, new mothers and fathers feel their whole world—inside and out—has changed forever, and they need a little time to integrate the change. The Hopi of the Southwest, as well as people from many other cultures, traditionally isolate and protect new mothers and babies for twenty-one to thirty days to ensure a gentle transition into parenthood.

After the new mother has recovered enough to get up without dizziness, it is time to wash off the sweat, perhaps by tak-

Recipe for Mother Warming Soup[2]

Dang Gui Chicken Soup

2 lbs. organic chicken

1 c. water

4 c. organic chicken stock

5 spring onions, thinly sliced

1 stalk celery, sliced

2 carrots, sliced into ¼-inch rounds

5 slices ginger

½ tsp. sea salt

pepper to taste

¼ c. rice wine

5 very thin slices dang gui (available from Asian grocery stores or online)

20 goji berries

Rinse the chicken and add it to the water and broth in a heavy stockpot. Bring to a boil. Add the onions, celery, carrots, and ginger, then cover and reduce heat. Simmer for 1 hour. Remove the chicken from the broth and shred the meat into small pieces. Strain the broth through a strainer or sieve, and pour it back into the stockpot. Add the sliced carrots, herbs, salt, pepper, and rice wine. Bring to a boil, cover, and reduce heat. Simmer for 25 minutes. Add the chicken and the dang gui and gogi berries and cook for 10 minutes more. Remove the dang gui before serving.

Note: Dang gui is not recommended for women who are pregnant or menstruating.

ing a refreshing ceremonial herbal bath with flower petals. If she has had a cesarean birth, she might enjoy receiving a ritual sponge bath scented with essential oils. Massaging the mother will soothe the muscles that strained to bring her child into the world and the feet that crossed many inner thresholds to complete this journey.

Even with tender care, the transition between the two worlds can continue for hours, days, even weeks. Other than excitement about the new baby, most everyone around the mother carries on as usual because nothing extraordinary happened to them. Even if they witnessed the birth, this is not the same rite of passage as experiencing birth in the body and mind.

Generally speaking, we have no customs of seclusion to aid birthing women during this time of integration. Within minutes of giving birth, a woman is expected to reenter the world. Before she has even had time to bond with her baby, contemplate her experience, or clean up, her space is invaded. A flurry of social media messages may be sent and received through texts, phone calls, and digital photos. Visitors will likely trail in and out of her room to see the baby and make mindless comments about the labor. Nurses, following protocols, will ask long lists of questions and give routine, hurried instructions — even late in the night when an exhausted new mother should be resting (and can barely absorb the information). It is a good idea to be aware and advise others of the new mother's need for integration.

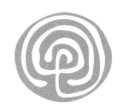

WELCOMING YOUR BABY

It's the strangest feeling at the end of pregnancy: you look down at this huge belly and try to imagine how some little person, whom you haven't even met, is going to emerge from it any day and completely change your lives.

—LISE ELIOT

How your baby experiences being born is unknowable. But allowing yourself to imagine your baby's experience and what he needs will help you welcome him to the world. In preparation, close your eyes and picture your baby's life in the womb:

Warm

Floating

Curled up in a soft, snug world

Silence visited by muted voices

And the drumming of your heartbeat.

Rhythmic rocking

Peaceful.

Now imagine your whole life had been this meditative dream. After being curled up snug in a warm womb, you are abruptly thrust into an environment of bright light, cold air, loud voices, and new sensations such as fabric against your velvety soft skin, and the extension of limbs into unbounded space. Now that you, as a parent, sense how startling these changes can be for a newborn, you can begin to intuit ways to welcome your baby. Following are a few ideas.

Near the end of labor, warm up the room: turn off the air conditioner, stoke the fire. While pushing, have someone warm baby blankets in a dryer or on a heating pad. Dim the lights. When your baby is born, speak softly. Receive your wet, wriggly baby skin to skin. Cradle him against the left side of your chest, allowing him to continue hearing the familiar sound of your heartbeat. Babies who snuggle skin to skin right after birth (not swaddled in a blanket or under a warmer) cry less, have more stable temperatures and blood sugars, and breastfeed longer.[1] Cover yourself and your baby with a soft blanket. Gently and rhythmically stroke your baby's back, simulating the familiar uterine contractions. Sing your baby's birth song.

Even though your baby is born, the cord will pulsate for a few minutes as it continues to send him oxygen while he takes his first breaths of air. If desired, your partner could cut the cord. Your birth attendant will assess your baby's well-being with a brief exam, which can be done while he is on your belly.

Let your baby slowly and quietly adjust to all the new sensations of this world. Spend as long as you wish seeing him for the first time. Take in the miracle and ordeal you just lived.

A newborn's eyes are usually wide open at birth and able to focus ten to twenty inches away—about the distance from his mother's face. When a newborn baby gazes into his mother's face, he tends to be quietly alert, getting to know her. Be-

Sing Your Baby's Birth Song

When a woman of the Himba African tribe knows she is pregnant, she goes to the jungle with other women, and together they pray and meditate until they find The Song of the Child. When the child is born, the community gets together and sings the child's song. When the child begins her education, people get together and sing her song. When she becomes an adult, the community gets together again to sing it. When it comes time for her wedding, she again hears her song. Finally, when her soul is going from this world, family and friends approach and, like at her birth, sing her song to accompany it on the journey.[2]

cause he already knows his mother's voice, he is soothed hearing it.[3] Newborns perceive sounds in the higher ranges; no wonder mothers instinctively speak in a higher pitch to their newborns.[4]

Another Little Lesson in Obstetric History

Immediately after birth, doctors used to hang babies upside down and slap their bottoms to make them cry, believing that intense crying was good for babies because it opened up their lungs. In *Mamatoto: A Celebration of Birth*, we learn that other cultures have similar rituals: "The Abron of the Ivory Coast splash their young with cold water, and in Haiti a large wooden bowl used to be inverted over the baby and beaten like a drum to wake it up!"[5]

The way babies were treated at birth was challenged by Frédérick Leboyer in his book *Birth without Violence*. Leboyer, an obstetrician who had delivered ten thousand babies in Paris during his forty years of practice, observed babies at birth. He believed their intense crying and dramatic body tension at birth were signs of terror, not healthy vigor. In an effort to make babies' transition from the womb to the outside world more gentle, he dimmed the lights in the delivery room and insisted on hushed voices. He massaged the newborn as she lay on her mother's belly. Sometimes he even murmured chants he'd learned in India. Wanting to return the newborn to her familiar watery environment, within the hour of birth Leboyer immersed her in a warm bath. Tender photographs capture the baby floating in water while held in Leboyer's hands, opening her eyes, looking around, sometimes even smiling or so deeply relaxed that she is falling asleep. This bath is a ritual of welcoming to her new world and is not used to wash the baby.[6]

THE GOLDEN HOUR

You have been bonding with your baby for many months before birth, feeling her move, talking to her, perhaps singing. There is a profound joy in meeting your wet, wriggly baby in the first hour after birth, sometimes called the golden hour. But if you are separated in the first hours or days there is no reason to believe you will not form a deep, lifelong bond.[7]

Here is what happened after my cesarean birth:

I was separated from my cesarean-born son for three long hours due to routine nursery protocol. I had read that missing the first hour could interfere with maternal-infant attachment, but for me it strengthened my maternal protectiveness and bond. After we were reunited, I made the nurses and doctors come to my room to do all baby checks. I told them, "My baby's weight and vital signs are not important to me. If it is important enough to you to do the check, you must come to my room. I had a cesarean surgery, so I am not coming to you. My baby and I are not going to be separated."

Apparently my maternal-infant bonding caused a stir in the change-of-shift report. Several nurses opened my door to look at me and said things like, "We heard about you in the report. We just wanted to see what you look like." Were they expecting a mother tiger?

If you and your baby are separated or the postpartum routines were disruptive, all is not lost. When you get home and settle in, create your own golden hour. Immerse yourself in seeing and feeling your baby without distractions or being rushed. Relish this memory.

HOSPITAL NURSERY

In a home birth and in baby-friendly hospitals, the newborn exam is done in the mother's room; mother and baby are only separated when there is a medical concern. However, in many hospitals, after an hour or two even a healthy baby is routinely separated from her mother for an hour or more after birth to satisfy nursery protocol. To find out what to expect from your hospital before you are in labor, ask during your prenatal tour of the facility. Even if it is hospital protocol to separate healthy babies from their mothers, inquire how an exception might be made for you. If separation cannot be avoided, delay it as long as you can during these precious hours, allowing breastfeeding to get off to a good start.

Here are a few more important things about newborns.

- A newborn baby is very alert during the first two hours after birth, with eyes wide-open and dreamy. So this is an ideal time to get to know your baby.

- The customary bath—a hasty sponge bath or a "shower" under a running tap, followed by brisk toweling—is neither necessary nor soothing. To a newborn who has just come from her warm, dark, watery world, this hurried bath under bright lights in a cold nursery is startling and stressful. Babies invariably get chilled after a bath as they lose body heat through "evaporative cooling."[8] Consequently, it is best to decline the baby bath.

- When a newborn gets cold, her blood sugar drops. So the phase following the standard baby bath involves rewarming the baby by putting her under electric lights in a baby warmer until her temperature returns to normal, which usually means another hour or two away from her mother. If the baby does get chilled, skin-to-skin contact with the mother helps regulate temperature more effectively and humanely than a hospital warmer.[9] Washing a newborn before she has had lots of skin-to-skin time and opportunities to nurse can also interfere with breastfeeding.[10]

  When you consider a lifetime with your child, a few more hours of separation for nursery rituals such as bathing does not seem very long, but when you have just given birth it can feel like an eternity.

- In utero, from around 25 weeks' gestation on, a baby's skin is coated with a creamy layer of vernix caseosa, which protects and moisturizes the skin while the fetus is immersed in amniotic water. Usually called "vernix," this white waxy substance, which looks like cream cheese, is filled with antimicrobial substances necessary to protect the hairless fetus's skin. Vernix, made by no other mammal, serves many purposes, including temperature regulation, immunity, and prevention of water loss. It is also a moisturizer high in vitamin E and has a unique scent that is part of mother-infant bonding.[11] The coating of vernix on your baby's body, designed to protect her from infection in utero and immediately after birth, contains surfactants that keep the airway sterile during baby's first breaths after birth.[12] When briskly drying the newborn, hospital staff often rub the vernix off, which is unfortunate because it provides a barrier to bacteria often found in hospitals (Staphylococcus, Bacillus, and E. coli).[13] So if possible, don't let them rub off the vernix.

Baby Probiotics

Infant probiotic drops help to restore the gut flora in a baby who was treated with antibiotics. Baby probiotics can help prevent colic.[14, 15]

- A baby's first poops (called meconium*) are black and sticky. After your newborn poops, avoid rubbing her downy soft skin to get the meconium off; rather, put a little olive or coconut oil on her bottom the first day so the meconium slides off.

Baby Massage

There is an Indian tradition of giving the newly born baby a cleansing massage with a soft dough ball made of wheat flour, water, a dash of turmeric, and almond oil. Instead of using hands, the lemon-sized dough ball is dipped in almond oil just before it is gently rolled over the baby's body. This is done every day for the first six days. Then for the next three weeks the baby is given a dough-ball massage, using repetitive strokes with moderate pressure. Between four and six weeks, you can begin massaging with your hands. If you want to learn more, find an infant massage class in your community.[16] Your baby will receive many benefits from a soothing massage: it may help regulate sleep and wake cycles

An Ancient Aztec Water and Naming Ceremony

An ancient Aztec ritual (ca.1535–1550) of bathing and naming the newborn child was conducted on the fourth day after birth. The midwife invoked the goddess of water and performed four rituals with water: putting drops of water on the baby's mouth, she told him to receive the water he needed to live upon the earth; touching the baby's chest with her wet hand, she invoked the purifying property of water that cleans the heart; casting drops of water on the baby's head, she told the baby to let the water enter his body; then finally, she washed the baby's body to keep evil from him. Following the ceremony, the baby was given a name.[17]

so your baby sleeps more peacefully; boost immunity; and reduce fussiness. It may also increase serotonin and oxytocin production in both you and your baby.

PLACENTA CUSTOMS

In many cultures it is customary to bury the placenta near the family home. The burial might entail giving the placenta back to the earth to nourish the roots of a tree, which grows as the baby does.

Most land mammals eat the placenta immediately after birth (placentophagy), but humans never have—until a recent trend to cook or encapsulate dried placenta began to develop in the United States. A study of 179 societies determined that humans have neither an instinct nor tradition to eat the placenta.[18] Perhaps the recent trend is an evolutionary adaptation since the placenta contains enzymes that perform major processes of metabolism, including filtering toxins, which accumulate in the placenta during pregnancy.

Advocates of placenta encapsulation claim the human placenta provides many postpartum benefits, such as boosting energy, minimizing baby blues, improving mood, increasing breast milk production, and treating anemia. In fact, almost nothing is known about the biological effects of human consumption of the placenta. According to one source, "No one has tested dosages, or whether the preparation process (freezing, drying, cooking, sterilizing, radiating, or pickling) destroys the potentially beneficial components."[19]

Promoters of placenta encapsulation often refer to a centuries-old traditional Chinese medicine practice utilizing dried human placenta (*zi he che*). An account of men in China written over six hundred years ago describes ingesting *zi he che* to boost their energy.[20] In combination with other herbs, dried placenta is used on rare occasions to treat infertility, impotence, chronic cough, asthma, and other conditions, but not postpartum mood disorders.[21]

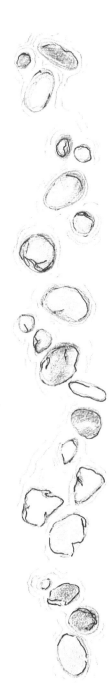

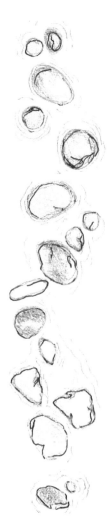

So what is inspiring the placental encapsulation trend in the United States? Is it that people have always looked for home remedies to treat postpartum mood disorders? Could it come from knowing we are out of touch with our bodies and life itself, and a longing to be natural? Although no scientific study or medical evidence exists that supports these claims, there are plenty of testimonials about positive results, which are promoted without regard to standardized preparation or dosage. The placebo effect can be a good thing: women who pay to have their placentas dried and encapsulated expect it to work, and it often seems to.

Dr. Andrew Weil, renowned author and director of the Arizona Center for Integrative Medicine, states: "I think there is probably little risk in eating...one's own placenta, but I frankly doubt there are many benefits, either. The modest quantities of beneficial substances that would survive cooking [and] freeze-drying would have virtually no effect. Instead, to alleviate the very real problem of postpartum depression, I strongly recommend eating cold-water fatty fish (wild-caught salmon, herring, and sardines) or supplementing with a quality fish oil. Two recent trials showed a 50 percent reduction in postpartum depression in women with relatively high intakes of omega-3 fatty acids. And 120 capsules of fish oil cost considerably less than $275."[22]

⑥

43

BREASTFEEDING FROM WITHIN

Breastfeeding is a journey that lasts longer than the journey of birth. More than a method of feeding, it is a dynamic and intimate relationship between you and your baby. Focusing on the connection with your baby and yourself is the heart of "breastfeeding from within."

A s humans, we are hardwired for breastfeeding, and the benefits for baby, mother, and the world are extensive and well documented.[1] While breastfeeding is instinctive and natural for a mother and baby, it is common for the first days and weeks to be a bit bumpy as you navigate a steep learning curve while also recovering from birth. Throughout this book, you have been learning how to awaken your inner Warrior and cultivate an attitude of being flexible, taking action, and practicing self-love, qualities that will serve you well as a breastfeeding mother. Persistence, patience, understanding the normal course of breastfeeding, and good support are essential in overcoming any challenges during the first month of breast-

**Tidbits for
Your Breastfeeding Basket**

Breastfeeding is a huge subject that cannot be covered fully in one chapter. To learn more, find a breastfeeding class or support group near you and refer to appendix C for recommended books and websites.

feeding. This chapter, written by Virginia Bobro, a breastfeeding counselor of twenty years, offers helpful tips based on current best practices.

Preparing for Breastfeeding

Mothers often tell us that they continue to use the mindfulness practices they learned in pregnancy to quiet the mind, decrease negative self-talk, and reduce stress during the first few months postpartum. Mindfulness also increases patience, resilience, and the flow of beneficial hormones.

Your Tasks of Preparation during pregnancy include learning about the normal course of breastfeeding, common problems and solutions, and local and online resources. Hanging out with breastfeeding mothers while pregnant (at La Leche League meetings, for example) allows you to learn firsthand about a variety of situations and solutions that will help you construct realistic expectations. And becoming part of the breastfeeding community provides you with a ready-made support system should challenges or questions arise.

When you hear breastfeeding stories that generalize, simplify, or are one-sided, restore balance by finding out more. If you hear a negative story, ask the storyteller: "How did you cope?" or "What was helpful or made things a bit easier for you?" When a woman is recounting how easy or wonderful her breastfeeding experience was, ask: "Were there any surprises or bumps in the road?" or "What was most helpful to you in the first few weeks?" The answers to these solution-focused questions can be gems of wisdom.

Within an hour of birth, your amazing newborn, when placed skin to skin on your belly, will begin crawling up toward your chest. Her reflexes and instincts will guide her, without any prompting or positioning, to latch on to and begin suckling at your breast.

GETTING OFF TO A GOOD START

A variety of factors can affect the start of your breastfeeding relationship, some of which are out of your control—for example, how your birth unfolds and your anatomy as well as your baby's, such as inverted nipples or tongue-tie.* Getting off to a perfect start is a rare occurrence (92 percent of women have breastfeeding concerns in the first three days[2]).

In the days, weeks, months, and even years that a mother is breastfeeding she may face numerous other obstacles, doubts, and unexpected events. Even the most optimistic, intelligent, healthy, and determined woman can struggle with breastfeeding, which is no reflection on her abilities as a woman or mother. While there are no guarantees, a natural birth, a supportive family, breastfeeding education, and good breastfeeding management will increase the likelihood of a positive experience. You can stack the odds in your favor by doing the following to the best of your ability and as circumstances allow:

- Initiate early and frequent skin-to-skin contact with your baby.

- Begin breastfeeding as soon after birth as you can, ideally within the first hour. If you miss that window, nurse your baby as soon as you can and hand-express or pump in the meantime.

- Delay bathing your newborn for at least twenty-four hours.

- Get help with good positioning and latch; try the "laid-back" position first.[3]

- Nurse ten to twelve times a day; newborns have tiny tummies and need frequent feeding.

- Hand-express or pump every two to three hours if your baby won't have access to you or isn't nursing well.

- Be aware of, and respond promptly to, your baby's feeding cues; watch your baby, not the clock.

- Avoid introducing a pacifier or bottle until breastfeeding is well established, meaning that baby is gaining weight well and your nipples are not sore.

Early Signs of Hunger in a Newborn

Being awake

Licking lips

Rooting

Late Signs of Hunger

Frantic fist-sucking

Fussing or crying

• Avoid swaddling in the first few weeks as it can decrease feeding frequency.

• Have the names and numbers of several experts you can call for help (WIC, La Leche League, a lactation counselor [IBCLC], and others).

MILK SUPPLY

While not common, some women, for a variety of reasons, are not physiologically able to produce a full supply of milk. However, most instances of low milk supply are actually due to poor understanding and management of breastfeeding, especially in the first week. Cultural messages about breastfeeding can subtly, or not so subtly, undermine your confidence in your body's ability to nourish your baby. Seeds of doubt can be planted soon after birth, when you are already feeling vulnerable and exhausted. Hearing women tell stories about "losing my milk" or using special lactation herbs or foods might

---

What's in a Name?

Anyone can call herself a "lactation consultant," so be sure to ask about your breastfeeding helper's credentials and training. Under the Affordable Care Act, breastfeeding classes, home visits, and pumps must be covered by insurance. The following resources may also be helpful:

LLL = La Leche League International: a mother-to-mother breastfeeding support organization run by trained volunteers who offer help by phone and at local meetings

WIC = Women, Infants, and Children: a special supplemental nutrition program for low-income families offering free breastfeeding help and pumps

IBCLC = International Board Certified Lactation Consultant: an allied healthcare professional who has extensive training and ongoing education in breastfeeding

lead you to believe that you cannot trust your body to know how to nourish your baby. Insufficient milk supply is often diagnosed incorrectly—for example, when a mother's breasts don't feel engorged anymore, or when normal newborn behavior is misinterpreted as hunger (wanting to nurse "all the time" or sleeping well after a supplemental bottle).

Excellent support and accurate information are essential ingredients for a good milk supply. (Refer to *The Breastfeeding Mother's Guide to Making More Milk* by Diana West and Lisa Marasco for good information on this topic.) Reach out for help (not lactation cookies) if you have concerns about your milk supply or baby's weight gain. Frequent breast stimulation by baby or a pump in the first three days is linked to a good milk supply at two months and beyond. Frequent skin-to-skin contact with your baby increases milk-making hormones and infant weight gain, decreases fussiness, and makes mothering more enjoyable. Treasure those moments of snuggling with your newborn baby as you fully awaken to your mother-self.

Your baby is getting enough milk in the first weeks if:

- She is nursing at least ten times in each twenty-four-hour period.

- She has vigorous jaw movements and you can hear swallowing during feeds.

- She has at least six wet diapers and two to four poops per day (after day four).

- She has quiet alert periods every day. (In the first two weeks, a baby who is very sleepy or very fussy may not be getting enough calories.)

- She is gaining weight. (It is normal for a newborn to lose up to 10 percent of her birth weight in the first week and catch up to her birth weight by two weeks.

WHEN BREASTFEEDING HURTS

In general, breastfeeding should not hurt; it is designed to be enjoyable for both mother and baby. Some tenderness as you adjust to new sensations is to be expected in the first few days, but if your nipples are cracked, pinched, bleeding, or raw, or if breastfeeding isn't going smoothly in the first few weeks, get help as soon as possible from a skilled lactation professional.

There are many causes of sore or damaged nipples. Prompt help can prevent infection, mastitis, low weight gain, low milk supply, and other problems. Most cases of sore nipples are quickly resolved by adjusting the positioning and latch of the baby; the baby should have a large mouthful of breast, not be nibbling on the nipple. It is to no one's benefit for you to "grin and bear it." When you are struggling with feedings, emotional support and encouragement is just as important as practical advice; at times this may mean that you will need a "village" of breastfeeding allies.

Alternative Feeding Methods

If the baby needs supplemental feeding, bottle feeding is a common choice. However, for short-term use, especially when the goal is to get the baby feeding exclusively at the breast, there are a number of better options, such as cup feeding, tube feeding with a syringe or finger, or using a supplemental nursing device.

SELF-CARE WHILE BREASTFEEDING

We've found that creating lots of "rules" can make breastfeeding seem more difficult and restrictive than it needs to be. However, here are a few tips that might help.

Causes of damaged or sore nipples:

Poor positioning and/or latch technique

Tongue mobility restriction (tongue-tie*)

Infant birth injury

Flat or inverted nipples

Bacterial or yeast infection

Solutions:

Get expert help with latch and positioning

Assess and treat tongue-tie

Assess and treat infections

Get some bodywork (craniosacral or chiropractic therapy)

Last resort—use a nipple shield short-term, with help from IBCLC

Paced Bottle-Feeding

If your baby is being given a bottle, try a paced bottle-feeding technique to slow down the rate of feeding and more closely imitate the pace of breastfeeding. This not only allows your baby to more easily move back and forth between breast and bottle but is a more relaxing and natural way for a baby to be fed. Check online for instructional videos.

Diet

There are lots of ideas and myths about what breastfeeding mothers should and should not eat, but there is no need to avoid certain foods unless and until there is a reason to do so. It's important during this time of intensive mothering that you enjoy nursing and eating instead of trying to be perfect or follow strict rules. Continue following your "pregnancy diet," aiming for healthful and nutrient-dense foods. Nursing burns about 500 calories a day—causing many mothers to find that they need a big snack in the middle of the night. Aim to drink about eight large glasses of water a day (overhydration isn't helpful). The let-down reflex at the start of feed can bring on a strong thirst, so always have a full water bottle in your "nursing corner." It's important during this time of intensive mothering that you are able to enjoy nursing and eating, instead of trying to be perfect or follow strict rules.

Sleep

Recent research shows that, despite assumptions to the contrary, breastfeeding mothers actually get more sleep than formula-feeding mothers.[4] Newborns tend to "cluster feed," nurse frequently for a few hours then take a long nap. Become sensitive to this natural rhythm and ensure that you are resting during that long nap, too, even if it is during the day. When you are nurtured and nourished emotionally and physically, and allowed time to recover from birth and your transition to motherhood, you will feel less depleted, even when you are nursing round the clock. Sometimes what is really needed is reducing other responsibilities and chores, as well as reassurance that you are not alone in the ups and downs of adjusting to your "new normal."

A Mother's Tasks
Compassion and Self-Love

Once you are have established a day-to-day experience with breastfeeding, continue to practice mindfulness, maintain self-care and flexibility, and reach out for emotional and practical support. If breastfeeding does not match your hopes and expectations, reach out for support to keep going instead of getting mired in regret, blame, or self-judgment about what "went wrong."

For a variety of reasons, some mothers who are passionate about breastfeeding supplement or wean earlier than they had hoped. Such outcomes are best viewed as opportunities to reenvision how to nurture and nourish their babies. The definition of a "successful" breastfeeding relationship can change over time. No matter how your breastfeeding journey unfolds, what you really need to tell yourself and hear from others is that you are doing your best. Seek out wise mentors and peers who listen with compassion and offer nonjudgmental support that reinforces your positive identity as a mother. In the long run, that is what is most important for your child.

FEEDING WITH LOVE

This mindfulness practice can be done while breastfeeding or bottle feeding. When sitting (or lying down) to feed your baby, try this:

Begin to notice all the sensations around you, beginning with your baby:
> *Look at her face, notice the touch of her skin, breathe in her smell, her sounds.*

Then begin to bring your attention to your own body:
> *Where does your body touch your baby's body?*
> *How is your breath moving in and out of your body?*
> *Where do you feel relaxed and open?*
> *Where does your body feel tight, tense, or closed?*
>> *Gently and mindfully breathe into those places,*
>> *softening and releasing any worries or concerns that are unneeded in this moment.*

As your body lets go of anything extra, feel your heart opening.

If feeding is difficult, do what needs to be done then, when you are ready, take another conscious breath. Return to opening your heart to your little one as you nourish her.

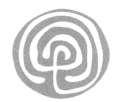

BIRTH STORY GATES

In the hours surrounding birth, most women are
so immersed in living the experience that they
cannot analyze it or tell a story about it. But soon
after the birth they begin developing a story about
it, both to remember it and to understand how
and why the events unfolded as they did.

While listening to women's birth stories over the years,
I began to see that they were not static but rather underwent
a somewhat predictable evolution over the postpartum year,
or longer. I subsequently identified nine modifications of birth
stories and theorized that a modern woman after giving birth,
like Inanna after her ordeal, returns from the underworld by
going back through the gates she entered during her descent
into Laborland plus two more to complete her rite of passage
to motherhood.

It helps to think of the postpartum return gates as birth
story gates. As you approach each gate, you will be remembering, sorting, putting events in order, gathering lost bits
of information, or forgiving yourself or others. Imagine
that there is a Gatekeeper at each one, asking you what
version of the story you are telling yourself now, what part

of it is a problem for you, and what you believe it means about you; then imagine the Gatekeeper lifting from your story one small piece that is no longer serving you and returning this piece to the underworld. In this way, your early account of the events that occur during labor will be transformed into a deeply personal story about your transition to motherhood.

Searching for meaning in an evolving birth story can be likened to the careful excavation of a buried treasure. If an archaeologist were quickly satisfied with the first shard discovered on the surface, the exploration would end before the hidden intact painted pot was found. Similarly, if a woman were satisfied with her first glimmering insight that explains what happened in labor or postpartum her search for deeper meaning might end. And when the search for new meaning stops, so does the journey "home."

As a "story archaeologist," let intuition guide you to where something important lies. Looking for meaning in your birth story, you might initially break ground with a shovel, then gradually work your way down to using a trowel and a soft brush to gently sweep away dust. During this patient process, you will eventually see how all the pieces and layers of your birth experience fit together. Following are some excavation tips to guide you through the nine story gates.

In the mythic story "Inanna's Descent," she descends and ascends through seven gates. However, in this book the Return is through nine gates to accommodate the nine birth stories.

FIRST GATE
No Birth Story

In numerology, the number nine symbolizes finality, spiritual awakening, global consciousness, a higher perspective, and service to humanity.

In the precious first hours after giving birth, a woman usually has few words with which to create a birth story. In Laborland, where time seems to stand still, you will probably float wordlessly through the Gate of No Story.

Then, before you've had time to form your own birth story people who witnessed your labor and birth might tell you their stories about your birth. Visitors who come later might also share their opinions about your birth, adding to the stories by others. Additionally, before being discharged you may be "de-briefed" by your birth attendant, who will tell you her story about your birth. Such stories by others leave a lasting impression that may eclipse your own memory of your birth.

This is what happened to Amy. When she told her story, she began by saying, "I hemorrhaged so badly I scared my midwife. She said it was the worst she ever saw."

"Amy, that is not your story, it is your midwife's story," I suggested. "If you could pretend your midwife had not told you her story, how would you begin telling *your* story?" After thinking about it for a moment, she told her story, which did not include any details of bleeding after birth.

SECOND GATE
Relief and Gratitude Story

Most women are initially relieved and grateful that labor is over and that they and their baby got through it. You will likely spend weeks to months at the Second Gate praising everyone and everything that helped you in any way, including technology, drugs, and intervention. This perspective dovetails with the joy that accompanies meeting your new baby and with your elevated oxytocin levels.

THIRD GATE
Relationships Story

At this gate, you review who was there, who wasn't, who helped in unexpected ways, and who, if anyone, abandoned you. You may also examine changes in your relationships with your mother, father, husband or partner, friends, birth attendants, older children, other mothers, and most importantly, your relationship with yourself as a result of events surrounding the birth.

Fourth Gate

Social Birth Story

The social birth story emerges with the first postpartum phone call, tweet, or visitor. Depending on who is listening, or what is emphasized or left out, it can change each time it is told. This story is the version most often told during "birth story swapping," a competitive ritual among women for purposes of bonding and bragging. Here is an example: A woman gave birth by cesarean because she had active herpes; social stigma influenced this story from the start so that in the recovery room the mother told a caller that she had to have a cesarean because the baby was too big.

"There is another way of breathing."

—Rumi[1]

Fifth Gate

Medical Birth Story

The medical birth story is the dominant birth story in our culture. It is considered the most valid account and the one new mothers are expected to share. Using medical jargon to justify, explain, or debate medical management can objectify what happened, thus creating emotional distance. At the same time, a detailed medical story can evoke strong emotional feelings. Understand the medical birth story and then try to progress beyond the Fifth Gate so you will know the deeper meaning of the birth.

Sixth Gate

Victim and Judge Story

When Inanna leaves the underworld, she passes by the judges. Women returning from Laborland also pass by judges—hearing not only self-judgments but also the opinions of others who question them about what happened and why.

Weeks, months, or even years after giving birth, you may begin to dwell on a few moments in the birth that you regret or wish you could do over. You begin to experience an internal dialogue between the archetypal voices called the Victim and the Judge. The Victim laments how what happened was not fair and not your fault, why it was someone else's fault, or why you were powerless to alter aspects of the birth. Instantly, the Judge answers the Victim, saying why and how aspects of the birth were the fault of the Victim, what the Victim could have done differently and should do in the future.

Then the Victim again explains how the way events unfolded were not her fault, spilling out her feelings, which are lost on the Judge, who reminds her of the things she could have done differently. In this way, the Sixth Gate becomes a revolving door in which the Victim and Judge go round and round, getting nowhere.

Many people never get past the Sixth Gate on their Return, remaining trapped in this revolving door for years, even for a lifetime. You cannot avoid this gate, so listen with compassion to what you are telling yourself about yourself; try to understand and embrace the Victim's feelings of powerlessness, betrayal, or having failed, and acknowledge the Judge's positive intention of trying to keep you strong and safe, and able to maintain your self-respect. One of the things you want at this gate is to be heard—by someone. That someone can be you. When you stop to listen to both voices in your head, the revolving door stops.

SEVENTH GATE
New Meaning Story

Eventually you gain new perspective on the birth and are able to ask yourself new questions and receive fresh answers that lead to sudden insights. This gate opens to compassion for yourself and others as you make connections between how your conditioning and everyone's conditioning (your partner's, your family's, and your birth attendants') influenced decisions made and other events that occurred during the birth. As you see how your birth story is connected to your past and the framework of birth in your culture, your story takes on new dimensions.

"If your compassion does not include yourself, it is incomplete."

—BUDDHA[2]

EIGHTH GATE
Huntress Story

As you function in the world, part of your attention is always turned inward, reflecting on your birth story. Instead of looking to others to affirm, validate, approve, or explain your experience, your Huntress begins to stalk your own habitual patterns of thinking and old assumptions. Passing through this gate, your mind opens to new words, phrases, images, and metaphors that appear unexpectedly to constantly rearrange the narrative of your story.

"The Warrior Sage dwells upon neither success nor failure, but rather just corrects her course as needed, even while moving on."

—G. BLUESTONE[3]

NINTH GATE
Wise Woman's Story

By the time you reach the Ninth Gate, you will have deconstructed, digested, and reconstructed your birth story. When you cross the threshold of the Ninth Gate, you will no longer need to tell your birth story to gain sympathy, advice, reassurance, or praise. Rather than telling your whole story from beginning to end, you will share with others only what might be helpful to them.

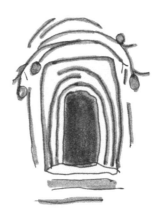

Burying Your Grief in Mother Earth

There is a time for grief, despair, or rage after a difficult experience or loss, and there is a time for healing and resolution. When grief, shame, blame, or feelings of powerlessness settle in and become familiar, we may be afraid to let go or not know how to. A ceremony to bury what has been lost may help you take another step toward healing. Find a place in nature that you love or that calls to you. Find three small objects (for example, a pebble, leaf, and feather) that represent something you want to release. Let your tears fall to Mother Earth; let her take your grief and transform it into healing, compassion, and a new perspective.

When you complete your journey through Laborland and the Return, a part of your map will always remain terra incognita. You can only have traversed a narrow swath of the infinite external and internal experiences possible during birth. It is humbling for a woman who births at home to acknowledge that, for her, many ways of giving birth, such as induction or cesarean birth, remain terra incognita. And for a woman who endured an induction, spontaneous labor remains terra incognita.

PERINATAL
MOOD DISORDERS

*Most people think that mood disorders associated
with birth only happen to others. However, they can
affect any new parent. There is much to be gleaned
in identifying and managing your perinatal* mental
health.*

Having a baby is a life-changing event that involves
a great deal of sudden change and loss—loss of the life you
used to have, loss of the body you once had, loss of sleep, autonomy, and free time. After you give birth, your relationships
with yourself, your partner, and others are in flux. Baby care
trumps and disrupts the routines that helped you stay on top
of things and count on a good night's sleep. Along with your
life being upended, exhaustion, the need for physical recovery,
and intense hormonal shifts can all contribute to causing mood
swings and irritability in the first few weeks and months postpartum.

At least 70 percent of new mothers experience some signs
of "baby blues" for part of each day during the first week or so
after birth. Symptoms, such as feeling sad, impatient, frustrated,
or having trouble sleeping even when exhausted, tend to coincide with milk coming in around day four or five. Baby blues

come to a natural end around fourteen days after birth; postpartum mood disorders, on the other hand, tend to increase in severity and duration after two to four weeks.

While everyone has heard of postpartum depression, there are several other mood disorders that can occur after birth, including anxiety, bipolar disorder, obsessive-compulsive disorder, PTSD*, psychosis, or a combination of these conditions. Such mood disorders first show up as personality or behavioral changes. Any new mother who exhibits these symptoms needs support as she takes her first steps toward identifying the disorder and learning to manage it.

Watchful Worrying or Full-Blown Anxiety?

You cannot fully anticipate the intensity of newly awakened parental instincts to protect your newborn. The overwhelming love for your infant is matched by an equal fear of losing him. With this comes the worry that is synonymous with parenting, which is especially noticeable when caring for an infant for the first time. In essence, watchful worrying is something every parent does.

Anxiety, on the other hand, may be symptomatic of a mood disorder. Often a woman who is developing a mood disorder does not realize it is happening. It may be others who are the first to notice changes in her personality or behavior. Since some degree of worry is normal, how do you know when to start worrying about the worrying? The following traits may indicate that a mood disorder is developing:

- Worrying obsessively about every little thing every day for weeks on end

- Catastrophic thinking about ordinary daily events

- Panic attacks

> "I was unexpectedly and thoroughly rearranged by childbirth in ways I could have never expected."
>
> —Kimberly

If your anxiety is mild to moderate, try the self-help tips described later in this chapter. If symptoms become severe or the self-help measures are not enough, talk to a professional trained to assess and treat perinatal mood disorders.

Prenatal and Postpartum Depression

Perinatal anxiety and depression are on the rise: nearly 20 percent of women in developing countries (and therefore their babies) are affected.[1] Depression in pregnancy can be missed because its symptoms, such as sleeping difficulties, tearfulness, anxiety, or moodiness, are common in pregnant women. To complicate matters, many doctors believe that women don't get depressed during pregnancy because they are naturally euphoric from the hormonal changes. However, a recent study found that a third of the women who would later have postpartum depression were already depressed during pregnancy.[2] Postpartum depression can also begin anytime during the first year postpartum, and generally lasts for three to six months. Half of women report mild symptoms that resolve without treatment, while the other half have serious symptoms that require treatment.[3] Severe postpartum depression is so distressing that women worry it will never end—but it will.

Scary thoughts

Scary thoughts, a very common symptom of postpartum depression and anxiety, are defined as negative, repetitive, unwanted thoughts parents have about the baby or themselves that come out of nowhere.[4] Just about every new mother and father has scary thoughts about their baby or themselves at some time. One study found 91 percent of new mothers and 88 percent of new fathers experience shocking, sometimes obsessive thoughts about accidentally or intentionally hurting their baby at some point,[5] but almost none act on it. Fortunately, if parents are worried about having scary thoughts it means they know the difference between right and wrong and therefore are not likely to hurt their baby.[6] Still, such parents don't know how they could be thinking such crazy thoughts, and they worry about acting on them. And because new mothers are often judged when they appear to be in any state other than maternal bliss they are naturally afraid of what others might think or do if they mention their scary thoughts. Sadly, at a time when such mothers need emotional support and assurance they often retreat, feeling isolated and lonely.

Even if a mother or the baby are not in immediate danger, when a mother believes she must be a "bad mother" because she has these thoughts it undermines a healthy self-image and her relationship with her infant. To avoid hurting her baby she may begin avoiding her baby, or to protect her baby from harm she may become hypervigilant.[7] In such instances, not only support but also information and counseling are important to help a woman separate symptoms of postpartum mood disorder from normal signs of coming to terms with her emerging mother-self.

Disturbing Postpartum Thoughts

Fleeting suicidal or homicidal thoughts

Thinking that another person is planning to hurt the mother or baby

Fantasies about accidentally or intentionally hurting the baby

In a study of one hundred parents between four and twelve weeks postpartum, unwanted thoughts of accidentally or intentionally harming the baby were universal.[8]

Causes of Postpartum Mood Disorders

Postpartum mood disorders are not new; Hippocrates documented postpartum mental illness as early as 400 BCE. However, recent studies reveal more about their causes, showing that they can arise from a combination of influences, many of which are uncontrollable and unforeseeable, such as a genetic predisposition; a sudden shift in hormones that affects brain chemistry; breastfeeding difficulties; emotional birth trauma; unsupportive family; a history of trauma, abuse, or PTSD; high expectations; perfectionism; socioeconomic stressors; sleep deprivation; poor diet; and thinking style (such as worrying, ruminating, or catastrophic thinking). Each factor can interact with the others, and they can activate or aggravate one another.[9]

Sudden shifts in hormonal levels

- During pregnancy, estrogen and progesterone levels increase more than a hundredfold. Immediately after birth, estrogen and progesterone levels plunge, a sudden drop that can decrease serotonin, disrupting brain chemistry. The precise influence that hormones have on perinatal mood disorders is not firmly established, but some women may be genetically predisposed to having increased sensitivity to shifts in hormones.

- While breastfeeding enhances bonding and feelings of well-being for many women, this is not true for all women. In one study, maternal oxytocin levels were measured in mid-pregnancy, and women with low oxytocin levels were later shown to be at greater risk for developing postpartum depression.[10] In another study, researchers found that breastfeeding mothers who had lower levels of oxytocin at eight weeks postpartum "were less happy and more stressed, depressed, irritated and overwhelmed during...feeding."[11]

- People with depression, anxiety, irritability, or insomnia have low levels of tryptophan, which leads to low levels of serotonin.[12] Serotonin stimulates the secretion of endorphins, which produce feelings of well-being and happiness. Until recently, women were blamed or judged for not being blissed out by motherhood, but in light of new research we are learning the hidden influence of hormones.

- Although it is rare, an abnormal thyroid level can contribute to postpartum anxiety or depression. It is diagnosed with a simple blood test and resolved with thyroid medication. Women with a previous history or family history of thyroid disease are at increased risk; women with type 1 diabetes have a three times higher risk and should be routinely screened postpartum.[13]

Stories limit perspectives and options

Every story a mother tells about her mental health shapes her self-image and perceptions about her situation. For example, if she says she is depressed because her baby went to the NICU or because she had an unwanted cesarean, and other contributing factors are not acknowledged, her narrative can lead her to feel regret and self-blame. A more helpful personal narrative would be one told with less certainty, allowing for more possibilities. For example, a mother might say, "Although I sense certain factors are contributing, I don't know exactly why I am feeling this way." The same holds true of stories others tell about a new mother's mental health.

Postpartum depression is no fun for mothers, fathers, or their babies

Babies flourish when they are held, smiled at, talked to, and played with. When parents thrive, baby thrives, too. A parent with postpartum depression often misses cues from the baby for nurturing or playing.[14] This is another reason to assess and treat postpartum depression as early as possible.

WHAT LOVED ONES CAN DO FOR A WOMAN SUFFERING FROM POSTPARTUM DEPRESSION

The need for loving and attentive support of the birth mother from partners, relatives, and friends does not end when the birth is over. A partner, relative, or friend of a new mother knows her personality and will probably be the first to notice if she is struggling.[15] Therefore, it is important to recognize signs of postpartum depression to guide the mother forward.

The pervasive negative stigma surrounding postpartum depression can make initial attempts to talk about the problem difficult. Many women cope on their own because, as noted earlier, they know that showing anything other than elation or strength could be viewed negatively. Some women fear being separated from their baby by social services. Liam, a concerned and persistent father, recounted how it took "a month of tears" before his distressed wife would agree to see a doctor. And if a woman finally asks for help from a doctor she may simply be pacified, told to take a nap or go for a walk. If her depression is mild to moderate, it is helpful to encourage her to implement the self-help measures appearing later in this chapter.

The sooner a postpartum woman with postpartum depression receives appropriate assessment and treatment, the sooner she can feel better, and the sooner the mother-baby bond is safeguarded. If you believe a mother's symptoms warrant professional attention, find a doctor or therapist who specializes in postpartum mood disorders. You may need to make the phone calls for her, go with her to the appointment and become informed. Severe postpartum depression can be caused by chemical or hormonal imbalances that require medication in addition to therapy. Restoring balance often requires patience while different drugs or combination of drugs are tried.

NEW FATHERS CAN ALSO EXPERIENCE POSTPARTUM DEPRESSION OR ANXIETY

Some new fathers experience symptoms of depression or anxiety, especially when the mother is experiencing a mood disorder.[16] During the first six months after the birth of their first child, many fathers report an increase in fatigue, irritability, headaches, difficulty concentrating, backache, colds, number of sick days, and a general decrease in vitality.[17] And, like mothers, their mental health and recovery depend on the support they receive.[18]

Partners who witness a difficult birth, especially when lots of unexpected things happen and they feel unprepared, unsupported, or unable to help, are at a higher risk of developing a mood disorder, particularly PTSD. They may benefit from a counseling or a Birth Story Medicine session to help them make sense of their experience.

POSTPARTUM PSYCHOSIS

Because the media sensationalize a rare condition called postpartum psychosis, whenever a woman is anxious or has scary thoughts about the baby or herself, people may immediately worry about postpartum psychosis, which occurs in only one or two women per thousand.[20] Symptoms begin in the first weeks after birth and include rapid speaking, racing thoughts, inability to concentrate, hyperactive behavior, bizarre thoughts, paranoia, suicidal fantasies, feeling detached from the baby, not wanting to nurse or care for the baby, and seeing or

Risk Factors for Postpartum Mood Disorders

Unplanned pregnancy

Teen pregnancy

Money worries

Short paid maternity/paternity leave

Marital conflict or unsupportive partner

A recent move or social isolation

Difficult or traumatic labor/birth

Cesarean birth

A baby in NICU; a preterm or sick baby[19]

Multiple birth

Breastfeeding difficulties

Sleep deprivation

A personal or family history of depression

hearing things others do not, such as warnings or instructions "from God" to hurt or kill the baby or older children.

What distinguishes normal "scary thoughts" from the extreme thoughts of postpartum psychosis? A psychotic mother does not worry about her "scary thoughts" because she believes them.

One final word: Don't abandon the new mother

If you suspect a new mother has postpartum psychosis, don't leave her alone, or alone with her baby or older children; seek professional help immediately from a psychiatrist, not a doula, herbalist, or placenta capsules. Psychosis is a medical emergency. With proper diagnosis, medication, hospitalization, counseling, and support, this condition usually improves within a few months and is resolved by the end of the first year postpartum.

◎

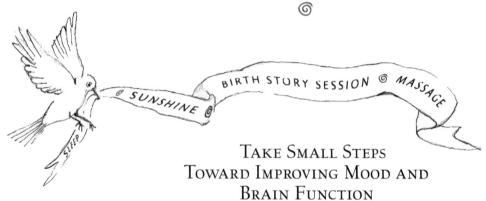

Take Small Steps Toward Improving Mood and Brain Function

One barrier to reaching out for and receiving help are the cultural and personal messages that women should be strong enough to deal with problems on their own and that needing or asking for help is a sign of weakness or failure. If you believe that smart, capable women don't get depressed, or that if you just try harder you will overcome the difficulties, then your belief could pose a significant obstacle in getting the help you need. Acknowledging that you are struggling and reaching out for support are signs of strength, good mothering, and compassionate self-care.

Think of worry, postpartum anxiety, scary thoughts, postpartum depression, and even postpartum psychosis as another turn in the Laborinth. The Birth Warrior's way through and out is by taking one small step at a time, doing the best she can. Following is a list of evidence-based suggestions for action.

Get more sleep

Within the first few weeks postpartum, like most new parents you may be exhausted from sleep interruption and deprivation. Four consecutive hours of sleep raises serotonin and melatonin levels, but an infant's need to feed and cuddle frequently makes it challenging to achieve this in the early postpartum period. As one father said, "You don't know the meaning of the word *tired* until you have a baby."

> *The most sound and timeless advice:*
> *Sleep when your baby sleeps. Leave the housework to others,*
> *and nap when your baby naps in the afternoon.*

To get to sleep and sleep more soundly:

- After feeding your baby, say good night and leave your baby with a loving caretaker in another room, giving them an opportunity to get to know each other a little better while you sleep.

- Eat protein with a simple carb before a nap or bedtime.

- Drink a cup of chamomile, skullcap, or tulsi tea.

- Put in earplugs, or turn on a fan or white noise machine. Wear a sleep mask or darken the room. In darkness, melatonin levels rise, which means the level of melatonin in your breast milk also increases, helping your baby sleep better, too.

- Turn off all electronic devices at least an hour before sleep. The blue light emitted by computer monitors inhibits normal sleep patterns.

Eat wholesome food

A study showed that people who ate a lot of processed foods were at higher risk of depression than those who consumed mostly whole foods.[21] Optimal brain function depends on a well-balanced diet. Aim for frequent small meals of high-quality fats, proteins, and complex carbs. Stay hydrated. Eat a diet rich in tryptophan. And enjoy dark chocolate, a proven and delicious mood-enhancer.

Boost your brain serotonin with foods rich in tryptophan:

Elk, seaweed, spirulina, spinach, chicken or turkey breast, shrimp, tuna, salmon or halibut, beef, pork, lamb, dark chocolate, milk, pumpkin seeds, yogurt, cottage cheese, eggs, bananas, and nuts (walnuts, almonds, cashews, peanuts). [22]

Supplement with omega-3 and B vitamins

Without supplementation of omega-3, maternal levels of this crucial fatty acid decrease during pregnancy and remain low for at least six weeks following birth. Numerous studies have linked low omega-3 levels and maternal depression.[23] Conversely, in one study, women who took 300 milligrams of DHA (a form of omega-3) beginning in their 24th week of pregnancy had significantly fewer symptoms of postpartum depression or anxiety.[24] High-quality fish oils are a good source of omega-3 and are now regularly recommended for pregnant women and new mothers.

To increase your serotonin level and improve your ability to cope with stress, get lots of B vitamins by eating foods high in B vitamins and folic acid (papaya, oranges, lentils and other legumes, avocado, dark leafy greens, corn, and beets) and by taking a supplement.

Consider sugar a downer

If sugar were a positive nutrient, we would all be healthier and happier. Unfortunately, sugar has an adverse effect on brain function and mood. Your brain depends on an even supply of glucose, but refined sugar, carbs, and processed food make blood sugar unstable, which contributes to mood swings.[25]

Compile a New-Parent Bliss List

Make a Bliss List of three activities you would like to start doing or do more of, activities that would be fulfilling, bring you joy, or create harmony in your life. Post your Bliss List where you can see it often, and write the following pledge on it: "I promise to do everything on my list at least once before my baby's first birthday." Here's what I did:

I was caught off guard by postpartum depression with my first child. During my second pregnancy, I made plans to "get ahead of it." I signed up for a six-week drawing class to start about six weeks after I gave birth. I looked forward to my two-hour class every week, and the drawings I made were pretty good; I still have them.

Vitamin D, produced when sunlight is absorbed through the skin, promotes serotonin production, boosts immune function, and reduces inflammation. Low levels of vitamin D are correlated with postpartum depression.[26] Talk with your healthcare provider about having your serum vitamin D levels tested and taking a supplement, especially in the winter.

Arrange weekend breakfast or brunch dates

To help Colleen recover from postpartum depression, I arranged weekly child care for our Sunday morning breakfast date. At first it was hard to get away, but soon we looked forward to reconnecting with each other free of distractions once a week.
—Sean

A lot of new parents find their weekly date nights are sabotaged because not only are they tired but babies tend to be fussy in the evenings. On weekend mornings, parents and their baby are more rested.

Find social and emotional support

Becoming a mother can mean an upheaval in your identity, your body image, your time management, and your relationships. However, social and emotional isolation can exacerbate a negative mood. So it's important to connect emotionally with other mothers in your community or online. But be discerning: groups that are judgmental or cling to rigid dogma about how to be a perfect mother may only increase your feelings of loneliness. Look for groups that are compassionate, accepting, and have experienced or older mothers rather than just peer support.

Meditate and do mindfulness practices

Quieting your mind through meditation or mindfulness practices can help you face the challenges of new mothering. It has been shown that meditation makes a positive difference in women with postpartum depression.[27] The mindfulness and pain-coping practices in this book can be effective in reducing the negative effects of mood disorders. Breath Awareness and Circular Breathing are particularly helpful in decreasing anxiety and signs of PTSD. Also, walking or tracing a labyrinth can be soothing and enjoyable.

Many women have found that meditation, exercise, and diet changes were enough to help them overcome depression without medication.

Get a massage

A study found that when pregnant women were massaged twice a week by their partners for four months their serotonin levels increased by 30 percent.[28] Your doula may offer this service; if not, find a massage therapist who specializes in mother massages.

Massaging the baby has been found to lessen postpartum depression. Lovingly touching and gazing at your baby during the massage does wonders for bonding and increases oxytocin in both you and baby.[29] One study found that when young babies were massaged for fifteen minutes twice a week for six weeks, their serotonin levels jumped 34 percent.[30] Massage benefits babies in other ways too, by reducing colic and increasing weight gain.

Exercise

A great deal of research documents the positive impact of physical activity on depression and anxiety. Exercise boosts mood and energy levels, producing mental and physical benefits that can last all day. Get some fresh air while taking walks or talking with other new mothers at the park. Interestingly, studies show that mothers are more likely to speak and laugh when their babies are facing them in the stroller rather than facing away.[31] You can also wear your baby in a soft carrier while you walk, which increases oxytocin and feelings of connection with your baby.

Keep a journal and create art

Journaling can provide an outlet for difficult thoughts and feelings, as well as allowing safe space to reflect on your experiences of becoming a mother. Creating art can also be therapeutic and enlightening, as well as enjoyable. Find twenty to thirty minutes a day to draw in your journal, perhaps sketching your baby sleeping or revisiting the assignment "Seeing Myself as a Mother" in chapter 7, or work with clay. You could also gather with other mothers to knit or make things together, such as cloth dolls, baby quilts, or toys.

Seek counseling

Counseling may help in clarifying the role and expectations of motherhood; integrating losses that are part of becoming a parent, such as changes in the marriage, finances, or career; and resolving underlying issues surrounding a new mother's own mother-daughter relationship. Look for therapists who have special training in and experience with the postpartum period.

Consider Birth Story Medicine

A difficult birth can contribute to depression, anxiety, low self-esteem, and lack of confidence in parenting. Of women who experience a traumatic birth, 2 percent to 6 percent develop post-traumatic stress disorder (PTSD*).[32] When postpartum depression and PTSD occur together, the resulting condition can interfere with mother-infant attachment and cause new mothers to worry about becoming pregnant or giving birth again. If you are blaming yourself for what happened during birth or having flashbacks, talk to someone trained in Birth Story Medicine to help you work through your birth story.

Recognize the limitations of antidepressants and other medications

Antidepressant medications came into widespread use in the late 1990s. The most commonly prescribed antidepressants are those that raise serotonin levels (SSRIs), but exactly how they work is not fully understood. A 2014 Cochrane report on antidepressants for postpartum depression explained: "Antidepressants are commonly used as the first treatment option . . . but there is little evidence on whether antidepressants are an effective and safe choice for the treatment of this disorder in the postnatal period. More trials are needed."[33]

Medications that stabilize brain chemistry should be reserved primarily for severe perinatal mood disorders. If you are taking medication, don't think the pills will do all the work of improving your outlook on life. Do your part: eat a well-balanced diet, get more sleep, learn how to change your thinking style, and become more solution-focused through cognitive therapy.

The Journey

Sometimes with
the bones of the black
sticks left when the fire
has gone out

someone has written
something new
in the ashes of your life.

You are not leaving.
Even as the light
fades quickly now.

—DAVID WHYTE[34]

Although mood disorders present additional challenges the first year after childbearing, it is helpful to realize that many women struggle with this problem and that the stigma surrounding such mental health issues is slowly decreasing. Compassion, accurate information, and loving support are essential in helping families cope with these disorders. Fortunately, due to their frequency and the toll they take on families, this subject is being extensively studied, so we can take heart that new treatments and perspectives are being explored.

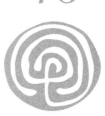

46

RITUALS OF THE RETURN

When the mother leaves the hut the first time after the birth, she emerges dressed specially, in her hand a staff such as is carried by the elders, followed by the child who cooks for her. Sedately they make their way to the market, where they are greeted with songs such as were sung to the warriors returning from battle.

— JUDITH GOLDSMITH

In the West, other than the six-week postpartum exam, few rituals mark the postpartum Return. Rituals are important, however, because they honor the initiate; they help her reflect on who she is becoming; and they mark milestones as she leaves the mystery of birth and reenters her ordinary everyday world. Since the modern birth map lacks meaningful rituals for new mothers, we must either seek inspiration from those of traditional cultures or invent our own.

ANNOUNCING YOUR "BIRTH" AS A MOTHER OR FATHER

After the birth, we announce, "Our baby has been born." After the birth, the Ticopia of the Solomon Islands say, "A mother has given birth."

—CLAUDIA PANUTHOS

Along with the announcements of your baby's birth, send a creative declaration of your "birth" as a mother or father to special people in your family or close friends, and preserve a copy of it for yourself. Your parent birth announcement should not detail the birth itself but rather describe the moment you first became truly aware of your new role as a parent. This may have occurred when your child was born, or perhaps at a later private, unforgettable moment, like the first time you soothed your baby to sleep. Your announcement could also highlight what you now know about yourself that you didn't know before you became a parent, or how being a parent is changing you.

Your parent birth announcement can be plain, poetic, funny, or artistic. You can make it by hand or on the computer, perhaps adding a photo or creating a collage of yourself as a new parent.

Closing of the Bones—A Mayan Ritual

The powerful energies of giving birth create a profound "opening" in a woman's body and soul. Hours, days, even weeks after birth many women describe a lingering sensation of feeling shattered, scattered, or left open. In parts of Mexico and Central America, around three days postpartum the new mother undergoes a Mayan healing ritual called the "closing of the bones" to help her gather her soul, release residual tension in the body, and feel contained on many levels.

To create sacred space and intention as the ritual begins, words are spoken to acknowledge that the new mother has journeyed far and crossed many thresholds; she has sacrificed something; and a part of her old self has died. Now a part of her feels shocked and shattered. Prayers invoke the Great Mother and call the mother's spirit back.

The ceremony begins with a ritual herbal bath (*baña de hierbas*) to help restore her warmth and relieve muscle fatigue. After the bath, the woman lies down and receives a massage or other body treatment. Next the mother lies flat on her back. Soft music, a scent of incense or aromatherapy wafting through the air, and dim lighting aid deep relaxation.

Then two support people get on either side of the mother. A rebozo is placed under her, beginning at her head and, with positioning, tightening, and releasing, moving down to her abdomen, hips and thighs, and finally her legs and feet. At each new level, after a few moments of rest the mother raises her head, shoulders, or hips slightly so the rebozo can be moved down. Old thoughts, judgments, grief, and mental tension around the birth and transition to motherhood are literally wrung out of her, and her body is realigned. When the closing of the bones ritual is complete, the mother lies quietly, feeling the new flow of energy in her body.[1, 2]

New Mother *Mehda*

In some traditional societies, when an initiate has experienced a change of heart or a healing, an elder marks the initiate in a special way so that the village recognizes and honors this change. Acknowledge yourself in this way by wearing a special piece of jewelry or item of clothing that represents the personal growth or internal healing you have experienced. You can also gather your "new mother *mehda*." One of the Tasks of Return is to retire your pregnancy clothes and buy a new outfit, or pretty new underwear, or earrings. After the baby begins pulling on long hair, a new haircut is often part of the "mommy makeover."

A Personal Inanna Ceremony

To maintain balance and harmony, there is an exchange in nature. Ripe fruit cannot just be harvested; it has to send seeds to the underworld to guarantee life in the future.

After making your ascent and returning "home" with your baby, you are consumed with new responsibilities as your role and daily life have changed dramatically. And yet a part of you may try to keep participating in all the activities and hobbies you value in addition to caring for your baby and yourself. But there are risks in trying

Upon her Return to the upper world,
Inanna had to send someone to the underworld in her place.

to balance too much—usually something will be neglected and fall off your overly full plate.

When you feel you have lost touch with something you value and enjoy, you may grieve that you no longer have time for it, compare your "sacrifice" to that of your partner or a friend, or complain that it's unfair. This negative response is heightened when a loss occurs without your agreement, often leading to resentment, anger, or guilt.

One new way of thinking about this is to imagine Bidu meeting you at each gate of your Return to take something of your old life from you so that you have more time and energy for mothering, adjusting, and healing. At each gate, you have a choice: hold on to everything and get into a tug-of-war with Bidu or willingly offer something up to leave in the underworld.

Sending something to the underworld

Choose one or two activities that you love but that your Warrior knows cannot be prioritized while you adjust to your first year of mothering. Choose an object to symbolize each of them, and decide on a specified period of time in which to give them up. To each object attach a tag bearing the date you plan to resume engagement, then bury the object (imagine sending it to the underworld), leaving the tag visible to serve as a reminder. Retrieve each object on its designated day and resume your participation in the sacrificed activity.

Here is how I perform this ritual in my classes. Mothers make a cutout of the Sumerian symbol for Inanna and write on it their promise to give up some activity and the date they plan to resume it. For example, one mother wrote:

> I, Asha-Inanna, agree to put "gardening" in the underworld
> for one year while I put "mothering my new baby" first.
> I promise to put in a garden by May 15 next year.

Asha then tied her Inanna card to a trowel she put in a potted houseplant, where she saw it often and remembered her promise. You can also do this ritual with your partner, with each of you choosing something to send to the underworld and perhaps choosing an additional activity that you enjoy as a couple (not sex).

This personal ceremony helps new parents compassionately and realistically prioritize, maintain a sense of control, and remember what gives their lives joy and meaning. Their "loss" is a temporary and mindful one, and they look forward to resuming what has given them bliss.

Seeing with New Eyes

By six weeks postpartum, you and your baby have both crossed many thresholds, so it is a good time to have a ritual of reconnection with your baby. Create a quiet space free from social media to see your baby with new eyes, as if for the first time. You might like to give your baby a flower petal bath or massage, or go for a walk in nature or in a labyrinth. If you had a difficult birth, your healing and your baby's are well underway, so begin letting go of thoughts that you or your baby are not okay or that bonding was impaired. Savor your baby's soft skin, sweet smell, and little sounds. Feel yourself fully inhabiting your new mother-shoes.

ONE YEAR
Looking Back

The first birthday can be a bittersweet threshold. I remember that anniversary of my birth-day as a mother:

> I did not expect to experience Sky's first birthday as my own first birthday as a parent. From morning until night, I relived the highlights of our labor and birth-day of a year ago. I also reflected on highlights that marked our first year together, including "bad mommy" moments and special events.

Celebrate yourself on this day, too. And if there is someone special who played an important part in your birth-day or first year as a parent, surprise them with a note of gratitude.

Examples of what parents have put in the underworld:

Surfing

Competing in marathons

Going to yoga retreats

Dressing up and dancing on Friday nights

Reading long novels or trashy magazines

Writing a first novel

Volunteer work

Home renovation

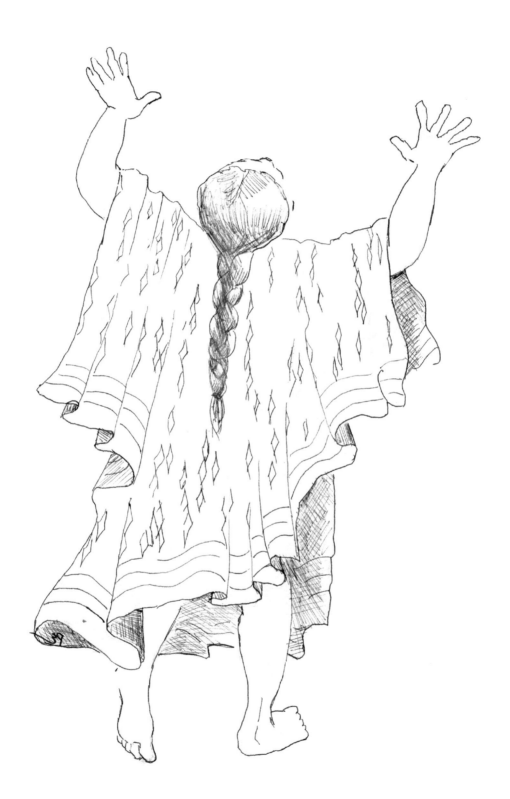

THE WARRIOR'S TREASURE

47

If it is hoarded it has no value. If it is squandered it has no legacy. When shared wisely for the benefit of all, it becomes worthy of the blood, sweat, and tears you shed to gain it.

— DAVID HARTMAN AND DIANE ZIMBEROFF

Your travels through the terrain of Laborland and back have brought you across thresholds, through gates, and into new parts of yourself. When you felt disoriented, your compass pointed to your heart and your deepest truth. Now, as you emerge from your Laborinth into the upper world, you are changed and carry newly garnered gifts with you in addition to your precious newborn.

What are the gifts your Birth Warrior receives when her Tasks of Return are complete? It is never what you expected. It is not the "prize" or reward that you sought, and it is not easily obtained. This soul-treasure is a deep knowing and a far-seeing compassion, as well as newfound inner strength, self-love, stamina, patience, humility, the capacity for deep listening, and a quiet wisdom.

Accepting these gifts is the beginning of a new way of being, which requires a surrender of what no longer works for you. The surrender is a disrobing, a leaving behind of what no longer fits, which is why grief and disorientation often accompany this heart-opening initiation. Embracing such gifts does not happen in six weeks; it takes years, even decades, to unearth their full potential.

In time, you will learn to share what you've learned in a language that others, especially the uninitiated, can understand. Your wisdom can guide and heal new mothers, whether preparing for their journeys or returning from them. Now that the topography of your wisdom is imprinted within you, it becomes a part of the collective map of birth in our culture. Remember, though, that no single map can show the way to a perfect birth; no one map can provide the answer to the complexities of birth in our culture. Inner maps can be shown to others but not replicated for the masses or even for generations to come. The terrain, borders, and lines on all maps are continually changing.

⑥

Although your birth journey is complete, the call to self-knowing is endless. Keep your ear open to the Great Below and continually answer the call to love yourself—exactly as you are unfolding and evolving. Potentially, your whole life can become the rewarding journey of a Warrior so that ultimately you can live vitally as your true self without any map.

So the end… becomes the beginning.

GRATITUDES

Many thanks to those who have taught, mentored, or inspired me—in person or through books—over four decades, whose influence is woven through the pages of this book. I want to pay special tribute to the birth professionals who gathered several times to advise me on message and accuracy of medical information, including but not limited to Rebecca Leeman, Lisa Bishop, Mary Rosanna Davis, Mary Lou Singleton, Nicole Lassiter, Siglinde Schewenzl, Tara Armijo-Prewitt, Rhonda Cox, and *mi amigas* Carolina Quintana de Oropaza and Leticia Loza. My sons, Sky and Lucien, excellent writers in their own right, encouraged me and enriched this book and me as a writer by enthusiastically reading many chapters and giving me warm, ardent feedback. I want to honor my lifelong friend Lyn Jones, who supported me as I crossed countless thresholds, for her enthusiastic co-writing and long editing of the chapter "Nourishing the Life Within," and for making sure all the food values were exactly right. Keeping my spirits up and believing

405

in this project, my dear friend Russ gave me eloquent and funny pep talks over many happy hours. And for her many trips to Albuquerque to keep me well during the long writing of this book, as well as for her encouraging voice at the other end of the line, I thank my sister Laura.

Special thanks to Manuel Casanova and David Blake, ultrasound researchers. for their generous telephone consultations; Elena Mitchel, for her stunning drawings of six archetypes of birth; and Anna Katherine, therapist and storyteller, for her generous recommendations for applying the symbolism of the story of Seal Woman to VBAC preparation. For the excellent digital reproductions of my paintings and illustrations in this book, I thank my friends Pat and Barbara Carr of Carr's Imagery. I also wish to thank Karen Stroker for the initial design of the book. My deepest gratitude, reaching back four thousand years, goes to priestess Enheduanna, who preserved the epic poem "Inanna, Queen of Heaven and Earth" on clay tablets so that we would have the "ancient map" upon which this book is based. I am equally beholden to my colleague Virginia Bobro, for her many talents and expertise, including her gifts for organization and languaging; her intimate knowledge of the influence of "Inanna's Descent" on birthing women; her expertise as a lactation consultant, as reflected in her contribution of chapter 43; and her collaboration on the book cover, especially her exquisite drawing of Topograph Woman.

Last but not least, I am indebted to the extraordinary and dedicated guidance from Blessingway Authors' Services in Santa Fe, New Mexico. What a blessing to have found this team! The masterful copyediting by Ellen Kleiner, with incredible attention to detail, made the manuscript sparkle. And the rare combination of artistic skill and meticulous focus of Angela Werneke graced the book's design inside and out.

Appendix A
ABOUT PAM'S PAINTINGS

MEXICAN LABYRINTH OF BIRTH
2013, acrylic and mixed media on Masonite, 20 x 30 inches

Mexican Labyrinth of Birth was inspired by a story my friend Alberto told me. Alberto is from Oaxaca, Mexico. Two of his *tias* (aunts) are *parteras* (midwives). One way they prepare a pregnant woman for birth is by telling her that when she is in labor she will have to be a warrior and go to the underworld, where spirits hold all the unborn babies. There she will have to find the spirit holding her baby and battle with that spirit to free her baby and bring him home. If the spirit gives up her baby easily, then labor will be short; if the spirit does not, labor will be long. Only the mother can bring her baby into the world, so she must be determined in labor and battle until she has her baby.

FAITH BASED BIRTH: CESAREAN
2004, acrylic on canvas, 36 x 24 inches

Birth customs reflect whatever a culture has faith in at the time. The lower third of this painting depicts buried matriarchal spirituality and culture. The Great Mother, ensconced in a pomegranate, a symbol of fertility, represents ancient knowledge and compassion. She hears the cries of birthing women, even as she is calling to all women, including women who have medical and surgical births. She is holding a large bowl, collecting the tears, amniotic fluid, and blood of birthing women. Buried in the earth, and our collective memory, are the primordial images of Inanna and goddesses.

The center panel shows the Inquisition (1400–1700), when untold thousands of women, including midwives and healers, were tortured, burned alive, or drowned by men of the Church. To survive, women made a tacit agreement to be silent and compliant. Centuries later, having never grieved this first war on women, we are still living their unconscious agreement.

The upper third of the painting portrays where modern Western culture has put its faith in birth: separation of the baby from its mother. The tiles falling off the wall suggest that this trend is not sustainable.

ROARING THE BABY OUT
1990, watercolor on paper, 18 x 24 inches

While giving birth to my second son, I had a fleeting moment of feeling like a roaring lion. Days later I wanted to capture that powerful inner experience in watercolor. A decade later I made a second painting of it in acrylic.

ARCHIVAL ART PRINTS (high-quality digital reproductions) of these and other paintings are available in a variety of sizes. Visit our store online.

Appendix B
CIRCUMCISION
Facts and Forethoughts on Your Baby's Foreskin

At one time in recent history, circumcision was done without informed consent. Today there are studies, conversations, expert opinions, and controversy about the procedure. An abundance of evidence is changing our culture's attitudes and assumptions about circumcision, and yet a taboo prevents many new parents from talking openly about this for fear they will be judged. Furthermore, when caregivers consider circumcision a preference instead of a medical concern, they fail to warn parents of the risks of unnecessary circumcision. This appendix presents evidence-based information about circumcision and your baby that can help you begin a thoughtful process of decision making about this controversial procedure.

Function of the Foreskin

The foreskin is not an extra flap of skin.

—Dan Bollinger, Founder of Boys' Health Advisory

Circumcision is the surgical removal of the foreskin. The foreskin is a retractable, double-layered fold of nerve-rich skin uniquely evolved to lubricate the glans, the head of the penis: it also helps protect the penis against constant abrasion from clothing. The foreskin is the most sensitive part of the penis; the glans is less sensitive. When the foreskin is removed, twenty thousand nerves are cut.[1] In addition, blood vessels are severed, forever disrupting the normal blood flow to parts of the penis.[2] Consequently, after circumcision it is estimated that 75 percent of sensation is permanently lost.[3] It is likely that some men's foreskins are more sensitive than others, which means that circumcision will affect men differently. In the words of one physician, "A man with a particularly sensitive foreskin has more to lose by cutting it off, and that's something you can't know in advance when you're looking at an infant."[4]

Intact Penis Hygiene

When bathing your baby, wash his bottom but leave the penis alone. Do not use Q-tips or retract the foreskin (remember, it is still attached to the glans, and forcibly separating it may cause it to scar and adhere to the glans). After the foreskin retracts naturally, just as your child learns to shampoo his hair and brush his teeth he will also learn to pull the foreskin back and rinse during showers or baths (soap is not needed).

What Is Circumcision?

Many parents erroneously think a circumcision is like having an ear pierced.

—Laurie Evans

Circumcision entails forcibly tearing the foreskin from the glans then cutting the foreskin off. In this regard, circumcision can be likened to removing a fingernail from its nail bed.[5] After circumcision, the glans is bloody and raw. Educator Laurie Evans describes the shock parents experience when hearing their baby boy's screams and seeing the blood and their baby's raw glans after the procedure.

In the womb, the foreskin is fused to the glans and is almost never retractable at birth. The fusion dissolves in childhood, usually by ten years of age, although it may take longer. When the penis is uncircumcised, the glans typically retains its original smooth, moist mucous membrane surface. After a circumcision, however, the glans eventually scars, dries out, and develops pitting where the foreskin was torn from it. Over time, the surface of the exposed glans continues to thicken, further reducing sensation.

Short-Term Complications

A recent analysis stated that the incidence of medical complications after newborn circumcision is 0.5 to 10 percent.[6,7] There are twenty potential complications, including hemorrhage, infection, permanent alteration of the length and shape of the penis, and, in rare cases, amputation of the penis. One hundred percent of newborn boys experience severe pain during and after the procedure and permanently lose sensitivity. Moreover, data suggest that severely painful experiences early in life may have long-term negative effects on the brain and sensitize boys to stronger pain responses in the future.[8]

In 1999, nurses at Kingston General Hospital in Ontario, Canada, noticed that newborns experienced excruciating pain and changes in behavior after being circumcised. After talking with these nurses, researcher Paul D. Tinari, PhD, used MRI and PET scans to observe changes in two babies' brains before, during, and after circumcision. Dr. Tinari explains the results as follows:

> Analysis of the MRI data indicated that the surgery subjected the infant to significant trauma. The greatest changes occurred in the limbic system concentrating in the amygdala and in the frontal and temporal lobes. A neurologist who saw the results postulated that the data indicated that circumcision affected most intensely the portions of the newborn's brain associated with reasoning, perception, and emotions. Follow-up tests on the infant one day, one week, and one month after the surgery indicated that the child's brain never returned to its baseline configuration.[9]

This research was suppressed and the researchers reprimanded before it could be published in medical journals. Further study in this area is needed.

Also, infant feeding, both at the breast and by bottle, is negatively impacted in the first twenty-four hours or so after the surgery. In fact, lactation consultants recommend that parents opting to circumcise their babies delay the procedure until breastfeeding is well established (at least a week after birth) to minimize disruption to feeding and the mother-infant bond.

Long-Term Complications

Some men who were circumcised as babies don't believe that circumcision affects them during sex, but they have no point of reference. Men who were circumcised as adults inform us that circumcision permanently altered their once pleasurable experience of sex, often dramatically. After being circumcised as an adult, one man compared the difference of experiencing orgasm without a foreskin to "sight without color... [like] only being able to see in black and white rather than seeing in full color. He concluded, "There are feelings you'll just never have without a foreskin."[10]

Leave his poor, little penis alone.

—Dr. Benjamin Spock

Why Male Newborn Circumcision Became Routine in the United States

The practice of routine circumcision in the United States originated from an antimasturbation and cleanliness hysteria in the late 1800s,[11] and its promotion continues to be reinforced. For decades, doctors told parents that their newborn's penis was not innervated at birth or that babies did not feel pain so the circumcision would be painless. Many of these doctors heard the screams and saw babies turn blue from not being able to catch their breath during the procedure, but knowingly deceived patients.

Globally, 80 percent of men are not circumcised. Many parents, after learning that circumcision is painful and medically unnecessary, decide to decline this procedure for their baby boy.

In fact, newborn circumcision in the United States has decreased from about 85 percent in 1979 to 32.5 percent in 2009, with rates varying widely from region to region.[12]

Are there medical benefits to circumcision?

Recent research indicates that circumcision may protect adult men from some sexually transmitted infections, such as HIV, and other urinary tract issues later in life. For some parents and medical professionals in the United States, this data seem to be enough to tip the balance in favor of newborn circumcision, a position underscored by the American Academy of Pediatrics (AAP) Circumcision Policy Statement in 2012.[13]

However, the populations studied, primarily in developing nations, do not necessarily translate to contemporary Western populations, so there is no conclusive evidence that the health benefits outweigh the short- and long-term risks, which are still being uncovered. See circumcision.org for a detailed discussion of the validity of research and list of studies that show few to no health benefits. As a result of the debate about the evidence regarding medical benefits, many insurance companies are reducing or eliminating coverage of routine newborn circumcision; Medicaid no longer pays for it in eighteen states.

Who should decide about circumcision?

The AAP states: "Parents ultimately should decide whether circumcision is in the best interests of their male child. They will need to weigh medical information in the context of their own religious, ethical, and cultural beliefs and practices. The medical benefits alone may not outweigh these other considerations for individual families."[14] Many considerations come into play. In one survey, parents reported that their decision not to circumcise their infant son was based on knowing that circumcision is elective surgery and that by leaving him intact they allow him choice about his own body.[15]

Overall in the United States, the most prevalent reasons for circumcision are social and cultural. Men who were circumcised tend to favor having their sons circumcised as well, usually without doing research on the potential risks and side effects.

As for mothers, fears of having their sons teased in the locker room for looking "different" or not looking "like Dad" can overpower their concerns about risks and their babies' pain and autonomy. While a generation ago it was less common to have an intact penis and therefore be at risk of standing out, today it's about a fifty-fifty split, meaning an uncircumcised boy will fit in just fine.

> *There is a growing movement to leave the "circumcision decision" to the individual who will be affected by it, so that he can decide— when he's old enough to understand what's at stake—if he'd rather experience sex and masturbation with an intact penis (however sensitive his particular foreskin turns out to be), or with a modified one (if he wants to go for surgery).*
> — BRIAN D. EARP

Ethical considerations

There are sound moral reasons for challenging routine newborn circumcision. Some physicians refuse to do routine circumcision based on their ethical pledge to "do no harm."[16] In their paper about the changing politics of circumcision, Fox and Thompson suggest:

> As with female genital cutting, male circumcision ought to be debated within a paradigm of social justice which gives adequate weighting to the interests of all affected parties (including women whose health may actually be compromised by the procedure) and which renders visible the socioeconomic dimensions of the issue. In line with a social justice approach, we argue that public health initiatives must comply with international ethico-legal standards and be attentive to the emergence of an international human right to health.[17]

New perspectives regarding religious circumcision

Religious arguments for circumcision are familiar, particularly in the Jewish and Islamic traditions. However, within religions scholars and experts disagree on the merits and religious importance of ritual circumcision.

In the spirit of *tikkum olam* (repairing the world from old, harmful patterns), many Jewish parents are opting not to have the *bris milah*, or circumcision. Instead, they are choosing a non-cutting *brit shalom*, a naming ceremony performed by a rabbi that has all the joy of ritual without the pain of the circumcision. Jewish couples who disagree on circumcision may experience resentment in their marriage. If this is true for you, read Laurie Evans's article "Counseling Couples in Disagreement about Circumcision: A Jewish Perspective."[18]

In the Islamic tradition, circumcision is typically done when the boy approaches puberty, at which point it tends to have more risks than after birth. The Qur'an does not explicitly mention circumcision, yet the procedure is customary and expected. In fact, the majority of circumcised men in the world are practicing Muslims. It is up to each family, no matter what their spiritual practice, to balance their religious beliefs with sound information about medical procedures.

Uncircumcised boys can have a Bar Mitzvah.

Rabbis don't "check."

Still undecided?

Some parents who are ambivalent but "go ahead" with the surgery to avoid conflict or to conform to tradition may later regret it. Before giving consent, arrange to watch a newborn circumcision, talk to other parents, and read about the risks, benefits, and complications (see Appendix C).

IF YOU DECIDE TO HAVE YOUR BABY'S FORESKIN CIRCUMCISED...

Many parents who now choose to circumcise decide to delay the surgery for several weeks after birth, rather than having it done before hospital discharge, to reduce the risk of interrupting breastfeeding. In either case, your son will need you to stay with him and talk to him during the procedure. Although a few babies withdraw into themselves and don't cry (perhaps they are in shock from the pain and slip into a semi-comatose state to survive the pain and trauma[19]), your baby will likely scream in pain and be difficult to console. Afterward, he may be limp, exhausted, agitated, and have trouble feeding, even following the use of anesthesia.[20] Evidence that the procedure is excruciating shows up in one study where, thirty minutes after circumcision, the stress hormone cortisol in newborns was elevated three to four times those of pre-circumcision levels.[21]

Over the first week or two following your male baby's circumcision, you may notice increased irritability, screaming when his diaper is wet, varying sleep patterns, and a change in infant-maternal interaction.[22] In his discomfort while healing, he will need extra patience and soothing. Also keep in mind that boys who were circumcised have stronger pain responses to later painful experiences, such as immunizations.[23]

Appendix C
SELECTED REFERENCES ON BREASTFEEDING AND CIRCUMCISION

Breastfeeding

Books and Articles

Colson, Suzanne. *An Introduction to Biological Nurturing*. Plano, Texas: Hale Publishing, 2010.

Mohrbacher, Nancy, and Kathleen Kendall-Tackett. *Breastfeeding Made Simple: Seven Natural Laws for Nursing Mothers*. Oakland, CA: New Harbinger Publications, 2010.

Newman, Jack, and Teresa Pitman. *Dr. Jack Newman's Guide to Breastfeeding* (Kindle ed.). New York: HarperCollins, 2014.

West, Diana, and Lisa Marasco. *The Breastfeeding Mother's Guide to Making More Milk*. New York: McGraw-Hill Education, 2008.

Wiessinger, Diane, Diana West, and Teresa Pitman. *The Womanly Art of Breastfeeding*, 8th ed. (La Leche League International Book). New York: Ballantine Books, 2010.

Websites

biologicalnurturing.com—Laid-back breastfeeding by Dr. Suzanne Colson and Joelle Temurcin, of England and Wales

breastfeeding.com— A series of teaching videos

breastfeedinginc.ca—Breastfeeding Inc., Canada

drghaheri.com—Tongue-tie and breastfeeding information from Bobak Ghaheri, MD

ilca.org—International Lactation Consultant Association information and directory

kellymom.com—Evidence-based information and support

lalecheleague.org—Mother-to-mother help and support groups

YouTube.com/watch?v=zrwflcPB1u4—Breast crawl video by UNICEF

Circumcision

Books and Articles

Earp, Brian D., "Does Circumcision Reduce Penis Sensitivity? The Answer is Not Clear Cut." *Huffpost Science* (blog), April 21, 2016, http://www.huffingtonpost.com/brian-earp/does-circumcision-reduce-_b_9743242.html.

Evans, Laurie. "Counseling Couples in Disagreement about Circumcision: A Jewish Perspective." *Journal of Prenatal and Perinatal Psychology and Health* 17, no. 1 (Fall 2002): 85–94.

Fleiss, Paul. "Protect Your Uncircumcised Son." *Mothering Magazine* 103 (June 29, 2002): 40–47, http://www.mothering.com.

Goldman, Ronald. *Circumcision: The Hidden Trauma*. Boston: Vanguard Publications, 1997.

Simelane, Musa. "More Circumcised Men Are HIV Positive: Circumcision Program a Failure." *Times of Swaziland* (September 2010), http://www.times.co.sz/index.php?news=20909.

Wallerstein, Edward. "Circumcision: The Uniquely American Enigma." *Urology Clinics of North America* 12, no. 1 (1985): 123–32. Accessed February 2011, http://www.cirp.org/library/
general/wallerstein/.

Websites

circumcision.org—Jewish Associates of the Circumcision Resource Center

cirp.org—Circumcision Information and Resource Pages

doctorsopposingcircumcision.org—Doctors Opposing Circumcision (DOC)

icgi.org—International Coalition for Genital Integrity

icgi.org/medicalization/—History of circumcision slide show (no images)

NOTES

INTRODUCTION

1. Marian F. MacDorman, T.J. Mathews, and Eugene Declercq, "Home Births in the United States *1990–2009," National Center for Health Statistics Data Brief* (January 2012): 84.

2. Jinsong Zhang et al., *"U.S. National Trends in Labor Induction, 1989–1998," International Reproductive Medicine* 47, no. 2 (February 2002): 120–24.

3. Joyce A. Martin et al., "Births: Final Data for 2010," *National Vital Statistics Reports* 61, no. 1 (August 28, 2012).

4. Lewis Richard Farnell, *Greek Hero Cults and Ideas of Immortality* (Oxford, UK: Claredon Press, 1921).

CHAPTER 3: "INANNA'S DESCENT": A MYTHIC STORY

Tribute (p. 14): Diane Wolkstein and Samuel Noah Kramer, *Inanna, Queen of Heaven and Earth: Her Stories and Hymns from Sumer* (New York: Harper and Row, 1983).

1. N. Scott Momaday, "Plains Ways," in Kenneth Lincoln, *Speak Like Singing: Classics of Native American Literature* (Albuquerque, NM: University of New Mexico Press), 125.

2. Keith H. Basso, *Western Apache Language and Culture: Essays in Linguistic Anthropology* (Tucson, AZ: University of Arizona Press, 1992), 124–25.

CHAPTER 4: YOUR CALL IS AN INVITATION

Epigraph (p. 21): Carlos Castaneda, *The Teachings of Don Juan: A Yaqui Way of Knowledge* (Berkeley, CA: University of California Press, 1968), 22.

Epigraph (p. 21): James Hillman in David Hartman and Diane Zimberof, "The Hero's Journey of Self-Transformation," *Journal of Heart-Centered Therapies* 12, no. 2 (2009): 8.

CHAPTER 5: THREE WAYS OF KNOWING

Epigraph (p. 27): Mark Twain, quotes/keywords/facts.html.

Epigraph (p. 27): Kahlil Gibran, Sand and Foam (CreateSpace, 2014).

1. Liz Wiseman, *Rookie Smarts: Why Learning Beats Knowing in the New Game of Work* (New York: HarperBusiness, 2014).

2. Thich Nhat Hanh, *Miracle of Mindfulness: An Introduction to the Practice of Meditation* (Boston: Beacon Press, 1976), 15.

Epigraph (p. 30): Rumi, http://www.quotegarden.com/rumi.html.

CHAPTER 6: INNOCENCE AND TRUST

1. Meryl Streep, Barnard College Commencement Speech (May 16, 2010).

CHAPTER 7: THE MOTHER

Epigraph (p. 37): M. Esther Harding, *The Way of All Women* (Boston: Shambhala Publications, 1970).

Epigraph (p. 37): Tony Crisp, "Archetype of the Great Mother," http://dreamhawk.com/dream-encyclopedia/archetype-of-the-great-mother/.

Epigraph (p. 40): Helen Walsh, *Go to Sleep* (Edinburgh, Scotland: Canongate Books, 2012).

1. Joshua Schriftman, "History and Interpretations of the Labyrinth Motif in Native North American Cultures," www.ashlandweb.com/labyrinth/laby.hist.html.

CHAPTER 8: PLACENTAL CLOCK

1. Sophia N. Kalantaridou and Antonis Makrigiannakis et al., "Stress and the Female Reproductive System," *Journal of Reproductive Immunology* 62, nos. 1, 2 (June 2004): 61–68.

2. Pablo Nepomnaschy and Kathleen Welch et al., "Cortisol Levels and Very Early Pregnancy Loss in Humans," *Proceedings of the National Academy of Sciences* 103–110 (February 22, 2006): 3938–42.

3. Gwen Dewar, "Pregnancy Stress Hormones: How a Natural Rise in Hormone Levels May Benefit Baby . . . and Re-program Mom's Brain," accessed July 2012, http://www.parentingscience.com/Stress-hormones-during-pregnancy.html.

4. Ibid.

5. Ibid.

6. Graham C. Liggins, "The Role of Cortisol in Preparing the Fetus for Birth," *Reproduction, Fertility and Development* 6, no. 2 (1994): 141–150.

7. Murray Thompson, "The Effects of Placental Corticotrophin Releasing Hormone on the Physiology and Psychology of the Pregnant Woman," *Current Women's Health Reviews* 4 (2008): 270-79.

8. Gwen Dewar, "Pregnancy Stress Hormones: How a Natural Rise in Hormone Levels May Benefit Baby . . . and Re-program Mom's Brain, accessed July 2012, http://www.parentingscience.com/Stress-hormones-during-pregnancy.html.

9. Ibid.

10. Petra C. Arck et al., "Early Risk Factors for Miscarriage: A Prospective Cohort Study in Pregnant Women," *Reproductive Biomedical Online* 17 no. 1 (2008):101–113.

11. Patricia H. C. Rondó and Rute F. Ferreira et al., "Maternal Psychological Stress and Distress as Predictors of Low Birth Weight, Prematurity and Intrauterine Growth Retardation," *European Journal of Clinical Nutrition* (2003).

12. Calvin Hobel et al., "Psychological Stress and Pregnancy Outcome," *Clinical Obstetrics and Gynecology* 51, no. 2 (2008): 333–48.

Epigraph (p. 43): David Mamet, *Boston Marriage* (New York: Vintage, 2002).

13. Gwen Latendress and Roberta J. Ruiz, "Maternal Coping Style and Perceived Adequacy of Income Predict CRH Levels at 14–20 Weeks of Gestation," *Biological Research Nursing* 12, no. 2 (2010): 125–36.

Epigraph (p. 43): Dennis Merritt Jones, *Your Redefining Moments: Becoming Who You Were Born to Be* (New York: Jeremy P. Tarcher, 2014), 15.

14. Shamanthakamani, Narendran et al., "Efficacy of Yoga on Pregnancy Outcome," *Journal of Alternative & Complementary Medicine* 11 (2005): 237–44.

15. Jeannette R. Ickovics, et al., "Group Prenatal Care and Perinatal Outcomes: A Randomized Controlled Trial," *Obstetrics and Gynecology* 110, no. 2 (August 2007): 330–39, doi:10.1097/01.AOG.0000275284.24298.23.

Chapter 9: Is Ultrasound Safe for My Baby?

1. Mattias Martensson et al., "High Incidence of Defective Ultrasound Transducers in Use in Routine Clinical Practice," *European Journal of Echocardiography* 10, no. 3 (May 2009): 389–94.

2. Tahereh Ashrafganiooei and T. Naderi et al., "Accuracy of Ultrasound, Clinical and Maternal Estimates of Birth Weight in Term Women," *Mediterranean Health Journal* 16, no. 3 (2010): 313–17.

3. Junu Bajracharya et al., "Accuracy of Prediction of Birth Weight by Fetal Ultrasound," *Kathmandu University Medical Journal* 10, no. 38 (April–June 2012): 74–75.

4. Eugene R. Declercq et al., *Listening to Mothers II* (New York: Childbirth Connection, 2013).

5. Dana Sadeh-Mestechkin et al., "Suspected Macrosomia? Better Not Tell," *Archives of Gynecology and Obstetrics* 278, no. 3 (2008): 225–30.

6. Ashrafganiooei and Maderi et al., "Accuracy of Ultrasound," 74–75.

7. Susan London, "Ultrasound Diagnosis of Fetal Macrosomia Found Inaccurate," *Family Practice News Digital Network* (2011).

8. Sadeh-Mestechkin et al., "Suspected Macrosomia?" 225–230.

9. Ibid.

10. Eugene R. Declercq et al., *Listening to Mothers III: Pregnancy and Childbirth* (New York: Childbirth Connection, 2013).

11. Sadeh-Mestechkin et al., "Suspected Macrosomia?" 225–230.

12. Susan London, "Ultrasound at Term Overestimates Macrosomia," *Family Practice News* (Aug 8, 2011), accessed November 2014, http://www.familypracticenews.com/search/search-single-view/ultrasound-diagnosis-of-fetal-macrosomia-found inaccurate/36fa34152db3bcf39aaa0bbe33ecc2ff.html.

13. David Blake, personal correspondence.

Epigraph (p. 48): Beverly Beech, "Ultrasound: Weighing the Propaganda against the Facts," *Midwifery Today* 51 (1999).

14. Aubrey Milunsky et al., "Maternal Heat Exposure and Neural Tube Defects," *Journal of the American Medical Association* 268, no. 7 (1992): 882–85.

15. Marshall J. Edwards, "Hyperthermia and Fever During Pregnancy," *Birth Defects Research Part A: Clinical and Molecular Teratology* 76, no. 7 (2006): 507–16.

16. Silvana Haddad et al., "Low-Intensity Ultrasound Energy Applied to Testes of Aged Rats," *Journal of Histology & Histopathology* 13 (1998): 385–89.

17. Claire Doody et al., "In Vitro Heating of Human Fetal Vertebra by Pulsed Diagnostic Ultrasound," *Ultrasound in Medicine & Biology* 25 (1999): 1289–94.

18. Juriy Wladimiroff and Sturla Eik-Nes, *European Practices in Gynecology and Obstetrics: Ultrasound in Obstetrics and Gynecology* (Philadelphia: Elsevier, 2009), 30.

19. Stanley B. Barnett, "Can Diagnostic Ultrasound Heat Tissue and Cause Biological Effects?" in S.B. Barnett and G. Kossoff, eds., *Safety of Diagnostic Ultrasound* (Carnforth, UK: Parthenon Publishing,1998).

20. Stanley B. Barnett et al., "The Sensitivity of Biological Tissue to Ultrasound," *Ultrasound in Medicine & Biology* 23 (1997): 805–12.

21. Judy S. Cohain, "Prenatal Ultrasound Does Not Improve Perinatal Outcomes," *Midwifery Today* 102, nos. 46–47 (2012): 68–69.

22. Sylvie Viaux-Savelon et al., "Prenatal Ultrasound Screening: False Positive Soft Markers May Alter Maternal Mother-Infant Interaction," *PLOS One* 7, no. 1 (2012), accessed November 2014, doi: 10.1371/journal.pone.0030935.

23. Calvin M. Chama et al., "From Low-Lying Implantation to Placenta Praevia: A Longitudinal Ultrasonic Assessment," *Obstetrics* 24, no. 5 (2004): 516–18.

24. Stephen Wolstenhulme, "Does the Ultrasound Diagnosis of Low-Lying Placenta in Early Pregnancy Warrant a Repeat Scan?" *Journal of the Royal Army Medical Corps* 137, no. 2 (June 1991): 84–87.

Epigraph (p. 50): Barbara Katz Rothman, *The Tentative Pregnancy: How Amniocentesis Changes the Experience of Motherhood* (New York: Norton), 1993.

25. Chama, "From Low-Lying Implantation," 516–18.

Epigraph (p. 51): Wendell Berry, *Life Is a Miracle* (Washington DC: Counterpoint, 2000).

26. Barnett et al., "Sensitivity of Biological Tissue," 805–12.

27. Gail ter Haar, "Ultrasonic Imaging: Safety Considerations," *Interface Focus*, no. 4 (August 2011): 686–97.

28. David A. Toms, "Safety Issues in Fetal Ultrasound," http://www.fetalultrasoundsafety.net/Downloads/fetalultrasoundsafety.pdf.

29. Jennifer Margulis, "Are Ultrasounds Causing Autism in Unborn Babies?" *The Daily Beast* (April 2013).

30. Ibid.

31. Angela Warner, "Cell Division, Autism and Ultrasound," *Age of Autism* (blog), http://www.ageofautism.com/2008/10/cell-division-a.html.

32. Ousseny Zerbo et al., "Is Maternal Influenza or Fever during Pregnancy Associated with

Autism or Developmental Delays?" *Journal of Autism and Developmental Disorders* 43, no. 1 (January 2013): 25–33.

33. Emily L. Williams and Manual Casanova, "Potential Teratogenic Effects of Ultrasound on Corticogenesis: Implications for Autism," *Medical Hypothesis* 75, no. 1 (July 2010): 53–58.

34. Lisa J. Rudy, "Is Autism on the Rise?" *About Health*, accessed October 2014, http://autism.about.com/od/causesofautism/p/ontherise.htm.

35. Centers for Disease Control and Prevention, http://www.cdc.gov/ncbddd/autism/data.html.

36. Irva Hertz-Picciotto, "Diagnostic Change and Increased Prevalence of Autism," *International Journal of Epidemiology* 38, no. 5 (2009): 1239–41.

37. Marissa King and Peter Bearman, "Diagnostic Change and Increased Prevalence of Autism," *International Journal Epidemiology* 38, no. 5 (2009): 1224–34.

38. Sara Jane Webb et al., "Severity of ASD Symptoms and their Correlation with the Presence of Copy Number Variations and Exposure to First Trimester Ultrasound," *Autism Research* (September 1, 2016), doi:10.1002/aur.1690.

Epigraph (p. 54): Ann McDonald, "A Development: The Dana Guide to Brain Health by Floyd E. Bloom et al.," accessed November 2014, https://www.dana.org/news/brainhealth/detail.aspx?id=10050.

Epigraph (p. 54): Wendell Berry, *Life Is a Miracle* (Berkeley, CA: Counterpoint Books, 2001), 137.

39. Anthony J. DeCasper and Melanie J. Spence, "Prenatal Maternal Speech Influences Newborns' Perception of Speech Sounds," *Infant Behavior and Development* 9, no. 2 (June 1986): 133–50.

Chapter 10: Nourishing the Life Within

Epigraph (p. 57): David Stewart, *Five Standards for Safe Childbearing: Good Nutrition, Skillful Midwifery, Natural Childbirth, Home Birth, Breastfeeding* (Marble Hill, MO: NAPSAC, 1981), 105–106.

1. Gail S. Brewer and Tom Brewer, *What Every Pregnant Woman Should Know* (New York: Penguin, 1977), 92.

2. Julie A. Mennella, "Exploring the Beginnings of Food and Flavor Learning," *Pediatrics for Parents* (February 2002), www.pedsforparent.com/articles/2857.shtml.

3. Salt Institute, "Human Salt Requirements," http://www.saltinstitute.org/Issues-in-focus/Food-salt-health/Human-salt-requirements.

4. Peter Gluckman et al., "Effect of in Utero and Early-life Conditions on Adult Health and Disease," *New England Journal of Medicine* 359 (July 2008): 61–73.

5. Joseph C. Jimenez-Chillaron et al., "Intergenerational Transmission of Glucose Intolerance and Obesity in Utero Undernutrition in Mice," *Diabetes* 58, no. 2 (February 2009): 460–68.

6. "Without Miracles: 5 Brain Evolution and Development: The Selection of Neurons and Synapses," http://faculty.education.illinois.edu/g-cziko/wm/05.html.

7. Judith Graham, "Children and Brain Development: What We Know about How Children Learn," *University of Maine Bulletin* 4356 (2011), http://umaine.edu/publications/4356e/.

8. Brenda Patoine, "The Vulnerable Premature Brain: Rapid Neural Development in Third Trimester Heightens Brain Risks," *The DANA Foundation News* (May 24, 2010), http://www.dana.org/News/Details.aspx?id=43496.

9. J. Summer, "Flavored Fish Oil—Why Do They Add Flavor?" http://www.articlesdic.com/flavored-fish-oil-why-do-they-add-flavor.html.

10. "Mercury in Your Environment," *United States Environmental Protection Agency News*, http://www.epa.gov/hg/effects.htm.

11. Ingrid B. Helland et al., "Maternal Supplementation with Very-Long-Chain n-3 Fatty Acids during Pregnancy and Lactation Augments Children's IQ at 4 Years of Age," *Pediatrics* 111, no. 1 (2003): 33–44.

12. John Colombo et al., "Maternal DHA and the Development of Attention in Infancy and Toddlerhood," *Child Development* 75 (2004): 1254–67.

13. Joseph Hibbeln, "Seafood Consumption, the DHA Content of Mothers' Milk and Prevalence Rates of Postpartum Depression," *Journal of Affective Disorders* 69, no. 1 (2002): 15–29.

14. Werner Knoepp, "National Sugar Epidemic Killing Us—Sugar Consumption at Lethal Levels," *Health and Fitness Nutrition* (April 25, 2010), http://ezinearticles.com/?National-Sugar-Epidemic-Killing-Us---Sugar-Consumption-at-Lethal-Levels&id=4175267.

15. Raakel Luoto et al., "Impact of Maternal Probiotic Supplemented Dietary Counseling on Pregnancy Outcome and Prenatal and Postnatal Growth," *British Journal of Nutrition* 103, no. 12 (June 2010): 1192–199.

16. Richard Cohen, "Sugar Love (A Not-So-Sweet Story)," *National Geographic* (August 2013), http://ngm.nationalgeographic.com/2013/08/sugar/cohen-text.

17. David DiSalvo, "What Eating Too Much Sugar Does to Your Brain," *Forbes* (April 1, 2013), http://www.forbes.com/sites/daviddisalvo/2012/04/01/what-eating-too-much-sugar-does-to-your-brain/#2399a257a208.

18. John Casey, "The Hidden Ingredient That Can Sabotage Your Diet," *US Department of Agriculture News* (2005–2014), http://www.medicinenet.com/script/main/art.asp?article key=56589.

19. Heather B. Patisaul and Wendy Jefferson, "The Pros and Cons of Phytoestrogens," *Frontiers in Neuroendocrinology* 31, no. 4 (2010): 400–419.

20. Sally Fallon Morell, "Phytoestrogens in Diets of Infants and Adults," Weston A. Price Foundation News (October 2002), http://www.westonaprice.org/soy-alert/soy-formula-birth-control-pills-for-babies.

21. A. Leung et al., "Concerns for the Use of Soy-Based Formulas in Infant Nutrition," *Paediatric Child Health* 14, no. 3 (2009): 109–113.

22. Patisaul and Jefferson, "Pros and Cons of Phytoestrogens," 400–419.

23. Marcia Herman-Giddens et al., "Secondary Sexual Characteristics and Menses in Young Girls Seen in Office Practice," *Pediatrics* 99, no. 4 (April 1, 1997): 505–512.

24. Oqba Al-Kuran et al., "The Effect of Late Pregnancy Consumption of Date Fruit on Labour and Delivery," *Journal of Obstetrics and Gynaecology* 31, no. 1 (2011): 29–31, accessed July 2015, doi: 10.3109/01443615.2010.522267.

25. N. Khadem et al., "Comparing the Efficacy of Dates and Oxytocin in the Management of Postpartum Hemorrhage," *Shiraz E-Medical Journal* 8, no. 2 (April 2007): 64–71, accessed July 2015, https://www.researchgate.net/publication/264384650_Comparing_the_efficacy_of_dates_and_oxytocin_in_the_management_of_postpartum_hemorrhage.

26. Fred Hageneder, *The Meaning of Trees: History, Healing, Love* (San Francisco: Chronicle Books, 2005), 138–146.

27. "Dates Nutrition Facts," http://nutrition-and-you.com/dates.html.

Chapter 11: Incubation Rituals

1. James Hollis, *The Middle Passage* (Toronto: Inner City Books, 1993), 102.

2. Eileen London and Belinda Recio, *Sacred Rituals: Creating Labyrinths, Sand Paintings, and Other Traditional Arts* (Gloucester, MA: Fair Winds, 2004), 20.

3. Monica Sjöö and Barbara Mor, *The Great Cosmic Mother: Rediscovering the Religion of the Earth* (New York: Harper and Row, 1987), 84.

4. Erich Neumann, *The Great Mother: An Analysis of the Archetype* (New York: Bolligen Foundation, 1963), 96.

5. Sjöö and Mor, *Great Cosmic Mother*, 17.

Epigraph (p. 74): Marjory Zoet Bankson, *The Soulwork of Clay: A Hands-On Approach to Spirituality* (Woodstock, VT: SkyLight Paths Publishing, 2008), prologue.

6. Paulus Berensohn and True Kelly, *Finding One's Way with Clay: Pinched Pottery and the Color of Clay* (Dallas, TX: Clay Biscuit Books, 1997).

Chapter 12: The Gatherer

1. http://nanact.org/encounter-the-people/navajo/navajo-basketry.html.

Chapter 13: Leaving "Home"

1. Mantak Chia, *Awaken Healing Energy through the Tao* (Santa Fe, NM: Aurora Press, 1983), 2.

2. Ibid., 7, 73–75.

Chapter 14: Birth Attendants

1. Debra J. Jackson et al., "Outcomes, Safety, and Resource Utilization in a Collaborative Care Birth Center Program Compared with Traditional Physician-Based Perinatal Care," *American Journal of Public Health* 93, no. 6 (June 2003): 999–1006, doi: 10.2105/AJPH.93.6.999.

Epigraph (p. 88): James Hollis, *The Middle Passage* (Toronto: Inner City Books, 1993), 77.

2. Jamie Passaro, "Who Will Heal the Healers? Pamela Wible on What's Missing from Healthcare Reform," *The Sun* (2009), 407.

3. Ibid.

4. Katy Backes Kozhimannil et al., "Doula Care, Birth Outcomes, and Costs Among

Medicaid Beneficiaries," *American Journal of Public Health* 103, no. 4 (April 2013): e113-e121, doi: 10.2105/AJPH.2012.301201.

5. Ibid.

CHAPTER 15: BIRTHPLACE

1. Larry Leeman and Rebecca Leeman, "A Native American Community with a 7% Cesarean Delivery Rate," *The Annals of Family Medicine* 1, no. 1 (May 2003): 36–43.

2. Nancy C. Sorel, *Ever Since Eve* (New York: Oxford University Press, 1984), 114–115.

3. Adrian E. Feldhusen, "The History of Midwifery and Childbirth in America: A Time Line," *Midwifery Today* (2000), http://www.midwiferytoday.com/articles/timeline.asp.

4. Susan Stapleton et al., "Outcomes of Care in Birth Centers," *Journal of Midwifery & Women's Health* 58, no. 1 (January/February 2013): 3–14.

5. Marian F. MacDorman, T.J. Mathews, and Eugene Declercq, "Trends and Characteristics of Home and Out-of-Hospital Births in the United States, 1990–2005," *National Center for Vital Statistics Data Brief* 56, no. 11 (2010).

6. Rondi E. Anderson and Patricia A. Murphy, "Outcomes of 11,788 Planned Home Births Attended by Certified Nurse-Midwives," *Journal of Nurse Midwifery* 40, no. 6 (1995): 483–92.

7. MacDorman, Mathews, and Declercq, "Trends and Characteristics."

8. Kathleen Kennedy Townsend, "Giving Birth at Home: A Good Idea?" *The Atlantic* (July 2011).

9. Katy B. Kozhimannil et al., "Cesarean Delivery Rates Vary Ten-Fold among US Hospitals; Reducing Variation May Address Quality and Cost Issues," *Health Affairs* 32, no. 3 (2013): 527–35.

10. "Maternal Decision Making Ethics and the Law," *American Congress of Obstetricians and Gynecologists Committee Opinion*, no. 321 (November 2005).

CHAPTER 16: RELAXIN' AND OPENIN' YOUR PELVIS

1. Jean Sutton and Pauline Scott, *Understanding and Teaching Optimal Fetal Positioning* (Tauranga, New Zealand: Birth Concepts, 1996).

2. Liz Koch, "The Psoas Is Not a Hip Flexor," *Pilates Digest* (September 2009), http://www.pilatesdigest.com/the-psoas-is-not-a-hip-flexor/.

3. L. Koch, "The One Muscle That Does Not Need Strengthening," http://www.coreawareness.com/articles/the-one-muscle-that-does-not-need-strengthening/.

4. Jan Mens et al., "The Mechanical Effect of a Pelvic Belt in Patients with Pregnancy-Related Pelvic Pain," *Clinical Biomechanics* 21, no. 2 (Oct. 2005): 122–27.

5. http://wordscribe43.hubpages.com/hub/Pregnancy-Belt-Maternity-Girdle.

CHAPTER 17: MAPS THROUGH LABOR PAIN

1. Grantly Dick-Read, *Natural Childbirth* (London: Heinemann, 1933), 86.

2. Patrick Wall, *Pain: The Science of Suffering* (New York: Columbia University Press, 2000), 67-68.

3. Ibid., 71.

4. Naomi Wolf, *Vagina* (New York: HarperCollins, 2013), 19, 20–21.

5. Thierry Postel, "Childbirth Climax: The Revealing of Obstetrical Orgasm," *Sexologies* (May 3, 2013), http://www.improbable.com/2013/06/26/counting-on-childbirth-and-orgasm/.

6. Michael S. Kramer, "Aerobic Exercise for Women during Pregnancy," *Cochrane Pregnancy and Childbirth Group* (April 22, 2002), http://onlinelibrary.wiley.com/doi/10.1002/14651858.CD000180/full.

7. Caroll Dunham, *Mamatoto: A Celebration of Birth* (New York: Viking, 1991), 88.

8. Helen Akinc, "The Pain of Childbirth: Differing Cultural Perceptions" (blog), *Kybele*, April 10, 2013, http://www.kybeleworldwide.org/041013-the-pain-of-childbirth-differing-cultural-perceptions.html.

9. Josephine M. Green, "Expectations and Experiences of Pain in Labour: Findings from a Large Prospective Study," *Birth* 20 (1993): 65–72.

10. Tetsuo Koyoma, "The Subjective Experience of Pain: Where Expectations Become Reality," *Proceedings of the National Academy of Sciences of the United States* 102, no. 36 (September 2005): 12950–55, doi: 10.1073/pnas.0408576102.

Chapter 18: Ceremony and Celebration

Epigraph (p. 140): Corita Kent and Jan Steward, *Learning by Heart: Teachings to Free the Creative Spirit* (New York: Bantam Books, 1992), 198.

1. Eileen London and Belinda Recio, *Sacred Rituals: Creating Labyrinths, Sand Paintings, and Other Traditional Arts* (Gloucester, MA: Fair Winds, 2004), 61.

2. Ibid., 31–32.

Chapter 20: Worry Is the Work of Pregnancy

1. Rebecca Solnit, *A Field Guide to Getting Lost* (New York: Viking, Penguin Group, 2006), 165.

Chapter 21: Birth Tiger Safari

1. David Hamilton, "Visualization Alters the Brain & Body," *Using Science to Inspire* (blog), April 2015, http://drdavidhamilton.com/visualisation-alters-the-brain-body/.

2. "Stress Management for Health Course: The Fight Flight Response," http://stresscourse.tripod.com/id11.html.

3. Damien Pearse, "Lion Reported to Be on the Loose Near Clacton," *The Guardian*, accessed August 26, 2012, http://www.guardian.co.uk/world/2012/aug/26/lion-on-the-loose-in-essex?INTCMP=SRCH.

4. Megan Gambino, "What Animal is the Best Mother?" *Smithsonian* (May 2011), http://www.smithsonianmag.com/science-nature/what-animal-is-the-best-mother-158591597/?no-ist .

CHAPTER 22: THE BIRTH WARRIOR

1. Shunryu Suzuki, *The Beginner's Mind* (Boston, MA: Shambhala Publications, 2006).

2. Emily Lee, et al., *The Healing Art of Tai Chi* (New York: Sterling Publishing, 1996), 22–23.

Epigraph (p. 164): Robert Moore and Douglas Gillette, *King, Warrior Magician Lover* (San Francisco, CA: Harper San Francisco, 1990), 127.

3. Modified phrase from the original "I'm good enough, I'm smart enough, and doggone it, people like me," coined by comedian Al Franken's character, Stuart Smalley, that aired on *Saturday Night Live*'s "Daily Affirmations with Stuart Smalley."

4. Michael Meade, *Fate and Destiny* (Aurora, CO: Mosaic Multicultural Foundation, 2010), 259.

CHAPTER 23: THE BIRTH PLAN OF A WARRIOR

Epigraph (p. 172): Kelli Way, "Effective Birth Plans," *International Journal of Childbirth* (March 31, 1996).

CHAPTER 24: INFORMED CONSENT IS A DIALOGUE

1. The Childbirth Connection, "Understanding and Navigating the Maternity Care System: Informed Decision Making," accessed February 2012, http://www.childbirthconnection.org/article.asp?ck=10081.

2. Solace for Mothers, "Questions to Consider When Interviewing a Doctor or Midwife" (2009), accessed February 2014, http://www.solaceformothers.org/informed_consent_tool.html.

3. Nancy Rhoden, "Informed Consent in Obstetrics," *Western New England Law Review* 9, no. 67 (1987): 67–68.

4. Annie Brewster, "Patient Angst: When You Just Have to Say 'No' to the Doctor," WBUR's *Common Health* (August 21, 2012).

5. Nancy Rhoden, "Informed Consent in Obstetrics," *Western New England Law Review* 68.

6. Rebecca M. D. Smyth et al., "Amniotomy for Shortening Spontaneous Labour," *Cochrane Database of Systemic Reviews* 4 (2007).

7. "Hurricane Reconnaissance," www.washingtonpost.com/wp-srv/weather/hurricane/info/recon.htm.

8. www.usatoday.com/weather/hurricane/2003-07-16-flying-hurricanes_x.htm.

9. Ingrid Michaelson, "Keep Breathing" (song), 1989.

CHAPTER 25: PREPARING FOR YOUR RETURN

1. Joanna H. Raven et al., "Traditional Beliefs and Practices in the Postpartum Period in Fujan Province, China: A Qualitative Study," *BioMed Central Pregnancy and Childbirth* series 7, no. 8 (2007), doi: 10.1186/1471-2393-7-8.

2. Svea Boyda-Vikander, "Mothering the Mother: 40 Days of Rest," *Birth Without Fear* (October 21, 2012), http://birthwithoutfearblog.com/2012/10/21/mothering-the-mother-40-days-of-rest/.

3. Frank Waters, *Book of the Hopi* (New York: Ballantine Books, 1963), 9–10.

CHAPTER 26: CROSSING THE THRESHOLD

1. Hermann Kern, *Through the Labyrinth: Designs and Meanings over 5,000 Years* (London, UK: Prestel, 2000), 294.

2. Ibid.

CHAPTER 27: MAPS FOR NAVIGATING LABORLAND

Epigraph (p. 203): Kabir Helminski, *The Knowing Heart: A Sufi Path of Transformation* (Boston: Shambhala, 2000).

Epigraph (p. 206): Helen Curry, *The Way of the Labyrinth: A Powerful Meditation for Everyday Life* (New York: Penguin, 2000).

1. Sarah Buckley, "Pain in Labour: Your Hormones Are Your Helpers," http://sarahbuckley.com/pain-in-labour-your-hormones-are-your-helpers.

2. Ruth Feldman, "Level of Oxytocin in Pregnant Women and Mother-Child Bond," *Association Psychological Science* (2007), http://www.psychologicalscience.org/index.php/news/releases/level-of-oxytocin-in-pregnant-women-predicts-mother-child-bond.html.

3. Ikka Räisänen, "Pain and Plasma Beta-Endorphin Level during Labor," *Obstetrics and Gynecology* 64, no. 6 (December 1984): 783–86.

4. Sarah Buckley, "Hormones in Labour and Birth—How Your Body Helps You Birth," accessed September 2005, http://www.bellybelly.com.au/birth/ecstatic-birth-natures-hormonal-blueprint-for-labor/.

5. Regina P. Lederman, "Anxiety and Epinephrine in Multiparous Women in Labor: Relationship to Duration of Labor and Fetal Heart Rate Pattern," *American Journal of Obstetrics and Gynecology* 153, no. 8 (1985): 870–77.

6. Michel Odent, "The Fetus Ejection Reflex," *The Nature of Birth and Breastfeeding* (Sydney, Australia: Ace Graphics, 1992), 29–43.

7. Sachiyo Nakamura and S Shigeko Horiuchi, "Relationship between Advanced Maternal Age, Hiesho (Sensitivity to Cold) and Abnormal Delivery in Japan," *The Open Nursing Journal* 7 (2013): 142–48.

8. ACOG and SMFM Consensus Statement, "Safe Prevention of the Primary Cesarean Delivery," accessed March 2014, http://www.acog.org/Resources-And-Publications/Obstetric-Care-Consensus-Series/Safe-Prevention-of-the-Primary-Cesarean-Delivery.

9. Rachel Reed, "Early Labour and Mixed Messages," *Midwife Thinking* (blog), accessed 2014, http://midwifethinking.com/2012/09/22/early-labour-and-mixed-messages/.

10. Penny Armstrong and Sheryl Feldman, *A Midwife's Story* (New York: Arbor House, 1986), 59–62.

11. Carl O. Simonton et al., *Getting Well Again* (New York: Bantam, 1992).

Epigraph (p. 216): Jeremy L. Neal et al., "Outcome of Nulliparous Women with Spontaneous Labor Onset Admitted to Hospitals in Preactive versus Active Labor," *Journal of Midwifery and Women's Health* 59, no. 1 (January/February 2014): 28–34.

12. H. Cheyne et al., "Should I Come in Now? Women's Early Labour Experiences," *British Journal Medicine* 15, no. 10 (2007): 604–609.

13. Ingmarie M. Carlsson et al., "Swedish Experiences of Seeking Care and Being Admitted during the Latent Phase of Labour," *Midwifery* 2 (2009): 172–80.

14. Sherry Boschert, "Use 6-cm Dilation to Judge Labor Progress," *Ob. Gyn. News* (June 2013), http://www.obgynnews.com/single-view/use-6-cm-dilation-to-judge-laborprogress/37a4f40e561fe33b3aa7594c00de6622.html?tx_ttnews[sViewPointer]=1.

15. Leeanne Lauzon and Ellen D. Hodnett, "Labour Assessment Programs to Delay Admission to Labour Wards," *Cochrane Pregnancy and Childbirth Group* (John Wiley & Sons, January 30, 2004).

16. Ingmarie M. Carlsson et al., "Maintaining Power: Women's Experience from Labour Onset before Admittance to Maternity Ward," *Midwifery* 28, no. 1 (2012): 86.

17. A. Kavitha et al., "A Randomized Controlled Trial to Study the Effect of IV Hydration on the Duration of Labor in Nulliparous Women," *Archives of Gynecology and Obstetrics* 285, no. 2 (February 2012): 343–46.

18. Rebecca Dekker, "Are IV Fluids Necessary during Labor?" *Evidence-Based Birth* (blog), May 24, 2012, evidencebasedbirth.com.

19. Ibid.

20. Dekker, "Are IV Fluids Necessary during Labor?"

21. Nancy C. Sharts-Hopko, "Oral Intake during Labor: A Review of the Evidence," *American Journal of Maternal Child Nursing* 35, no. 4 (2010): 197–203.

22. Ibid.

23. Mandisa Singata et al., "Eating and Drinking in Labor," *Cochrane Collaboration: Pregnancy and Childbirth Group* (August 2013), http://www.cochrane.org/CD003930/PREG_eating-and-drinking-in-labour.

24. Ibid.

25. Caroline J. Chantry et al., "Excess Weight Loss in First-Born Breastfed Newborns Relates to Maternal Intrapartum Fluid Balance," *Pediatrics* 127, no. 1 (2011), http://pediatrics.aappublications.org/content/127/1/e171?variant=abstract&sso=1&sso_redirect_count=1&nf-status=401&nftoken=00000000-0000-0000-0000-000000000000&nfstatusdescription=ERROR%3a+No+local+token.

26. Joy Noel-Weiss et al., "An Observational Study of Associations among Maternal Fluids during Parturition, Neonatal Output, and Breastfed Newborn Weight Loss," *International Breastfeeding Journal* 6 (August 2011): 9, doi: 10.1186/1746-4358-6-9.

27. Valerie J. Flaherman, et al., "Early Weight Loss Nomograms for Exclusively Breastfed Newborns," *Pediatrics* (2014), http://pediatrics.aappublications.org/content/early/2014/11/25/peds.2014-1532.

28. Dekker, "Are IV Fluids Necessary during Labor?"

Epigraph (p. 224): Emily Lee et al., *The Healing Art of Tai Chi: Becoming One with Nature* (New York: Sterling, 1996), 22–23.

29. M. Valiani et al., "Massage Therapy Reduces Labor Pain," *Iranian Journal of Nursing and Midwifery Research* 15, Supplement 1 (2010): 302–10.

30. Siw Alehagen et al., "Fear, Pain and Stress Hormones during Childbirth," *Journal of Psychosomatic Obstetrics and Gynaecology* 26, no. 3 (2005): 153–65.

31. Seyedeh Hamideh Mortazavi et al., "Effects of Massage Therapy and Presence of Attendant on Pain, Anxiety and Satisfaction during Labor," *Archives of Gynecology and Obstetrics* 286, no. 11 (July 2012): 19–23.

32. Lawrence Williams and John A. Bargh, "Experiencing Physical Warmth Promotes Interpersonal Warmth," *Science* 322, no. 5901 (2008) 606-607, doi: 10.1126/science.1162548.

33. Elizabeth R. Cluett et al., "Randomised Controlled Trial of Labouring in Water Compared with Standard of Augmentation for Management of Dystocia in First Stage of Labour," *British Medical Journal* 328 (February 2004): 314.

34. Yu-Hsiang Liu, Mei-Yueh Chang, and Chung-Hey Chen, "Effects of Music Therapy on Labour Pain and Anxiety in Taiwanese First-Time Mothers," *Journal of Clinical Nursing* 19 nos. 7, 8 (2010): 1065–072.

35. Jayne M. Standley, "Music Research in Medical Dental Treatment," *Journal of Music Therapy* 23, no. 2 (1986): 56–122.

36. Mimi M. Tse et al., "The Effect of Music Therapy on Postoperative Pain, Heart Rate, Systolic Blood Pressures and Analgesic Use Following Nasal Surgery," *Journal of Pain and Palliative Care Pharmacotherapy* 19, no. 3 (2005): 21–9.

37. "Harriet Beecher Stowe," *Ohio Reading Road Trip*, Greater Dayton Public Television (2004), http://www.orrt.org/stowe/.

Chapter 28: Through the Seven Gates

1. Joseph Campbell, *The Power of Myth* (New York: Doubleday, 1988), 37.
Epigraph (p. 230): Ibid.

Chapter 29: The Gatekeeper

1. Paul B. Courtright, *Ganesa: Lord of Obstacles, Lord of Beginnings* (New York: Oxford University Press, 1985).

2. Zora Neale Thurston, *Their Eyes Were Watching God* (New York: Harper Collins: 2006), 67–68.

Chapter 30: Optimal Positions in Labor

1. Pamela Vireday, *The Well-Rounded Moma* (blog), March 2015, http://wellroundedmama.blogspot.com/2015_03_01_archive.html.

2. Gail Tully, "How Do You Do Walcher's?" Spinning Babies, http://spinningbabies.com/learn-more/techniques/other-techniques/walchers-open-the-brim/.

3. Ana Hill, "The Peanut Ball and Its Effect on Laboring Women" (2012), http://www.cappa.net/documents/Articles/Peanut%20Ball.pdf.

4. Ricardo López Méndez, "*El Rebozo de Mi Madre,*" *Artes de México* no. 20 (August 2008): 43.

5. Guadalupe Trueba, "Comfort Measures for Childbirth," *The Rebozo Way* (Mexico City: Instituto Nacional Indigenista, 1994).

CHAPTER 31: WHAT TO DO FOR STALLED LABOR AND BACK LABOR

1. Ella Peregrine et al., "Impact on Delivery Outcome of Ultrasonographic Fetal Head Position Prior to Induction of Labor," *Obstetrics & Gynecology* 109, no. 3 (2007): 618–25.

2. "In Celebration of the OP Baby" (June 2015), http://midwifethinking.com/2010/08/13/in-celebration-of-the-op-baby/.

3. Claire M. Andrews and Edward C. Andrews, "Nursing, Maternal Postures, and Fetal Position," *Nursing Research* 32, no. 6 (1983): 336–41.

4. Azar Karaminia et al., "Randomised Controlled Trial of Effect of Hands and Knees Posturing on Incidence of Occiput Posterior Position at Birth," *British Medical Journal* 328, no. 7438 (2004): 490.

5. Christina Tussey and Emily Botsois, "Decrease the Length of Labor with the Use of a Labor Ball with Patients That Receive an Epidural," Presentation at AWHONN, Denver (2011), https://awhonn.confex.com/awhonn/2011/webprogram/Paper6986.html.

6. Janie McCoy King, *Back Labor No More!! What Every Woman Should Know before Labor* (Dallas, TX: Plenary Systems, 1993).

7. Ibid.

8. Gail Tully, *The Belly Mapping Workbook* (Bloomington, MN: Maternity House Publishing, 2005), 44.

9. W. J. Carsedine et al., "Does Occiput Posterior Position in the Second Stage of Labour Increase the Operative Delivery Rate?" *Australian and New Zealand Journal of Obstetrics & Gynaecology* 53, no. 3 (June 2013): 265-70, doi: 10.1111/ajo.12041.

10. Henci Goer, "Does Epidural Analgesia Predispose to Persistent Occiput Posterior?" *Science & Sensibility* (blog), Lamaze, March 2016, https://www.scienceandsensibility.org/p/bl/et/blogid=2&blogaid=556.

11. Ellice Lieberman, et al., "Changes in Fetal Position during Labor and their Association with Epidural Analgesia," *Obstetrics & Gynecology* 105, no. 5, pt. 1 (May 7, 2005): 974–82.

CHAPTER 32: PUSHING BABY OUT

1. Sheila Kitzinger, *Complete Book of Pregnancy and Childbirth* (New York: Alfred A. Knopf, 2003), 260.

2. Cara F. Natterson, "Babies and Their Head Shapes and Other Info," http://www.pregnancyandbaby.com/baby/articles/941853/changes-to-your-babys-head.

3. Elizabeth G. Baxley, Ellen L. Sakornbut, and Matthew K. Cline, *Family Medicine Obstetrics* (Philadelphia: Mosby Elsevier, 2008), 419, referring to article by G. Hamilton, "Classical Observations and Suggestions in Obstetrics," *Edinburgh Medical Journal* 7 (1861): 313–21.

4. Aaron B Caughy et al., "Safe Prevention of Primary Cesarean Delivery," *ACOG Obstetric Care Consensus* (March 2014).

5. Ibid.

6. Ibid.

7. Susan Tucker Blackburn, *Maternal, Fetal, Neonatal Physiology: A Clinical Persepective*, 4th ed. (Maryland Heights, MO: Elsevier Sanders, 2013), 131.

8. Thomas H. Kuntz et al., "Alloparental Care: Helper-Assisted Birth in the Rodrigues Fruit Bat Pteropus Rodicensis," *Journal of Zoology* 232 (1994): 691–700.

9. "Use of Surgical Procedure to Facilitate Child Birth Declines," *Journal of American Medical Association Network* (January 13, 2015), http://media.jamanetwork.com/news-item/use-of-surgical-procedure-to-facilitate-child-birth-declines/.

10. Petra Petrocnik and Jayne E. Marshall, "Hands-Poised Technique," *Midwifery* 31, no. 2 (February 2015): 274–79.

11. Roberto Caldeyro-Barcia, "The Influence of Maternal Bearing-Down Efforts during Second Stage on Fetal Well-Being," *Birth and the Family Journal* 6, no. 1 (March 2008): 17–21.

12. Gulay Yildirim and Nezihe Kizilkaya Beji, "Effects of Pushing Techniques in Birth on Mother and Fetus," *Birth Issues in Perinatal Care* 35, no. 1 (March 2008): 25–30.

13. Roger P. Goldberg, "Effects of Pregnancy and Childbirth on the Pelvic Floor," www.springer.com.

14. Rachel Reed, "Pushing: Leave It to the Experts," *Midwife Thinking* (blog), https://www.google.com/search?client=safari&rls=en&q=midwifethinking.com+pushing&ie=UTF-8&oe=UTF-8.

15. James O. Drife, "History of Medicine: The Start of Life: A History of Obstetrics," *Postgraduate Medical Journal* 78, no. 919 (2002): 311–15, doi:10.1136/pmj.78.919.311.

Epigraph (p. 271): Lauray Yule, *Coyotes* (Tuscon, AZ: Rio Nuevo Publishing, 2004), 5.

16. Susan Diamond, *Hard Labor: Reflections of an Obstetrical Nurse* (New York: Forge, 1996), 58.

17. Richard Stephens, "Swearing as a Response to Pain—Effect of Daily Swearing Frequency," *Journal of Pain* 12, no. 12 (2011): 1274–81.

18. Frederik Joelving, "Why the #$%! Do We Swear? For Pain Relief," *Scientific American* (July 12, 2009), http://www.scientificamerican.com/article/why-do-we swear/.

19. Ibu Robine Lim, "Midwives Sing the Babies Earthside," *Midwifery Today* 96 (2010), https://www.midwiferytoday.com/articles/SingTheBabies.asp.

CHAPTER 33: THE FOOL

1. Arnold Mindell and Amy Mindell, *Riding the Horse Backwards: Process Work in Theory and Practice* (London, UK: Arkana, 1992), 20.

Epigraph (p. 278): Margaret Wheatley, *Leadership and the New Science* (San Francisco: Berrett-Koehler, 1992), 20–21.

Epigraph (p. 279): John L. Brown and Cerylle A. Moffitt, *The Hero's Journey: How Educators Can Transform Schools and Improve Learning* (Alexandra, VA: Association for Supervision and Curriculum Development, 1999), 21.

Chapter 34: When the Unexpected Happens—Get Back on Your Horse!

Epigraph (p. 281): Judith Goldsmith, *Childbirth Wisdom: From the World's Oldest Societies* (New York: Congdon & Weed, 1984), 86.

Chapter 35: Epidural

1. Treya Killam Wilber and Ken Wilber, *Grace and Grit: Spirituality and Healing in the Life and Death of Treya Killam Wilber* (Boston: Shambhala, 1993), 253.

2. McCallum R. Hoyt, "Patient Controlled Epidural Analgesia during Labor," talk presented at 2012 Sol Shnider Meeting held by SOAP in San Francisco (March 23, 2012).

3. Society for Maternal-Fetal Medicine, "Women Used 30 percent Less Analgesia during Labor When Self-Administered," *Science Daily* (February 10, 2011).

4. Ellen D. Hodnett, "Pain and Women's Satisfaction with the Experience of Childbirth," *American Journal of Obstetrics and Gynecology* 186 (May 2002): S160–72.

Epigraph (p. 289): Ellise Lieberman and Carol O'Donoghue, "Unintended Effects of Epidural Analgesia during Labor: A Systematic Review," *American Journal of Obstetrics and Gynecology* 185, no. 5 (May 2002): S31–68.

5. Michelle J. K. Osterman and Joyce A. Martin, "Epidural and Spinal Anesthesia Use in Labor: 27-State Reporting Area, 2008," *National Vital Statistics Reports* 59, no. 5 (April 5, 2011).

6. Peter H. Pan, T. D. Bogard, and M. D. Owen, "Incidence and Characteristics of Failures in Obstetric Neuraxial Analgesia and Anesthesia: A Retrospective Analysis of 19,259 Deliveries," *International Journal of Obstetric Anesthesiology* 13, no. 4 (October 2004): 227–33.

7. Angela Bader et al., "Maternal and Neonatal Fentanyl and Bupivacaine Concentrations after Epidural Infusion during Labor," *Anesthesia & Analgesia* 81, no. 4 (1995): 829–32.

8. Abha A. Shah and Grace H. Shih, "Epidural Anesthesia and Maternal Fever: Real or Fiction?" *Anesthesiology Clinics* 31 (2013): 559–70, doi: http://dx.doi.org/10.1016/j.anclin.2013.03.004

9. Elisabeth Greenwell et al., "Intrapartum Temperature Elevation, Epidural Use and Adverse Outcome in Term Infants," *Pediatrics* 129, no. 2 (February 2012): e447–e454. doi:10.1542/peds.2010-2301.

10. Shah and Shih, "Epidural Anesthesia," 559–70.

11. Nebojsa Sindik et al., "Vaginal Delivery and Continuous Epidural Analgesia: Should We Change Clinical Approach?" *Collegium Anthropologicum* 36, no. 2 (2012): 499–504.

12. Marco Caruselli et al., "Epidural Analgesia during Labor and Incidence of Cesarean Section," *The Journal of Maternal-Fetal and Neonatal Medicine* 24, no. 2 (February 2011): 250–52.

13. Barbara L. Leighton and Stephen H. Halpern, "The Effects of Epidural Analgesia on Labor, Maternal, and Neonatal Outcomes," *American Journal of Obstetrics and Gynecology* 186, no. 5 (2002): S69–S77.

14. Fiona Fouhy et al., "High-Throughput Sequencing Reveals the Incomplete, Short-Term Recovery of Infant Gut Microbiota Following Parenteral Antibiotic Treatment with

Ampicillin and Gentamicin," *Antimicrobial Agents and Chemotherapy* 56, no. 11 (November 2012): 5811–20.

15. William Murk et al., "Prenatal or Early-Life Exposure to Antibiotics and Risk of Childhood Asthma: A Systematic Review," *Pediatrics* 127 (2011): 1125–38.

16. Petri Volmanen, Jukka Valanne, and Seppo Alahuhta, "Breast-Feeding Problems after Epidural Analgesia for Labor: A Retrospective Cohort Study of Pain, Obstetrical Procedures and Breast-Feeding Practices," *International Journal of Obstetric Anesthesia* 13, no. 1 (January 2004): 15–19.

17. Yaakov Beilin et al., "Effect of Labor Epidural Analgesia With and Without Fentanyl on Infant Breast-Feeding: A Prospective, Randomized, Double-Blind Study," *Anesthesiology* 103, no. 6 (2005): 1211–17.

Chapter 36: Induction

1. Michelle J. K. Osterman and Joyce A. Martin, "Recent Declines in Inductions of Labor by Gestational Age," *NCHS Data Brief* 155 (2014).

2. Michael Kramer, quoted by Andre Seaman in "Induced Labors May Be Tied to Rise in Preterm Births," *Reuters Health* (August 31, 2010): 31, http://whtc.com/news/articles/2012/aug/31/induced-labors-may-be-tied-to-rise-in-preterm-births/.

3. Alabama Perinatal Excellence Collaborative, "APEC Guidelines: Scheduling Deliveries Prior to 39 Weeks Gestation," *Protocol* 2, version 3 (September 26, 2010), http://medicaid.alabama.gov/documents/4.0_Programs/4.4_Medical_Services/4.4.7_Maternity_Care/4.4.7.5_APEC/4.4.7.5_Delivery_Guidelines_pre-39-weeks_Final.pdf.

4. Andrew Seaman, "Induced Labors May Be Tied to Rise in Preterm Births," *Reuters Health*, accessed November 15, 2010, http://www.reuters.com/article/2012/08/31/us-induced-labors-preterm-idUSBRE87U18420120831.

5. ACOG Committee Opinion, "Definition of Term Pregnancy," no. 579 (November 2013), https://www.acog.org/About_ACOG/ACOG_Departments/~/media/Committee%20Opinions/Committee%20on%20Obstetric%20Practice/co579.pdf.

6. Nicette Jukelvics, "Labor Induction: Exposed," *Mother's Advocate* (blog), November 15, 2010, http://mothersadvocate.wordpress.com/2010/11/15/labor-induction-exposed/.

7. Carole R. Mendelson, "Fetal-Maternal Hormonal Signaling in Pregnancy and Labor," *Molecular Endocrinology* 23, no. 7 (July 2009): 947–54.

8. Catherine Limperopoulos, "Late Gestation Cerebellar Growth is Rapid and Impeded by Preterm Birth," *Pediatrics* (2005): 688–95.

9. Kate Johnson, "Elective Labor Induction May Soon Be Medical History," *Medscape News*: ACOG's 61st Annual Clinical Meeting (May 23, 2013), http://www.medscape.com/viewarticle/804700.

10. "Your Mind Can Keep You Well," PSI Tek (blog), http://www.psitek.net/pages/PsiTek-creative-visualization12.html.

11. S. Katherine Laughton et al., "Using a Simplified Bishop Score to Predict Vaginal Delivery," *Obstetrics & Gynecology* 117 (2011): 805–11.

12. http://perinatology.com/calculators/Bishop%20Score%20Calculator.htm.

13. Michael Boulvain, Catalin M. Stan, and Olivier Irion, "Membrane Sweeping for Induction of Labour," *Cochrane Database System Review* (2001), http://www.cochrane.org/CD000451/PREG_membrane-sweeping-for-induction-of-labour.

14. E. de Miranda and J. van der Bom et al., "Membrane Sweeping and Prevention of Prolonged Pregnancy in Low-Risk Pregnancies," *British Journal of Obstetrics and Gynaecology* 113 (2006): 402–08, www.ncbi.nlm.nih.gov/pubmed/16489935.

15. Marta Jozwiak et al., "Foley Catheter versus Vaginal Prostaglandin E2 Gel for Induction of Labour at Term," *The Lancet* 378, no. 9809 (December 2011): 2095–2103.

16. George Agnew and M. J. Turner, "Vaginal Prostaglandin Gel to Induce Labour in Women with One Previous Caesarean Section," *Journal of Obstetrics and Gynaecology* 29, no. 3 (April, 2009): 209–11.

17. Jefferson H. Harman and Andrew Kim, "Current Trends in Cervical Ripening and Labor Induction," *American Family Physician* 1:60, no. 2 (1999): 477–83, http://www.aafp.org/afp/990800ap/477.html.

CHAPTER 37: CESAREAN BIRTH

1. Luz Gibbons et al., "The Global Numbers and Costs of Additionally Needed and Unnecessary Caesarean Sections Performed Per Year: Overuse as a Barrier to Universal Coverage," *World Health Report, Background Paper* 30 (2010), http://www.who.int/healthsystems/topics/financing/healthreport/30C-sectioncosts.pdf.

2. http://www.cdc.gov/nchs/fastats/delivery.htm.

3. Ibid.

4. Luz Gibbons et al., "The Global Numbers."

5. Fay Menacker and Brady Hamilton, "Recent Trends in Cesarean Delivery in the United States," *National Center for Health Statistics Data Brief* 35 (2010), www.cdc.gov/nchs/data/databriefs/db35.htm.

6. "Cesarean Section: A Brief History, Part 2," *National Library of Medicine* (July 13, 2013), http://www.nlm.nih.gov/exhibition/cesarean/part2.html.

7. Robert W. Felkin, "Notes on Labour in Central Africa," *Edinburgh Medical Journal* 20 (April 1884): 922–30.

8. http://www.britannica.com/EBchecked/topic/103746/cesarean-section.

9. Nancy Caldwell Sorel, *Ever Since Eve: Reflections on Childbirth* (Oxford, UK: Oxford University Press, 1985), 109–110.

10. Adam Wolfberg, "The C-Section Boom," *Boston Globe* (October 30, 2011).

11. http://www.acog.org/Resources-And-Publications/Obstetric-Care-Consensus-Series/Safe-Prevention-of-the-Primary-Cesarean-Delivery.

12. Kristin Bole, "Patience during Stalled Labor Can Avoid Many C-sections," *Obstetrics and Gynecology*, http://www.ucsf.edu/news/2008/10/4158/patience-during-stalled-labor-can-avoid-many-c-sections-ucsf-study-shows.

13. Coalition for Improving Maternity Services, "The Risks of Cesarean Section," accessed 2010, http://www.motherfriendly.org/resources/documents/therisksofcesareansectionfebruary 2010.pdf.

14. Joann Romano-Keeler and Jorn-Hendrik Weitkamp, "Maternal Influences on Fetal Microbial Colonization and Immune Development," *Pediatric Research* 77 (2015): 189-195.

15. Rachel Ehrenberg, "Baby's First Bacteria Depends on Birth Route," *US News* (June 22, 2010), http://www.usnews.com/science/articles/2010/06/22/babys-first-bacteria-depend-on-birth-route.

16. Mette C. Tollanes et al., "Cesarean Section and Risk of Severe Childhood Asthma: A Population-Based Cohort Study," *The Journal of Pediatrics* 153, no. 1 (2008): 112–16.

17. Minna-Maija Grölund et al., "Fecal Microflora in Healthy Infants Born by Different Methods of Delivery: Permanent Changes in Intestinal Flora after Cesarean Delivery," *Journal of Pediatric Gastroenterology Nutrition* 28, no. 1 (1999): 19–25.

18. Liza Gross, "Microbes Colonize a Baby's Gut with Distinction," *PLOS Biology* 5, no. 7 (2007): e191.

19. Jesse Johnson-Cash, "The Human Microbiome," *Midwife Thinking* (September 9, 2015), http://midwifethinking.com/2014/01/15/the-human-microbiome-considerations-for-pregnancy-birth-and-early-mothering/.

Chapter 38: Birthin' Again after Cesarean

1. Clarissa Pinkola Estés, *Women Who Run with the Wolves* (New York: Random House, 1992).

2. Martin MacIntyre, "MacCodrum and His Seal Wife," in *Scotland's Stories* (2012), http://www.educationscotland.gov.uk/scotlandsstories/aselkiestory/maccodram/index.

3. Eugene R. Declercq et al., *Listening to Mothers II* (New York: Childbirth Connection, October 2006).

4. Jen Kamel, "Response to OB: Scare Tactics vs. Informed Consent," http://vbacfacts.com/2009/10/19/response-to-ob-scare-tactics-vs-informed-consent-aka-why-i-started-this-website/.

5. Jen Kamel, "Another VBAC Consult Misinforms," http://vbacfacts.com/2010/03/16/another-vbac-consult-misinforms/.

6. "ACOG Practice Bulletin No. 115: Vaginal Birth After Previous Cesarean Delivery," *Obstetrics and Gynecology* 116 (August 2010): 450–63, doi: 10.1097/AOG.0b013e3181 eeb251.

7. Salma Imran Kayani and Zarko Alfirevic, "Uterine Rupture after Induction of Labour in Women with Previous Caesarean Section," *British Journal of Gynecology* 112, no. 4 (April 2005): 451–55.

8. David M. Stamillio et al., "Short Interpregnancy Interval: Risk of Uterine Rupture and Complications of Vaginal Birth after Cesarean Delivery," *Obstetrics and Gynecology* 110, no. 5 (November 2007): 1075-82.

CHAPTER 39: DEATH OF THE MAIDEN, BIRTH OF THE MOTHER

Epilogue (p. 341): Kathryn Allen Rabuzzi, *Motherself: A Mythic Analysis of Motherhood* (Bloomington, IN: Indian University Press), 204.

1. Rajneesh, http://thinkexist.com/quotation/the_moment_a_child_is_born-the_mother_is_also/224601.html.

CHAPTER 40: YOUR JOURNEY HOME: TASKS OF THE RETURN

1. Nayyereh Khadem et al., "Comparing the Efficacy of Dates and Oxytocin in the Management of Postpartum Hemorrhage," *Shiraz E Medical Journal* 8, no. 2 (2007): 64–71.

2. Fred Hageneder, *The Meaning of Trees* (San Francisco: Chronicle Books, 2005), 138.

3. Noori Waili et al., "Honey for Wound Healing, Ulcers, and Burns," *Scientific World Journal* 11 (2011): 766–87.

CHAPTER 41: WARMING THE MOTHER

Epigraph (p. 353): Carroll Dunham, *Mamatoto: A Celebration of Birth* (New York: Viking Penguin, 1991), 129.

1. William Hutchinson Murray, *The Scottish Himalayan Expedition* (London, UK: Dent, 1951).

2. Recipe from Christina Gabbard, http://carolinaplacentalady.com/2011/01/mother-warming.

CHAPTER 42: WELCOMING YOUR BABY

Epigraph (p. 359): Lise Eliot, *What's Going On in There?* (New York: Bantam Books, 2000).

1. Nancy Mohrbacher, "Rethinking Swaddling," *International Journal of Childbirth Education* 25, no. 3 (2010): 7–12.

2. Phanem Tolba, "Your Song," *The Sun Chaser* (blog), May 30, 2012, https://jackysun chaser.wordpress.com/2012/05/30/your-song-by-tolba-phanem-african-poet/.

3. Barbara Kisilevsky et al., "Effects of Experience on Fetal Voice Recognition," *Psychological Science* 14, no. 3 (2003): 220–23.

4. Jose Ashford and Craig W. LeCroy, *Human Behavior in the Social Environment* (Belmont, CA: Brooks/Cole, 2010), 253.

5. Carroll Dunham, *Mamatoto: A Celebration of Birth* (New York: Viking, 1992).

6. Frédérick Leboyer, *Birth without Violence*, 4th ed. (Rochester, VT: Healing Arts Press, 2009).

7. Raylene Phillips, "The Sacred Hour: Uninterrupted Skin-to-Skin Contact Immediately after Birth," *Newborn Infant Nursing Review* 13, no. 2 (2013): 67–72.

8. Diane V. Lipka and Marcia K. Schulz, "Wait for Eight: Improvement of Newborn Outcomes by the Implementation of Newborn Bath Delay," *Journal of Obstetric, Gynecologic, & Neonatal Nursing* 41 (2012): S46–S47.

9. Nils Bergman et al., "Randomized Controlled Trial of Skin-to-Skin Contact from Birth versus Conventional Incubator," *Acta Paediatrica* 93 (2004): 779–85.

10. Genevieve Preer, "Delaying the Bath and In-Hospital Breastfeeding Rates," *Breastfeeding Medicine* 8, no. 6 (2013): 485–90.

11. Johan N. Lundstrom et al., "Maternal Status Regulates Cortical Status to the Body Odor of Newborns," *Frontiers in Psychology* 4 (2013): 597.

12. Gurcharan Singh and Gayatri Archana, "Unveiling the Mystery of Vernix Caseosa," *Indian Journal of Dermatology* 53, no. 2 (2008): 54–60.

13. Henry T. Akinbi et al., "Host Defense Proteins in Vernix Caseosa and Amniotic Fluid," *American Journal of Obstetrics and Gynecology* 191 (2004): 2090–96.

14. Valerie Sung et al., "Probiotics to Prevent or Treat Excessive Infant Crying," *Journal of American Medical Association Pediatrics* 167, no. 12 (August. 2013): 1150–57.

15. Ajitha Thanabalasuriar, "Neonates, Antibiotics and the Microbiome," *Nature Medicine* 20 (2014): 469–70.

16. Harish Johari, *Ayurvedic Massage* (Rochester, VT: Healing Art Press, 1996).

17. "Birth Rituals-Codex Mendoza in Children and Youth in History, #305," accessed August 21, 2015, https://chnm.gmu.edu/cyh/primary-sources/305.

18. Sharon M. Young, Daniel C. Benyshek, and Pierre Lienard, "The Conspicuous Absence of Placenta Consumption in Human Postpartum Females: The Fire Hypothesis," *Ecology of Food and Nutrition* 51, no. 3 (2012): 198–217.

19. Mark B. Kristal, in Susan Amorusco, "Can Eating Your Placenta Cure Postpartum Depression?" *Everyday Health*, http://www.everydayhealth.com/depression/can-eating-your-placenta-cure-postpartum-depression.aspx.

20. Sharon Young and Daniel Benyshek, "Eating the Placenta: How Do the Nutritional and Hormonal Profiles of Unprepared Human Placental Tissue Compare with Processed Human Placenta Capsules?" a talk cosponsored by Biological Anthropological Section and Biological Anthropology Section, University of Nevada, Las Vegas, http://www.aaanet.org/mtgs/dev/viewDetail.cfm?itemtype=paper_poster&matchid=24586.

21. Wah-Yun Low and Hui-Meng Tan, "Asian Traditional Medicine for Erectile Dysfunction," *The Journal of Men's Health and Gender* 4, no. 3 (2013): 245–250.

22. Andrew Weil, "Eating Your Placenta—Really?" http://www.drweil.com/drw/u/WBL02154/Eating-Your-Placenta-Really.html.

Chapter 43: Breastfeeding From Within

1. Bernardo L. Horta and Cesar G. Victora, "Long-Term Effects of Breastfeeding" (Geneva, Switzerland: World Health Organization, 2013).

2. Erin A. Wagner et al., "Breastfeeding Concerns at 3 and 7 Days Postpartum and Feeding Status at 2 Months," *Pediatrics* 132, no. 4 (2013): e865–75.

3. Suzanne D. Colson, Judith Meek, and Jane M. Hawdon, "Optimal Positions Triggering Primitive Neonatal Reflexes Stimulating Breastfeeding," *Early Human Development* 84, no. 7 (2008): 441–49.

4. Hawley E. Montgomery-Downs et al., "Infant Feeding Methods and Maternal Sleep and Daytime Functioning," *Pediatrics* 126, no. 6 (2010): 1562–568.

Chapter 44: Birth Story Gates

1. Coleman Barks, trans., *The Illuminated Rumi* (New York: Broadway Books, 1997), 40.

2. Jack Kornfield, *Buddha's Little Information Book* (New York: Bentam, 1994), 28.

3. G. BlueStone, *Light of the Kensei: Guide to the Way of the Warrior Sage* (Durango, CO: Avant Press, 1991).

Chapter 45: Perinatal Mood Disorders

1. Pauline Anderson, "Postpartum Depression, Anxiety, May Affect Infant Development," *Medscape Medical News* (August 2009), http://www.medscape.com/viewarticle/707719.

2. Michael W. O'Hara and Katherine L. Wisner, "Perinatal Mental Illness: Definition, Description and Aetiology," *Best Practice & Research Clinical Obstetrics Gynaecology* 28, no. 1 (January 2014): 3–12.

3. Pam Belluck, "Thinking of Ways to Harm Her," *New York Times* (June 15, 2014).

4. Karen Kleiman, *This Isn't What I Expected* (New York: Bantam, 2011).

5. Karen Kleiman, *Dropping the Baby and Other Scary Thoughts* (New York: Taylor and Francis Group, 2011), 38.

6. Ibid.

7. Jonathan S. Abramowitz, Maheruh Khandker, et al., "The Role of Cognitive Factors in the Pathogenesis of Obsessive Compulsive Symptoms," *Behavior Research and Therapy* 44 (2006): 1361–74.

8. Nichole Fairbrother and Sheila Woody, "New Mothers' Thoughts of Harm Related to the Newborn," *Archives of Women's Mental Health* 11, no. 3 (July, 2008): 221-29.

9. Kleiman, "Dropping the Baby," 40.

10. Marta Skrundz et al., "Plasma Oxytocin Concentration during Pregnancy Is Associated with Development of Postpartum Depression," *Neuropsychopharmacology* 36 (May 2011): 1886–93.

11. Ibid.

12. Joseph G. Reilly et al., "Rapid Depletion of Plasma Tryptophan," *Journal of Psychopharmacology* 11, no. 4 (1997): 381–92.

13. Katherine Pereira and Ann J. Brown, "Postpartum Thyroiditis," *Journal of Nurse Practitioners* 4, no. 3 (2008): 175–82.

14. Charles Stanley, Lynne Muray, and Alan Stein, "The Effect of Postnatal Depression on Mother–Infant Interaction, Infant Response to the Still-Face Perturbation, and Performance on an Instrumental Learning Task," *Developmental Psychopathology* 16, no. 1 (March 2004): 1–18.

15. James F. Paulson and Sharnail D. Bazemore, "Prenatal and Postpartum Depression in Fathers and Its Association with Maternal Depression: A Meta-Analysis," *Journal of American Medical Association* 303, no. 19 (May 2010): 1961–69.

16. Katherine Harmon, "Fact or Fiction: Fathers Can Get Postpartum Depression," *Scientific American* (2010), http://www.scientificamerican.com/article/fathers-postpartum-depression/.

17. Nicole Letourneau et al., "Identifying the Support Needs of Fathers Affected by Postpartum Depression," *Journal of Psychiatric Mental Health Nursing* 18, no. 1 (February 2011): 41–47.

18. Eleonora Bielawska-Batorowicz and Karolina Kossakowska-Petrycka, "Depressive Mood in Men after the Birth of Offspring in Relation to a Partner's Depression, Social Support, Personality and Expectations," *Journal of Reproductive and Infant Psychology* 24, no. 1 (2006): 21–29.

19. Anat Cohen Engler et al., "Breastfeeding May Improve Nocturnal Sleep and Reduce Infantile Colic," *European Journal of Pediatrics* 171, no. 4 (April 2012): 729–32.

20. R. E. Kendall, K. C. Chalmers, and C. Platz, "Epidemiology of Puerperal Psychoses," *British Journal of Psychiatry* 150 (1987): 662–73.

21. Tasnime N. Akbaraly et al., "Dietary Pattern and Depressive Symptoms," *British Journal of Psychiatry* 195, no. 5 (2009): 408–13.

22. C. Chih-chiang Chiu et al., "The Use of Omega-3 Fatty Acids in Treatment of Depression," *Integrative Psychiatry*, www.psychiatrictimes.com/integrative-psyhiatry/usega-3-fatty-acids-treatment-depression#sthash.Mmg2naaz.dpuf.

23. Joseph R. Hibbeln and Nicholas Salem, "Dietary Polyunsaturated Fatty Acids and Depression," *American Journal of Clinical Nutrition* 62, no. 1 (July 1995): 1–9.

24. Lisa M. Bodnar and Katherine L. Wisner, "Nutrition and Depression," *Biological Psychiatry* 58, no. 9 (November 2005): 679–85.

25. Ibid.

26. Pamela K. Murphy et al., "An Exploratory Study of Postpartum Depression and Vitamin D," *American Psychiatric Nurses Association* 16, no. 3 (May 2010): 170–77.

27. S. Dimidjian and S. Goodman, "Nonpharmacologic Intervention and Prevention Strategies for Depression during Pregnancy and the Postpartum," *Clinical Obstetrics and Gynecology* 52, no. 3 (September 2009): 498–515.

28. Tiffany Field, Nancy Grizzle, Frank Scafidi, et al., "Massage Therapy for Infants of Depressed Mothers," *Infant Behavioral Development* 19 (1996): 107–112.

29. M. O'Higgins, "Postnatal Depression and Mother and Infant Outcomes after Infant Massage vs. Support Group," *Journal of Affective Disorders* 109, nos. 1, 2 (July 2008): 189–92.

30. T. Field et al., "Cortisol Decreases and Serotonin and Dopamine Increase Following Massage Therapy," *International Journal of Neuroscience* 115 (2005): 1397–413.

31. Suzanne Zeedyk, "One Ride Forward, Two Steps Back," op ed, Dundee, Scotland *New York Times* (March 1, 2009).

32. Susan Garthus-Niegel, Tilmann von Soest, Margarete E. Vollrath, et al., "The Impact of Subjective Birth Experience on Post-Traumatic Stress Symptoms," *Archives of Women's Mental Health* 16, no. 1 (2012): 1–10.

33. Emma Molyneaux et al., "Antidepressant Treatment for Postnatal Depression," *Cochran Depression, Anxiety, and Neurosis Group* (July 2014).

34. David Whyte, *The Journey House of Belonging* (Langley, WA: Many Rivers Press, 1997).

Chapter 46: Rituals of the Return

Epigraph (p. 397): Judith Goldsmith, *Childbirth Wisdom: From the World's Oldest Societies* (New York: Congdon & Weed, 1984), 9.

Epigraph (p. 397): Claudia Panuthos, *Transformation through Birth: A Woman's Guide* (S. Hadley, MA: Bergin and Garvey, 1984), 132.

1. http://plantspirit.massagetherapy.com/benefits-of-the-closing-of-the-bones-ritual.

2. http://thefullmooneffectppc.weebly.com/closing-the-bones-ceremony.html.

Chapter 47: The Warrior's Treasure

Epigraph (p. 403): David Hartman and Diane Zimberoff, "The Hero's Journey of Self-Transformation," *Journal of Heart-Centered Therapies* 12, no. 2 (2009): 3–93.

Appendix B: Circumcision

Epigraph (p. 410): Dan Bollinger, "Lost Boys: An Estimate of U.S. Circumcision-Related Infant Deaths," *Journal of Boyhood Studies* 4 (2010): 78–90.

1. William Morgan, "The Rape of the Phallus" *Journal of the American Medical Association* 193 (1965), 123–129.

2. Dan Bollinger, www.circumcisiondecisionmaker.com.

3. Morris L. Sorrells et al., "Fine Touch Pressure Thresholds in the Adult Penis," *British Journal of Urology* 99 (2007): 864–69.

4. Dean Edell, "Circumcision Report for Television News, "KGO, San Francisco (1984), jewishcircumcision.org.

Epilogue (p. 410): Laurie Evans, "Counseling Couples in Disagreement about Circumcision," *Journal of Prenatal and Perinatology Psychology and Health* 17, no. 1 (2002): 85–94.

5. Ibid.

6. Aaron Krill, Lane S. Palmer, and Jeffrey S. Palmer, "Complications of Circumcision," *Scientific World Journal* 11 (2011): 2458–68.

7. M. Williams and L. Kapila, "Complications of Circumcision," *British Journal of Surgery* 80 (October 1993): 1231–36.

8. Anna Taddio et al., "Effect of Neonatal Circumcision on Pain Response during Subsequent Routine Vaccination," *The Lancet* 349, no. 9052 (March 1, 1997): 599–603.

9. Paul D. Tinari, "Circumcision Permanently Alters the Brain" (blog), Circumcision Resource Center, http://www.circumcision.org/brain.htm.

10. Ronald Goldman, "Circumcision: A Source of Jewish Pain" (blog), Jewish Circumcision Resource Center, jewishcircumcision.org.

Epigraph (p. 412): Dr. Benjamin Spock, "Circumcision—It's Not Necessary," *Redbook* (April 1989), http://www.doctorsopposingcircumcision.org/info/spock.html.

11. Robert Darby, "The Masturbation Taboo and the Rise of Routine Male Circumcision: A Review of the Historiography," *Journal of Social History* 27 (Spring, 2003): 737–57.

12. "Circumcision Rates Plummet: 2 Out of 3 Boys Escape the Knife," accessed August 14, 2010, http://www.icgi.org/2010/08/circumcision-rates-plummet-2-out-of-3-boys-escape-the-knife/.

13. "Task Force on Circumcision," Circumcision Policy Statement, *Pediatrics* 130, no. 585 (August 27, 2012), doi: 10.1542/peds2012-1989.

14. Ibid.

Epigraph (p. 414): Brian D. Earp, "Does Circumcision Reduce Penis Sensitivity? The Answer is Not Clear Cut" (blog), *Huffpost Science* (April 21, 2016), http://www.huffingtonpost.com/brian-earp/does-circumcision-reduce-_b_9743242.html.

15. "Circumcision, Ethics, and Medicine: Circumcision Violates the Principles of Medical Ethics" (blog), Circumcision Resource Center, http://www.circumcision.org/ethics.htm.

16. Marie Fox and Michael Thomson, "The New Politics of Male Circumcision," *Legal Studies* 32 no. 2 (2012), http://onlinelibrary.wiley.com/doi/10.1111/j.1748121X.2011.00218.x/abstract.

17. Laurie Evans, "Counseling Couples in Disagreement about Circumcision," *Journal of Prenatal and Perinatology Psychology and Health* 17, no. 1 (2002): 85–94.

18. "Pain Response During Circumcision" (blog), Circumcision Resource Center, www.circumcision.org/response.htm.

19. Ibid.

20. Megan R. Gunnar et al., "The Effect of Circumcision on Serum Cortisol and Behavior," *Psychoneuroendocrinology* 6, no. 3 (1981): 269–75.

21. "Infant Responses to Circumcision: Behavioral Response Following Circumcision" (blog), http://www.circumcision.org/response.htm.

22. Ronald Goldman, "The Psychological Impact of Circumcision," *British Journal of Urology International* 83, no. S1 (January 1999): 93–102.

GLOSSARY

ACOG—American Congress of Obstetricians and Gynocologists.

AMNIOTIC FLUID EMBOLISM—A serious but rare complication that occurs when amniotic fluid enters the mother's bloodstream during childbirth.

ANTERIOR LIP—When the top half of the cervix is swollen while the lower half is completely dilated. This happens at about 9 centimeters dilation and is associated with occiput posterior position, rapid descent of the baby, or immobilization of the mother.

APGAR—A quick visual assessment of the newborn at one and five minutes after birth. Developed by Dr. Virginia Apgar, it includes breathing, pulse, muscle tone, reflexes, and color, and scores ranging from 1 to 10, with a score of 7 or higher indicating the baby is doing well.

ARREST OF LABOR—The absence of cervical dilations or descent of the baby for two or more hours in active labor.

ASYNCLITISM—Tilting of a baby's head toward the right or left shoulder during labor, which interferes with the fit and rotation in the pelvis. Babies usually move and correct asynclitism as they pass through the pelvis; however, when a tilt is persistent it can prolong labor.

BIOEFFECTS—Unintended biological changes resulting from ultrasound.

BIOPHYSICAL PROFILE (BPP)—A prenatal measurement of the health of the fetus, using ultrasound to assess heart rate, movement, muscle tone, breathing, and the amount of amniotic fluid.

BLOODY SHOW—Vaginal fluid tinged with blood that occurs when the cervix thins and begins to dilate, causing tiny capillaries in the cervix to break. This discharge is a positive sign that labor is nearing.

BRAXTON-HICKS CONTRACTIONS—A sporadic, painless tightening of the uterine muscle, that occurs naturally in late pregnancy, often when the mother gets up, changes position, or is dehydrated. Also called false labor or practice contractions because they do not cause the cervix to thin or dilate.

CATECHOLAMINE—Any chemical, such as epinephrine and norepinephrine, that is produced by the adrenal gland.

COCHRANE REPORTS—A synthesis of all research done on a particular health topic by a group of scientists.

CROWNING—During pushing, when the baby's head (or bottom if breech) is visible and remains fixed at the vaginal opening without receding back into the vagina after each push.

ECLAMPSIA—A life-threatening complication of pregnancy, usually associated with advanced preeclampsia, that causes women to develop seizures or coma.

EVAPORATIVE COOLING—Vaporizing of amniotic fluid from a newborn's skin surface that causes the baby's temperature to drop quickly. It generally occurs when a wet infant moves from a warm enclosed womb to a cold delivery room. This is why hospital-born babies are dried, covered, or swaddled immediately after birth.

HELLP SYNDROME.—A life-threatening condition of pregnancy thought to be an advanced stage or a variant of pre-eclampsia that occurs after 28 weeks of gestation. HELLP = H (hemolysis, or breakdown of red blood cells), EL (elevated liver enzymes), LP (low platelet count). Symptoms include fatigue, swelling, headache, nausea and vomiting, upper right abdominal pain (liver), blurry vision, and, rarely, seizures. Treatment involves immediate delivery of the baby, usually by induction or cesarean.

HERTZ—A measurement of the frequency of vibrations per second; 1 hertz equals 1 vibration per second.

HYPOXIC—Affected by insufficient oxygen supply.

ICE CONTRACTIONS—Inducing an unpleasant sensation by holding ice for a 60-second "contraction" while practicing pain-coping techniques prenatally.

LABOR ARREST—Prolonged labor without dilation or descent, caused by physical, psychological, or environmental factors.

LAPIS MEASURING ROD AND RING—A short handheld rod with a coil looped above; possibly an ancient Sumerian symbol of divine justice.

LITHOTOMY POSITION—Birthing orientation in which the patient is lying on her back, knees flexed, and thighs apart, sometimes with the legs and feet held in place by straps.

MAIDEN—One of the Triple Goddesses that make up the Great Goddess (Maiden, Mother, Crone) portrayed in Greek mythology. The Maiden is depicted as a youthful woman who either focuses on or ignores her beauty; she may be a dutiful daughter who, having not yet developed a sense of self-worth, may overcompensate in service and goodness to earn approval. Or she may be self-indulgent, pursuing her own pleasures and dreams for herself.

MECONIUM—The first dark green feces passed by a newborn baby, containing mucus, bile, and epithelial cells. Meconium is also passed into the amniotic fluid in the womb when an unborn baby is hypoxic.

MECONIUM ASPIRATION SYNDROME—A condition occurring when a fetus inhales meconium before or during birth. Because the bile salts and enzymes can cause serious complications to the baby's lungs, possibly requiring medical attention after birth, when meconium is present in labor women birthing at home should be transferred to the hospital.

MEHDA (PRONOUNCED MAY-duh)—A Sanskrit word referring to feminine wisdom and used in this book as a substitute for the ancient Sumerian word *me*, meaning mother wisdom or referring to sacred objects such as a throne, temple, drum, or crown.

MICROBIOME—The microorganisms in a particular environment, including the body or part of the body.

MICROBIOTA—The ecological community of symbiotic microorganisms present in the human body. The human body contains over ten times more microbial cells than human cells. For this reason, some scientists regard the microbiome, identified in the late 1990s, as a newly discovered organ.

MUCUS PLUG—Clear or pinkish mucus that moves through the vagina when the cervix starts to thin and dilate. Labor may or may not begin soon after the mucus plug is noticeable.

MULTIPAROUS—Having birthed more than one child.

NEONATAL INTENSIVE CARE UNIT (NICU)—A hospital unit for preterm or sick newborns who need intensive nursing and medical care.

NICU—Newborn intensive care unit.

NULLIPAROUS—Having not yet born a child.

PARADIGM SHIFT—A changed conceptual worldview that can impact people's thoughts, feelings, or behavior.

PERINATAL—Occurring in, concerned with, or being in the period around the time of birth, from five months before to one month after the birth.

POSTERIOR ARREST—In labor, a baby presenting with occiput posterior (OP or "sunny side up") often rotates or spins into the occiput anterior (OA) position which means the diameter of the head passing through the pelvis is smaller. However, if the baby's occiput gets stuck on the mother's sacral promontory, the baby's rotation arrests (usually around 6 centimeters dilation), resulting in maternal back pain and cervical swelling.

POST-TRAUMATIC STRESS DISORDER (PTSD)—A condition characterized by thoughts about a traumatic event, or hypervigilance or avoidance of situations and people reminiscent of the event. A woman may experience PTSD following childbirth, resulting in injury to herself or injury to, or death of, her infant.

PRE-ECLAMPSIA—A complication of malnutrition in pregnancy, occurring around 38 weeks and associated with high blood pressure; protein in the urine; severe headache; blurred vision or seeing spots; upper right abdominal pain (liver); nausea and vomiting; swelling of hands, feet, and face; and generally not feeling well.

PRODROMAL LABOR—Rounds of irregular, stop-and-go contractions coming as often as every three minutes and lasting less than forty seconds.

PSYCHE—From a Greek word meaning soul, spirit, mind; also the name of the Greek goddess of the soul and the wife of Eros, god of love.

SCARAB—Any of a family of stout-bodied beetles; a stone beetle used in ancient Egypt as a talisman, ornament, and symbol of resurrection. Used in this book as a prenatal Task icon, the beetle is shown concentrating on her task of rolling a dung ball from which her babies will later be born.

SEVEN—A number that symbolizes hardship, endurance, and determination, qualities integral to a rite of passage.

STATION—The level of descent of a baby's head in relation to the ischial spines. When the baby's head is "high" in the pelvis, it's above the ischial spine and referred to as station -1, -2, or -3; -1 means the head is 1 centimeter above the ischial spines. When the baby's head is level with the ischial spines, it is at 0 station. As the baby's head descends past the ischial spines, stations are referred to as +1 to +4.

TERRA INCOGNITA—An unknown or unexplored land, region, or subject.

TONGUE-TIE—A condition where a baby's tongue is tightly attached to the bottom of the mouth, impairing tongue mobility and the ability to latch on effectively to suck breast milk. There are four classes of this condition; therefore, getting accurate assessmen and treatment may be challenging. For more information, visit www.drghaheri.com.

TRANSCUTANEOUS ELECTRICAL NERVE STIMULATION (TENS)—A device that emits low-voltage currents used for pain relief in labor.

TRANSVERSE ARREST—A condition that occurs when the baby's head, while deep in the mother's pelvis, gets wedged behind ischial spines and cannot rotate to an anterior-posterior position. If rotation does not occur, cesarean birth becomes necessary.

ZAFU (PRONOUNCED ZAH-fu)—A Japanese word referring to a thick, firm, round cushion used for sitting meditation, primarily zazen.

ILLUSTRATION CREDITS

Topograph Woman by Virginia Bobro © 2015, pen-and-ink drawing (cover)

Archetypes of Birth: Mother (p. 36), Gatherer (p. 142), Warrior (p. 162), Huntress (p. 201), Gatekeeper (p. 232), and Fool (p. 276) by Elena Mitchel © 2015, pen-and-ink drawings

First Kiss by Amy Harderer © 2011, mixed media, 12 x 12 in. (p. 326); reprinted with permission

Birth art images reproduced from drawings made by parents (pp. 106, 301, 315, 316)

Sugar Baby by Pam England © 2014, acrylic, 9 x 12 in. (p. 86)

Mexican Labyrinth of Birth by Pam England © 2012, acrylic on Masonite, 18 x 36 in. (p. 169)

Pushing Lucien Out by Pam England © 1990, watercolor, 18 x 24 in. (p. 256)

Faith Based Birth by Pam England © 2004, 2010, acrylic on canvas, 36 x 24 in. (p. 312)

Ugandan Cesarean copied from the original by Pam England (p. 318)

Untitled illustrations throughout by Pam England © 2015, pencil, pen-and-ink drawing, or watercolor

Index

About the Author

*P*AM ENGLAND, CNM, MA, is the author of *Birthing From Within* and *Labyrinth of Birth*. She founded the international mentor training program Birthing From Within in 1999. Formerly a nurse-midwife, she worked in hospital, birth center, and home birth settings for eighteen years. Her interest in birth psychology and resolving emotional birth trauma led her to earn a master's degree and develop Birth Story Medicine, a popular long-distance birth story listening course that she is currently developing into a book. Pam, also an artist, lives in Albuquerque, New Mexico.

BIRTHING FROM WITHIN

Classes, Phone Consultations, Distance Learning, Workshops, and More

Birthing From Within and Birth Story Medicine
are changing the conversation about birth in our culture.
Join us!

Expectant Parents: Take a Birthing From Within childbirth class from one of our Childbirth Mentors. Go to "Find a Class Near You" on our website. There are Birthing From Within Mentors across the United States and in eighteen countries. If you can't find a class or Mentor near you, contact our office and we will connect you with a Mentor who offers sessions by phone or Skype.

Aspiring and Experienced Birth-Related Professionals: *Ancient Map for Modern Birth* is not just a book about childbirth; it is part of a social movement. Here are some ways to get involved in that movement.

Check our website for upcoming offerings

Sign up for a dynamic, transformative workshop or a distance learning course:

- Childbirth Mentor Training and Certification Program
- Doula Training and Certification Program
- Birth Story Medicine Course

Make an appointment with Pam England, Virginia Bobro, or one of the BFW Childbirth Mentors for a consultation or class in your area.

BirthingFromWithin.com
Contact@BirthingFromWithin.com
805-964-6611